CARDIOMYOPATHIES

Edited by **José Milei**
and **Giuseppe Ambrosio**

Cardiomyopathies
http://dx.doi.org/10.5772/56744
Edited by José Milei and Giuseppe Ambrosio

Contributors

Bas Van Dalen, Anwer Qureshi, Gohar Jamil, Ahmed Abbas, Abdullah Shehab, Jan Klimas, Joseph Isaac Shapiro, Joe Xie, Larry Dial, Maegen Ackermann, Aikaterini Kontrogianni-Konstantopoulos, Takahiro Okumura, Toyoaki Murohara, Aspazija Nikola Sofijanova, Olivera Jordanova, Akihiro Hirashiki, Yazaki, M. Obadah Al Chekakie, Luis Oscar Vernengo, Ann Anderson, McLeod, Carolyn Pierce, Mounsey, Prabhat Kumar

Published by InTech

Janeza Trdine 9, 51000 Rijeka, Croatia

Copyright © 2013 InTech

Notice

Publishing Process Manager Iva Simcic
Technical Editor InTech DTP team
Cover InTech Design team

Additional hard copies can be obtained from orders@intechopen.com

Cardiomyopathies, Edited by José Milei and Giuseppe Ambrosio
p. cm.
ISBN 978-953-51-1103-0

For EU product safety concerns:
IN TECH d.o.o., Prolaz Marije Krucifikse Kozulić 3, 51000 Rijeka, Croatia,
info@intechopen.com or visit our website at intechopen.com.

Meet the editors

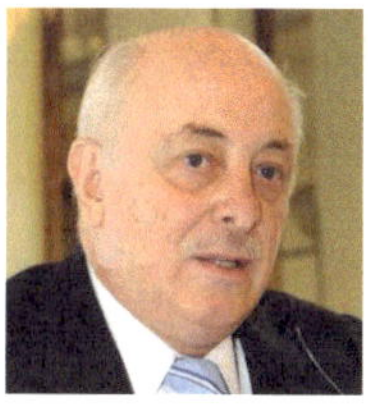

José Milei is Professor of Internal Medicine and Director of the Institute of Cardiological Investigations at the University of Buenos Aires (UBA) and the National Research Council for Science and Technology, Argentina. His thesis about the effects of isoproterenol on myocardium, has been extensively cited as well as his investigations in the '80 in NIH, National Heart, Lung and Blood Institute, USA under the guidance of his mentor, Victor Ferrans. Professor Milei is Chairman of the Module of Cardiology and Hypertension at the Argentine Medical Association devoted to South American general practitioners´ training. His research on early atherosclerotic lesions helped set up the basis for the importance of intimal thickenings in plaque genesis. He has authored over 140 papers in peer review journals, 4 books and over 10 invited chapters in books of cardiology. His treaty on Chagas' disease is a referent book in the last 20 years.

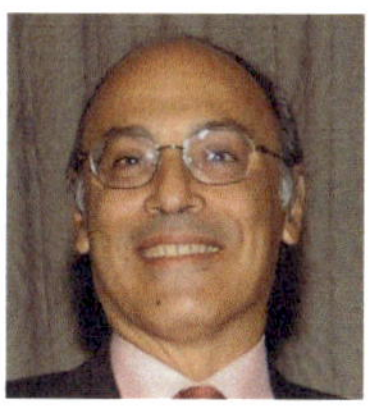

Dr. Giuseppe Ambrosio is Professor and Director at University of Perugia, School of Medicine, Division of Cardiology, Italy. He is Professor Honorario at the Institute of Cardiological Investigations at the University of Buenos Aires (UBA). He authored over 170 papers in peer review journals, has over 7000 citations in international literature and over 70 invited lectures and seminars at International Meetings. Dr. Ambrosio is a member of Committee on Heart Failure with Preserved Ejection Fraction (2008 -), at Heart Failure Association – European Society of Cardiology; a member of Committee on Prevention of Cardiovascular Disease, at American College of Cardiology. In addition, he is a member of Editorial Boards of several International Journals.

Contents

Preface

More than 50 years ago, in 1957, Bridgen the word "cardiomyopathy" has been used for the first time. One year later, Teare described nine cases of interventricular septal hypertrophy. In this book the broad aspects of cardiomyopathies are fully developed by renowned specialists. The book is divided in five sections – Cardiomyopathies - general aspects; pathophysiology and molecular mechanisms; genetics; sudden death and cardiomyopathies in special populations.

The disease of the heart muscle may develop secondarily to other cardiac alterations, such as ischemic, hypertensive, valvular and systemic, among others. However, there is also a group of conditions with intrinsic myocardial involvement of genetic or multifactorial etiology, characterized by high morbidity and mortality that represent a diagnostic and therapeutic challenge for the physician.

Cardiomyopathy (primary) is defined as a disease of the myocardium, which results in insufficient pumping of the heart. It is classified into four forms; dilated cardiomyopathy, hypertrophic cardiomyopathy, restrictive cardiomyopathy, and arrhythmogenic right ventricular cardiomyopathy.

The book is focused on these forms, its features, its pathophysiology, and its relationship to sudden death. Mention is made also on general aspects, like ecocardiographic findings and myocardial contractile reserve, specific as pathophysiology and molecular mechanisms. Special attention is deserved to cardiomyopathies in special populations, like pediatrics, diabetic patients, and women, as well as to cases of chronic heart failure and dilated cardiomyopathy.

Cardiomyopathies are characterized by extensive remodeling of the myocardium manifested as hypertrophy, due to enlarged myocyte size and interstitial fibrosis. With the progression of the disease, the heart turns to a dilated state, with increase of the intraventricular volume and a mild increase in ventricular wall thickness. These changes, apparently compensatory, ultimately become maladaptive.

Dilated cardiomyopathy is one of the most common types of cardiomyopathy worldwide. It is characterized by progressive chamber dilatation and myocardial systolic dysfunction and diagnosed by left ventricular enlargement and impaired systolic left ventricular function.

Regarding diagnosis, echocardiography is the most frequently used and readily available cardiac imaging technique. It has been established as the cardiac imaging modality of choice in diagnosis and longitudinal follow up of patients with cardiomyopathy.

In most patients suffering from cardiomyopathy and heart failure, symptoms are not present at rest but become evident with exercise. As said, the test universally used is echocardiography, but it is generally performed under resting conditions and left ventricular contractile function at rest is not reliable for the evaluation of the reversibility of myocardial contraction, that is contractile reserve. For this reason, it is important to evaluate functional response also under dynamic conditions by the use of pharmacological and/or exercise stress. Also, the prognostic value of dobutamine- and pacing- induced mechanical alterations in outpatients with idiopathic dilated cardiomyopathy and severe heart failure is discussed, with respect to clinical conditions and mechanisms of development.

In this connection, left ventricular twist is indispensable for proper left ventricular function. It originates from the dynamic interaction between oppositely wound subepicardial and subendocardial myocardial fibers. The direction of left ventricular twist is governed by the subepicardial fibers, mainly owing to their longer arm of movement. Measurement of left ventricular rotation by echocardiography has only recently become clinically feasible with the development of speckle tracking echocardiography. It has become clear that increased left ventricular twist, for example in hypertrophic cardiomyopathy, diabetes, and in healthy ageing population, may serve as a compensatory mechanism to preserve ejection fraction.

Also, it is emphasized that measurement of left ventricular untwisting may become an important element of diastolic function evaluation in cardiomyopathies.

Since 20 years, several mutations in genes encoding sarcomeric proteins have been causally linked to cardiomyopathies. There is a long list of affected sarcomeric proteins of striated muscles. Some selected proteins are described as to the molecular structure of their genes, as well as a comprehensive and up-to-date listing of the mutations that have been identified and directly linked to the development of cardiomyopathies is provided.

Most cardiomyopathies with primary myocardial pathology predispose to sudden cardiac death, especially in younger subjects. Although they account for a small fraction of population, a subset of these patients are at high risk and this justifies an aggressive preventive strategy. These include dilated cardiomyopathy, hypertrophic cardiomyopathy, left ventricular non-compaction and arrhythmogenic right ventricular cardiomyopathy. Sarcoidosis is a rare form of cardiomyopathy that affects young patients and put them at risk of sudden cardiac death. Early recognition and treatment of all these disease is mandatory. Regarding diagnosis, 123I-MIBG scintigraphy to evaluate myocardial sympathetic nerve activity may be useful in risk stratification of the risk of sudden death in heart failure patients without sustained VT and a history of ventricular fibrillation and dilated cardiomyopathy.

Implantable defibrillator therapy has emerged as the most important management strategy for prevention of sudden death in patients with cardiomyopathy. Whilst the use of beta-blocker therapy, angiotensin-converting enzyme inhibitors, angiotensin receptor blockers, as well as aldosterone antagonists have been shown to decrease the risk of sudden cardiac death especially in in patients with congestive heart failure.

Heart failure in women has a distinct phenotype; develops later in life, generally presents with preserved systolic function and it is less attributable to ischemic heart disease. In many women, an important event in heart failure is due to poor venous return resulting from inadequate calf muscle pump activity during upright posture. This explains that while women survival rate with heart failure is better, their quality of life with heart failure is far worse.

As shown, the broad spectrum of new aspects of "Cardiomyopathies" are developed in this book, with the hope to be useful to cardiologists.

Prof. Dr. José Milei
Director del Instituto de Investigaciones Cardiológicas
"Prof. Dr. Alberto C. Taquini"- UBA- CONICET (ININCA)

Prof. Giuseppe Ambrosio
Director of Cardiology
University of Perugia School of Medicine

Section 1

Cardiomyopathies - General Aspects

Chapter 1

Echocardiography Findings in Common Primary and Secondary Cardiomyopathies

Gohar Jamil, Ahmed Abbas, Abdullah Shehab and Anwer Qureshi

Additional information is available at the end of the chapter

http://dx.doi.org/10.5772/55036

1. Introduction

Cardiomyopathy is a heterogeneous group of disorders of varying etiology. Heart failure from systolic and/or diastolic cardiac dysfunction is common to all. Certain disorders are distinguished by life threatening arrhythmia. Onset of symptoms may be acute or progress from preclinical to symptomatic state over time and at a variable rate. Early recognition permits therapeutic intervention thereby retarding clinical progression and in some reversal or arrest of pathologic state. Echocardiography being the most frequently used and readily available cardiac imaging technique has established itself as the cardiac imaging modality of choice in diagnosis and longitudinal follow up of patients with cardiomyopathy. Complementary information from other imaging techniques, e.g., tissue characterization with cardiac MRI in iron overload states and evaluation of coronary anatomy with cardiac CT as in some cases of dilated cardiomyopathy, usually follows recognition of cardiomyopathy on echocardiogram.

An understanding of conventional echocardiogram and knowledge of novel applications of existing methods and emerging imaging echo techniques is important for effective clinical use of echocardiography.

1.1. Standard 2-D and M-mode echocardiogram

Standard echocardiogram includes analysis of myocardial and valvular structure, chamber quantification and estimation of function based on qualitative assessment and quantification by 2-D and M-mode echocardiography. Blood flow dynamics through different cardiac chambers and heart valves is assessed using spectral and color Doppler methods. Through prior work, pressure gradient across heart valves can be derived from measured flow velocity by using the modified Bernoulli equation ($4V^2$); flow velocity is directly measured from spectral Doppler display. Color Doppler techniques are useful in analyzing regurgitant valve lesions and in drawing attention to turbulent flow through stenotic valves as well as abnormal flow between cardiac chambers as in cases of atrial or ventricular septal defect.

1.2. Three Dimensional Echocardiography (3DE)

In patients with adequate imaging window, 3DE provides more accurate chamber quantification (Figure-1). Left ventricular end-diastolic and end-systolic volumes derived from 3DE has been validated against cardiac MRI [1], which is the current reference standard for such measurements. In routine clinical practice important use of 3DE derived chamber quantification is in establishing an accurate baseline, and in longitudinal follow up of patients. In addition to chamber quantification and determination of global left ventricular function, automated quantification also permits contractile assessment at regional and segmental level. The graphical display of this contractile information is plotted as segmental change in volume over time. Discrepant timing of this segmental volume change over time has been used to assess left ventricular dyssynchrony as that seen in patients with left bundle branch block (LBBB) pattern on ECG (Figure-1). However, concerns with reproducibility in patients with low left ventricular ejection fraction have compromised the diagnostic utility of this parameter in selecting patients for cardiac resynchronization therapy [2].

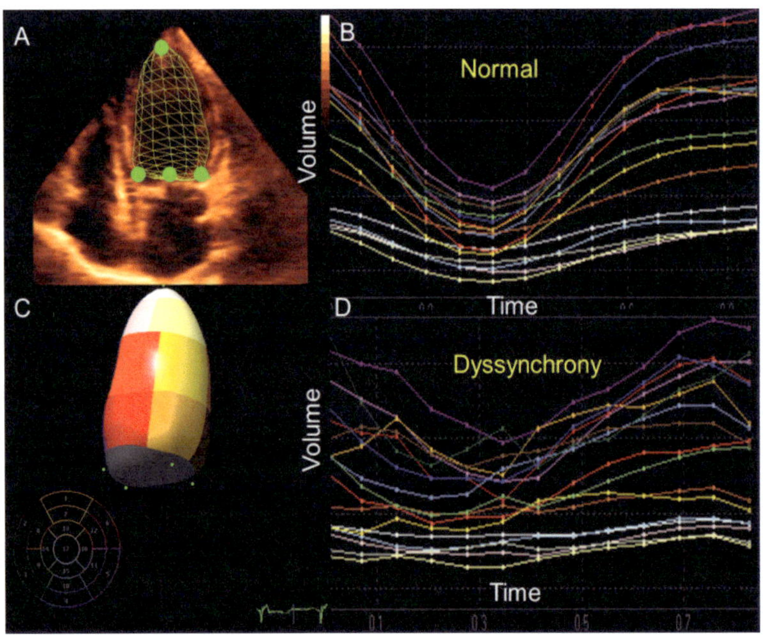

Figure 1. Panel-A: 3D data set of the heart is automatically cropped to display a 4-chamber and 2-chamber (not shown) projection of the heart. Left ventricular volume is tracked in end-diastole and end-systole from which volumetric LVEF is calculated. In panel-C segmental model of the heart is displayed. Each segment is color coded. Graphical display of the volume (y-axis) change over time (x-axis) is shown in panels-B and D. Each colored line corresponds to a segment of similar color in panel-C. In a normal heart all segments reach a minimum volume at the same time (panel-B). In panel-D there is a disarray of this time-volume curve signifying left ventricular dyssynchrony.

1.3. Doppler tissue velocity and doppler strain

Modification of the spectral tissue Doppler technique with filters that display high amplitude and low velocity signal permits segmental interrogation of myocardium for both systolic and diastolic function. Tissue Doppler at the mitral annulus level has long been used to assess myocardial diastolic function. Reversal of high early diastolic velocity (E′) with diastolic velocity coinciding with atrial systole (A′) is a flow independent marker of diastolic impairment. An elevated ratio of early mitral inflow Doppler velocity (E) with early tissue Doppler velocity (E′) is considered a reliable sign of elevated left ventricular end diastolic pressure [3-4].

Color encoded display of myocardial velocities on a 2-D image of the LV permits parametric assessment of myocardial contraction and Doppler based interrogation of multiple myocardial segments in the same frame. The latter is used for estimation of myocardial velocity and strain (Figure-2). Myocardial velocity in the long axis determines myocardial displacement, which may be active contraction or passive motion from contraction of adjacent segments [5]. Hence, its usefulness is limited when assessing segmental function. On the other hand, Doppler-derived longitudinal and circumferential strain measures segmental myocardial lengthening or shortening (deformation), signifying active contraction of the interrogated segment [5]. Strain is a dimensionless index (change in length/original length) of myocardial mechanics. The technique has been used for determination of cardiomyopathy in hereditary conditions,

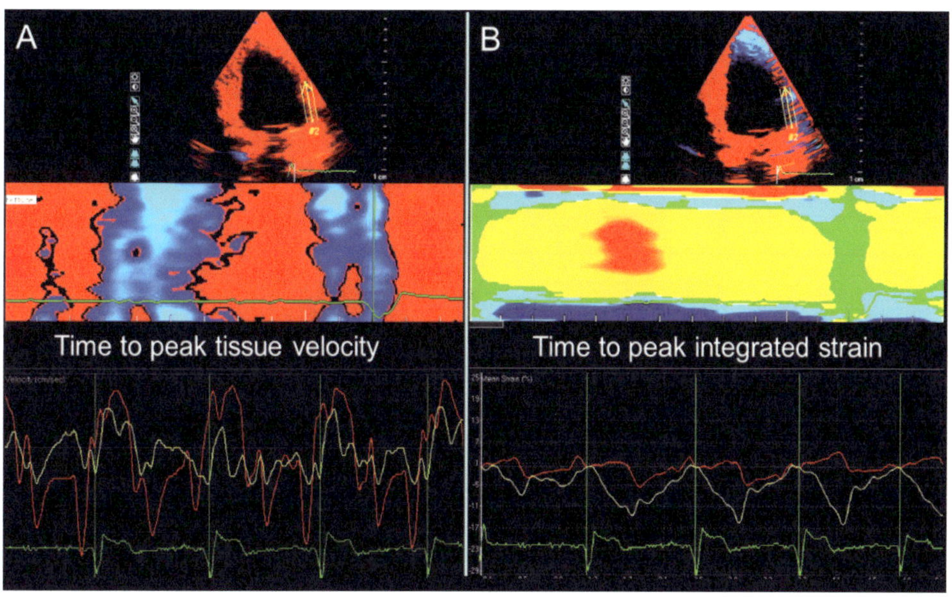

Figure 2. Color tissue Doppler derived tissue velocity (panel-A) and longitudinal strain (panel-B) is shown. Basal inferoseptum and lateral walls are interrogated. Panel-A: time (x-axis) to peak systolic tissue velocity (y-axis) measured from the onset of QRS (ECG displayed at the bottom of each panel in green color) of inferoseptum (red) is delayed when compared to the lateral wall (yellow). This signifies dyssynchrony. Longitudinal strain is shown in panel-B. Inferoseptum timing is again delayed. Note, however, that peak strain (strain is a negative value when measured in the long axis of the heart due to compression/shortening of the interrogated segment in systole) of inferoseptum is decreased signifying contractile dysfunction.

in differentiation of physiologic hypertrophy in elite athletes from pathologic variants [6, 23], in assessment of myocardial dyssynchrony [7], and in differentiating constrictive from restrictive physiology.

1.4. 2D or speckle strain and LV torsion

Doppler-based strain imaging is limited by angle dependency [8]. Innovation in imaging hardware and software now permit tissue-based measurement of segmental, regional and global myocardial function by determining tissue strain and torsion (Figure-3). The technique relies on good 2-D image quality for tracking tissue characteristics, termed "speckles", in regions of interest on a 2-D image through the entire cardiac cycle. To improve spatial resolution, image acquisition is performed at a slower frame rate contrasting with higher frame rate of Doppler-based techniques [9]. This may influence the accuracy of time dependent measurement of myocardial function as in milder forms of left ventricular dyssynchrony. Potentially valuable clinical information can be derived from speckle strain in a variety of cardiac disorders, including asymptomatic stages of cardiomyopathy [9].

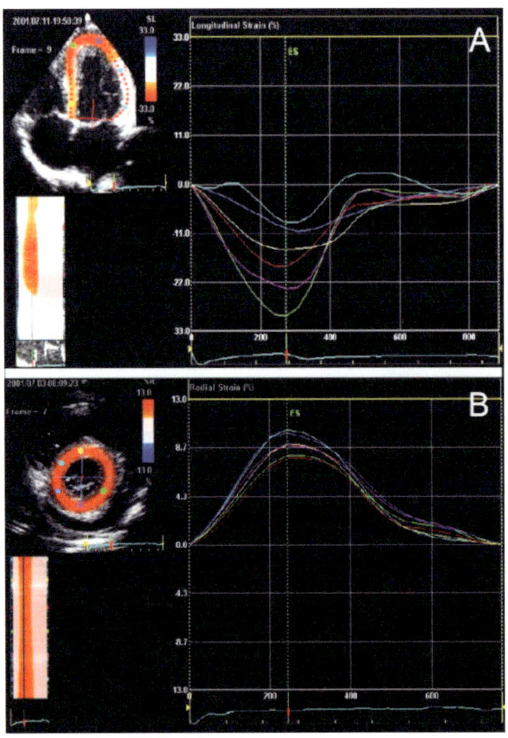

Figure 3. Speckle strain measurement inlongitudinal and radial direction is performed.In Panel-A, longitudinal strain is determinedat multiple levels from base to apex. Because contraction in longitudinal direction results in fiber shortening, strain values are negative. Segmental impairment of longitudinalstrain or contractility is present. In panel-B radial strain is depicted as a positive value due to fiber lengthening radially in systole. All segments at this level show normal contractility.LV torsion can be determined from the same data set.

Ratio of basal clockwise rotation to apical counterclockwise when viewed from the apex is as a measure of left ventricle twist or torsion. It is produced by contraction of helically oriented myofibers. Left ventricle torsion is affected in both systolic and diastolic myocardial dysfunction. When compared to a normal population, left ventricle torsion is decreased in dilated cardiomyopathy and increased in patients with hypertrophic cardiomyopathy [10].

2. Echo findings in cardiomyopathies

For this review a modification of 1995 World Health Organization /International Society and Federation of Cardiology (WHO/ISFC) Task Force on the Definition and Classification of Cardiomyopathies [11] and 2006 American Heart Association classification of cardiomyopathic disorders [12] is used. Discussion on echocardiographic findings will be limited to more frequently encountered disorders and to conditions with unique echo features.

2.1. Modified classification of primary and secondary cardiomyopathies

i. Genetic:

- Hypertrophic cardiomyopathy (HCM)
- Arrhythmogenic right ventricular cardiomyopathy/dysplasia (ARVC/D)
- Left ventricular non compaction (LVNC)

ii. Mixed (pre-dominantly non genetic):

- Dilated cardiomyopathy (DCM)
- Restrictive cardiomyopathy (non hypertrophied and non dilated) (RCM)

iii. Acquired Primary and Secondary Cardiomyopathy:

- Inflammatory myocarditis
- Stress provoked (takotsubo cardiomyopathy)
- Peripartum cardiomyopathy
- Tachycardia induced cardiomyopathy
- Ischemic cardiomyopathy
- Valvular cardiomyopathy
- Hypertensive cardiomyopathy
- Metabolic cardiomyopathy including amyloidosis and hemochromatosis
- Toxic cardiomyopathy: Alcohol and anthracyclines
- Connective Tissue Disorders: RA, SLE, PAN, scleroderma

- Muscular dystrophies: Duchenne, Becker-type and myotonic dystrophy
- Neuromuscular disorder: Friedreich's ataxia, Noonan's syndrome and lentiginosis

3. Genetic cardiomyopathies

Echocardiography remains the cornerstone for the detection and longitudinal follow up of patients with genetic cardiomyopathy. Inherited cardiomyopathies may have autosomal dominant pattern of inheritance. As such, surveillance echocardiogram of asymptomatic family members may allow early detection and life saving therapeutic intervention.

3.1. Hypertrophic Cardiomyopathy (HCM)

3.1.1. Introduction

HCM is the most frequently encountered inherited cardiomyopathy. Echocardiography plays a central role in diagnosis of HCM and in elucidating the pathophysiology of this disorder.

3.1.2. Features of HCM on standard echocardiogram:

Key diagnostic features of HCM are apparent on standard echocardiogram and are described below.

Distribution of left ventricular hypertrophy:

Several morphologic variants are known. Asymmetrical septal hypertrophy is the most frequently encountered (Figure-4). Hypertrophy of more than one region of left ventricular wall and at times of right ventricular wall is also seen. In the apical variant of HCM, myocardial hypertrophy is confined to the apical region of the left ventricle. This type is more frequently encountered in non-Caucasians.

Diagnostic criteria of Asymmetrical Septal Hypertrophy (ASH):

Septal thickness of >15 mm and a septal to posterior free wall ratio (interventricular septum/ posterior wall ratio) >1.3 are established echocardiographic criteria for the diagnosis of ASH [12]. However asymmetric left ventricular hypertrophy by itself is not pathognomonic of HCM as it may be encountered in a variety of congenital or acquired conditions, including systemic hypertension, aortic stenosis and cardiac amyloidosis [14].

Left ventricular function:

Systolic function is usually normal or above normal. Despite preservation of global left ventricular function [15], significant impairment of longitudinal contractile function is present with attenuation of annular velocities, longitudinal strain and strain rate (see below) [16]. Progressive myocardial fibrosis in advanced disease state is associated with impairment of systolic function, segmental myocardial thinning and left ventricle cavity enlargement [17]. Given myocardial characteristics, impaired myocardial relaxation is frequently observed [18].

Echo methods of estimating left ventricular end-diastolic pressure (E/E′ ratio) show heterogeneity and lack specificity in HCM [19].

Systolic Anterior Motion (SAM) of mitral valve:

Systolic anterior motion of the anterior mitral leaflet with or without obstruction to flow across the left ventricular outflow tract is highly suggestive of HCM (Figure-4). This finding has a specificity of > 90% [20]. Of note, SAM may also be encountered in hypercontractile states, following mitral valve repair, with anomalous papillary muscle insertion, in patients with anteroapical infarction, in takotsubo cardiomyopathy who have hyperkinesia of basal left ventricular segment and in elderly women with left ventricular hypertrophy and sigmoid shaped septum [21].

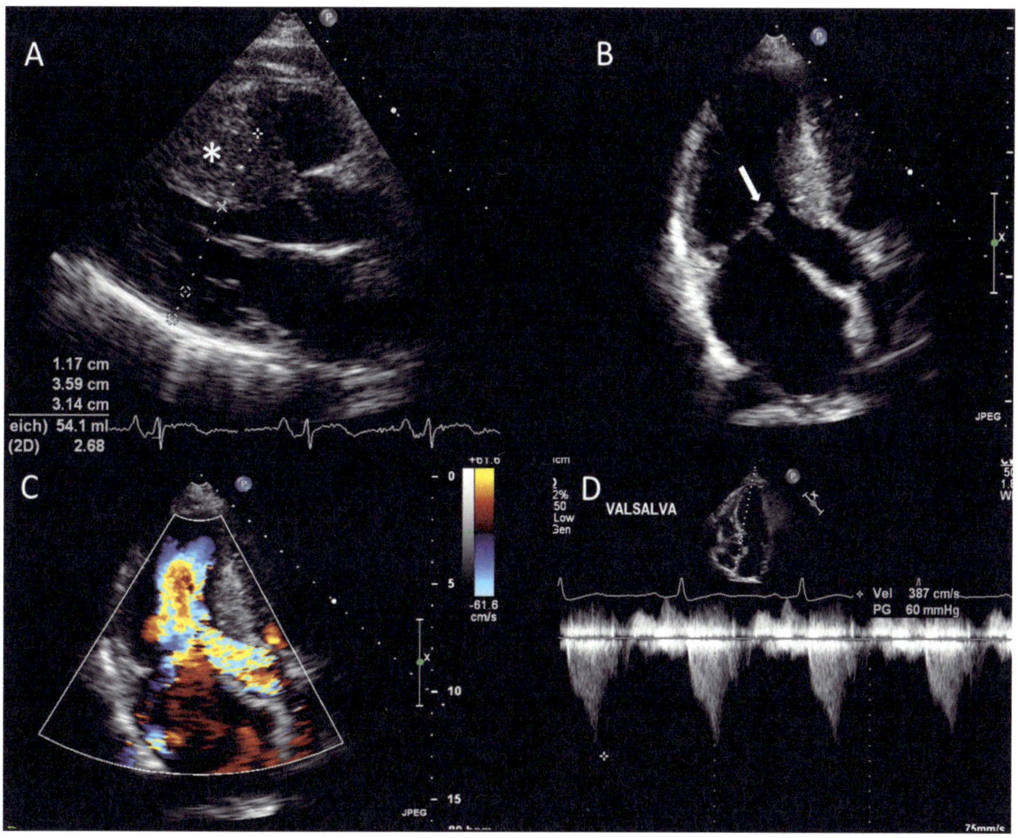

Figure 4. In panel A marked asymmetric septal hypertrophy (ASH) is noted (asterisk) in parasternal long axis display. Systolic anterior motion (SAM) of the mitral valve is seen in panel B (arrow). Turbulence of blood flow through the left ventricular outflow tract (LVOT) associated with posteriorly directed mitral regurgitation due to LVOT obstruction from SAM is present (panel C). Spectral Doppler through the LVOT confirms LVOT obstruction with a late peaking gradient of 60 mmHg (panel D). In this example Valsalva maneuver was used to confirm dynamic LVOT obstruction.

3.1.3. Tissue doppler imaging and speckle strain

Tissue Doppler and 2-D speckle techniques demonstrate impaired longitudinal velocity and strain even in non-hypertrophied myocardial segments. These indices of longitudinal fiber function are abnormal in inherited HCM even prior to grossly manifest left ventricular hypertrophy. The degree of functional impairment by these measures correlates with clinical outcome [22]. Furthermore, differentiation between pathologic and physiologic left ventricular hypertrophy is possible by documenting preserved longitudinal function in the latter which is impaired in HCM even when global left ventricular function is normal [23].

3.1.4. Three dimensional echo

A more accurate assessment of left ventricle mass and chamber volumes is made possible by 3DE. The clinical impact of this in routine clinical care is less apparent.

3.2. Arrhythmogenic right ventricular cardiomyopathy/dysplasia

3.2.1. Introduction

Arrhythmogenic right ventricular cardiomyopathy/dysplasia (ARVC/D) is a genetic cardiomyopathy with autosomal dominant inheritance. However, phenotypes with cutaneous manifestations have autosomal recessive inheritance. The disorder is pathologically characterized by fibrofatty infiltration of the right ventricle (RV) wall. In early stages, dysplasia is localized, affecting the RV inflow, RV outflow or RV apex. Progression to diffuse form is common. Clinical manifestation is with ventricular arrhythmias and RV systolic dysfunction [24-25].

3.2.2. Echo diagnosis of ARVC/D

Morphological and functional changes affecting the RV are divided into major and minor diagnostic criteria. In the proposed revision of ARVC/D task force document [26], right ventricle outflow tract (RVOT) long axis dimension of ≥ 32 mm (sensitivity/specificity: 75% and 95%, respectively), RVOT short axis dimension of ≥ 36 mm (sensitivity/specificity: 62% and 95%, respectively) and RV fractional area change of ≤33% (sensitivity/specificity: 55% and 95%, respectively) are considered as major criteria for the diagnosis of ARVC/D. Minor echo criteria are RVOT long axis dimension of ≥ 29 mm (sensitivity/specificity: 87% and 87%, respectively), RVOT short axis dimension of ≥ 32 mm (sensitivity/specificity: 80% and 80%, respectively) and RV fractional area change of ≤40% (sensitivity/specificity: 76% and 76%, respectively) [26]. Of interest, diastolic dimensions of the RV taken from the apical four-chamber view were least commonly enlarged [27]. Regional wall motion abnormality of the apex and anterior wall is seen in approximately 70% of patients [27]. Other frequent morphologic abnormality include trabecular derangement, occurring in 54%, hyper-reflective moderator band in 34% and sacculations of RV free wall in 17% [27]. Given its predominant autosomal dominant inheritance screening of family members is recommended.

3.3. Left ventricular non-compaction

3.3.1. Introduction

Left ventricular non-compaction (LVNC) is a distinct cardiomyopathy resulting from arrest of fetal development of the heart [28]. This leads to altered myocardial architecture that is seen as a two layered myocardium with a thin, compacted epicardial layer and a thick, non-compacted endocardial region (Figure-5). The non-compacted myocardial region is comprised of prominent trabeculations and deep intertrabecular recesses that directly communicate with the left ventricular cavity [29-30].The condition may present without any associated cardiac malformation and is then labeled isolated left ventricular non compaction (LVNC). Non compacted myocardium is also seen in conjunction with other cardiac abnormalities including cyanotic congenital heart disease, Ebstein's anomaly and other cardiomyopathies. Clinical presentation in LVNC is seen with congestive heart failure, ventricular arrhythmia and systemic thromboembolism.

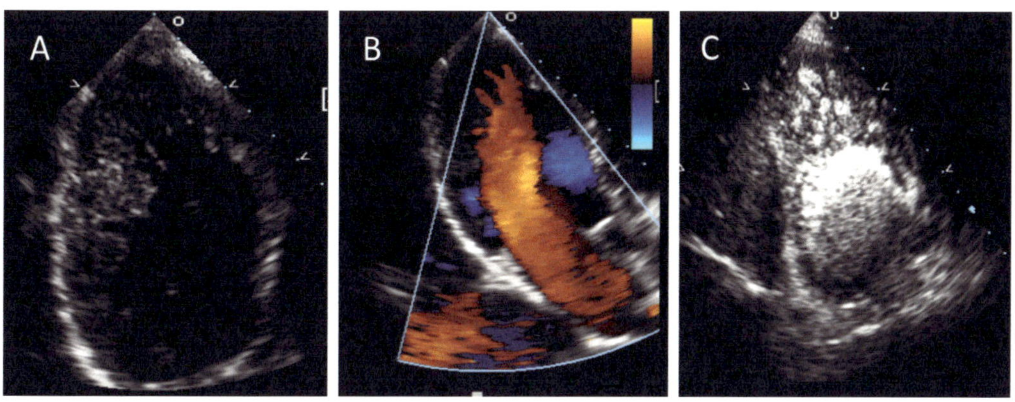

Figure 5. Marked trabeculation of LV myocardium is seen in the apical and inferolateral distribution (panel A) in this off axis projection of apical long axis of the heart. Ratio of non comapcted to compacted myocardium is consistent with the diagnosis of left ventricular non-compaction. Communication of deep intertrabecular recesses with LV cavity is noted on color Doppler (panel B) and following administration of echo contrast (panel C). Visual appearance of the non compacted myocardium is also enhanced following echo contrast.

3.3.2. Diagnostic criteria on cardiac imaging

Trabeculation in the left ventricle wall is seen even in healthy volunteers. To separate benign left ventricular trabeculation from pathological LVNC following diagnostic criteria is proposed.

- Echocardiogram: ratio of non-compacted to compacted myocardium in end-systole of > 2:1 [31]
- Cardiac MRI: ratio of non-compacted to compacted myocardium in end-diastole of > 2.3:1 [32]

The most frequently involved segments are apical, followed by the inferior and lateral mid-segments. Severity and distribution of non compacted segment is better appreciated with use of contrast echo.

Left ventricle contractile abnormality is present in patients with LVNC. The spectrum of myocardial function may range from normal to severe systolic dysfunction. Documentation of direct flow from ventricular cavity into inter-trabecular recesses either with color Doppler technique or following use of echo contrast is helpful in differentiating LVNC from other apical echocardiographic abnormalities such as apical hypertrophic cardiomyopathy and apical mural thrombus [31]. Information from 3DE is also helpful in identifying the extent of LVNC [33]. Screening of family members is advised.

4. Mixed genetic and non genetic cardiomyopathy

4.1. Dilated Cardiomyopathy (DCM)

4.1.1. Introduction

The prevalence of idiopathic dilated cardiomyopathy is not well understood but an estimate in the USA is ~40 per 100 000 persons [34]. DCM is the most common cardiomyopathy, accounting for 60% of all primary cardiomyopathies [35] and is a leading cause of heart failure and arrhythmia. Familial and sporadic forms of DCM are well described. Genetic factors are important, with 20% of cases having a familial basis with an autosomal dominant inheritance [36]. This has important implications for screening of first-degree relatives.

4.1.2. Features of DCM on standard echocardiogram

Wall motion abnormalities: Wall motion abnormality is global as opposed to regional abnormalities in ischemic cardiomyopathy. However, some regional variation in myocardial contractility may be encountered. Preservation of contractile function of basal inferolateral segment is not infrequent. Due to these overlapping features, ischemic cardiomyopathy should be conclusively excluded when appropriate.

Cardiac Chamber Enlargement: Left ventricular (LV) cavity enlargement and systolic dysfunction in the absence of valvular or ischemic heart disease are key diagnostic features of DCM. Dilatation of both left and right ventricles is encountered. Left ventricular cavity assumes a spherical shape in advanced cases (Figure-6). Chamber quantification is preferred over visual estimation for serial comparison. In addition to linear cavity dimension, which is increased in DCM, calculation of left ventricle volume and systolic function derived from modified biplane Simpson's method is recommended.

Low Flow State: Consequent to sluggish blood flow velocity, patients are at risk of developing LV mural thrombus. Low circulatory state can be appreciated by spontaneous echo contrast in left ventricle and by an increase in separation of mitral valve E point to ventricular septum and partial opening and early closure of aortic valve in systole. The latter is particularly important, as aortic stenosis may be overestimated on 2D echo (pseudo aortic stenosis) and underestimated by Doppler (low-gradient aortic stenosis) due to low flow state. Contractile augmentation with dobutamine is helpful in clarification in such situations [64].

Secondary Mitral Regurgitation: Altered mitral valve geometry from progressive LV cavity enlargement will lead to mitral regurgitation, which may be severe in advanced cases [37]. Presence of mitral regurgitation predicts poor outcome [38].

Diastolic Dysfunction: Presence of diastolic abnormality is established by Doppler interrogation of mitral inflow and mitral annular velocities. Severity of diastolic abnormality may be insightful and partly explanatory for the frequently observed discordance between degree of LV systolic dysfunction and severity of clinical symptoms. Patients with earlier stage of diastolic abnormality are less symptomatic when compared to those with more advanced diastolic dysfunction. Reduction in effective diastolic filling period is reflected by fusion of mitral diastolic E-wave and A-wave (Figure-6).

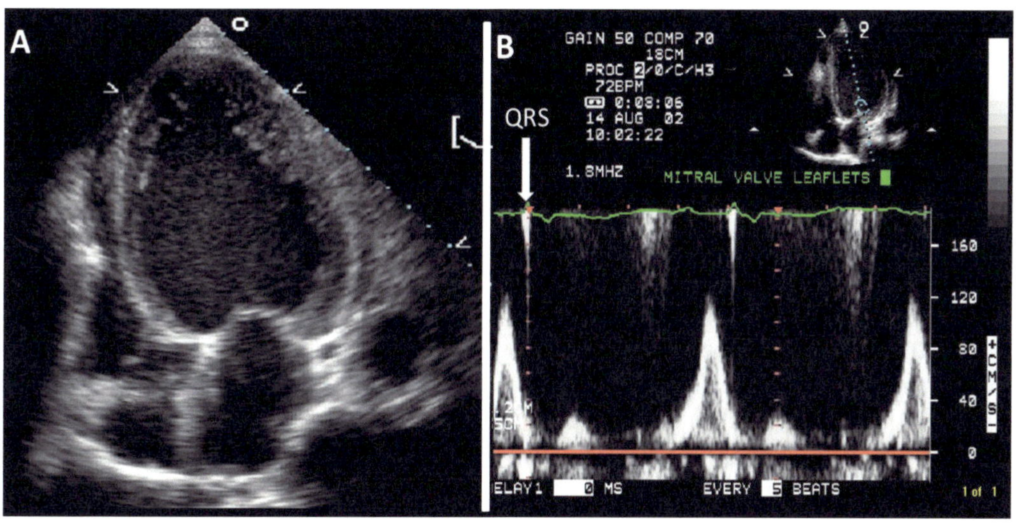

Figure 6. Apical four chamber view shows a dilated LV cavity with a spherical appearance. RV cavity is normal in this example. Pulse-wave Doppler at mitral leaflet tip shows fusion of diastolic E and A waves. Latter is a reflection of reduced diastolic filling period.

Right Ventricular (RV) Function: RV enlargement to a similar degree as the LV is associated with poor outcome [39]. RV systolic function can be measured by fractional area change or by tricuspid annular plane systolic excursion (TAPSE) [40]. TAPSE < 14 mm is associated with adverse prognosis [41]. In another study, 3DE derived measurement of RV volume and function was superior to conventional method [42].

4.1.3. Novel echo techniques

Routine use of Doppler-derived strain and 2D strain may have limited application in clinically manifest disease. Application of these techniques in preclinical state and in asymptomatic family members with inherited type of DCM may identify at risk subset of patients. Observation of intersegmental discordance in the timing of strain measures, particularly those of opposing segments identify a subset of DCM patients with LV dyssynchrony, who may benefit from cardiac resynchronization therapy.

4.2. Restrictive cardiomyopathy (non-hypertrophied and non-dilated)

4.2.1. Introduction

Primary restrictive cardiomyopathy (RCM) predominantly affects the elderly, with a slight female predominance [43]. Clinical presentation is with signs and symptoms of systemic and pulmonary venous congestion from diastolic heart failure and pulmonary HTN [43]. As opposed to other types of primary cardiomyopathies which have distinctive morphologic abnormalities, the diagnosis of RCM is largely dependent on an altered physiology of blood flow through the heart consequent to a non compliant ventricle. The condition has no distinctive histologic features [44]. RCM should be distinguished from infiltrative disorders of the heart where, in addition to restrictive physiology which may be indistinguishable from RCM, distinctive morphologic and histopathologic changes are present. Amyloid heart disease and endomyocardial fibrosis are typical examples of the latter.

4.2.2. Features of RCM on standard echocardiogram

Left ventricle (LV) appearance and contractility is usually normal. LV cavity size may be small. Biatrial enlargement in the absence of significant regurgitation of mitral and tricuspid valves or atrial fibrillation and with normal LV kinetics in patients with signs and symptoms of heart failure should prompt consideration of RCM (Figure-7). Impaired diastolic relaxation of the LV is encountered but a key diagnostic feature is the presence of restrictive physiology on Doppler as evidenced by an increase in E:A ratio >2 with rapid deceleration of early mitral inflow (E) velocity, usually to < 150 msec (Figure-7) [45]. This, in conjunction with reduced early mitral annular velocity (E') and elevated E/E' ratio, is confirmatory of elevated left ventricular end diastolic pressure (LVEDP). Reduced E' velocity, reflecting underlying myocardial disease, is useful in distinguishing RCM from constrictive pericarditis where mitral annular velocities are preserved [46-47]. Deformation of the LV on 2D speckle strain is constrained in the circumferential direction in constrictive pericarditis and in the longitudinal direction in RCM [48]. Flow propagation velocity on color M-mode of mitral inflow can provide additional insight into diastolic dysfunction of RCM.

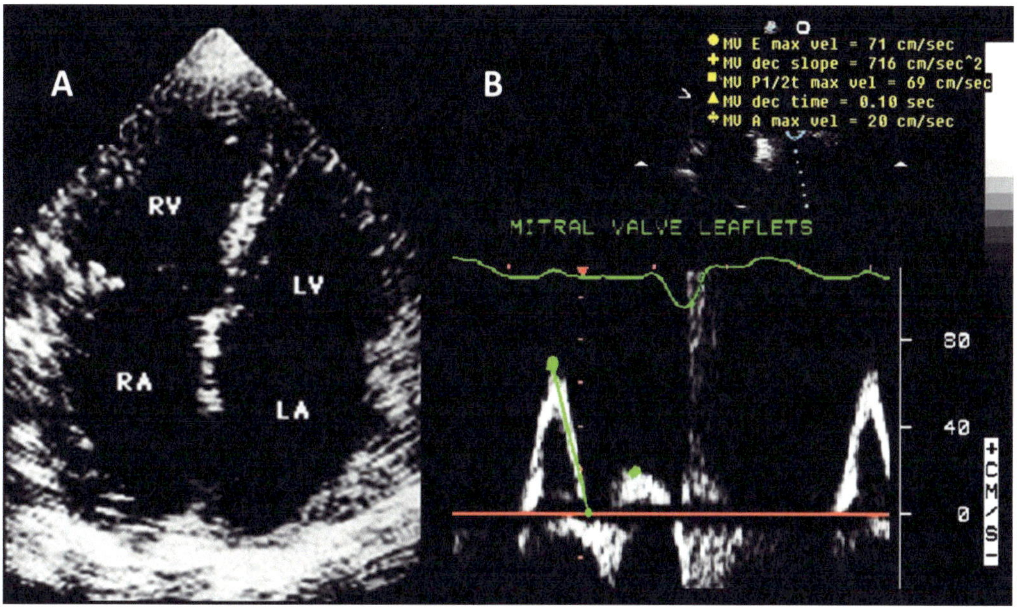

Figure 7. Morphologic and functional abnormality in restrictive cardiomyopathy is represented in this example. There is biatrial enlargement on apical four chamber view (panel A). Restrictive diastolic filling abnormality (E: A ratio of > 2 with rapid deceleration of early mitral inflow velocity) by Doppler is noted (panel B).

5. Acquired primary and secondary cardiomyopathy

For the purpose of this review, discussion will be limited to key features of commonly encountered acquired cardiomyopathy.

5.1. Inflammatory myocarditis

Inflammatory cardiomyopathy is defined by myocarditis in association with cardiac dysfunction [11]. Idiopathic, autoimmune, and infectious forms of inflammatory cardiomyopathy are recognized [11]. Echo findings are of non-specific LV cavity dilatation associated with global LV dysfunction similar to that seen in idiopathic dilated cardiomyopathy. Regional variation in LV contractility is not infrequently encountered.

5.2. Takotsubo cardiomyopathy (stress cardiomyopathy)

A transient and reversible cardiomyopathy first reported in Japan by Dote, et al., in 1991 [49]. Clinical presentation may be indistinguishable from acute coronary syndrome, invariably necessitating coronary angiography for exclusion of obstructive coronary artery disease. Prevalence is about 1-2% of patients undergoing coronary angiography for acute coronary syndrome. A precipitating emotional or physical stressor is typical. Complimentary imaging modalities including echocardiography and cardiac MRI are helpful in diagnosis and in monitoring clinical recovery. In fact, LV morphology at echocardiography is characteristic as it resembles a takotsubo (Japanese octopus trap) with dilatation of the apical region of the heart and preserved contractility of basal segments (Figure-8). About a fifth of patients will have hyperdynamic contractility of basal LV segments with consequent left ventricular outflow tract obstruction and systemic hypotension. Early recognition of this by echo has marked influence on therapeutic choice [50]. Reverse pattern of LV contractile dysfunction has been described. Right ventricular involvement in takotsubo is seen in 25-30% of patients and is associated with a more complicated clinical course [51]. It is encountered in patients with more severe LV involvement [52]. However, isolated right ventricular takotsubo has been reported [53]. The condition is prone to formation of LV apical mural thrombus which should be carefully excluded in all.

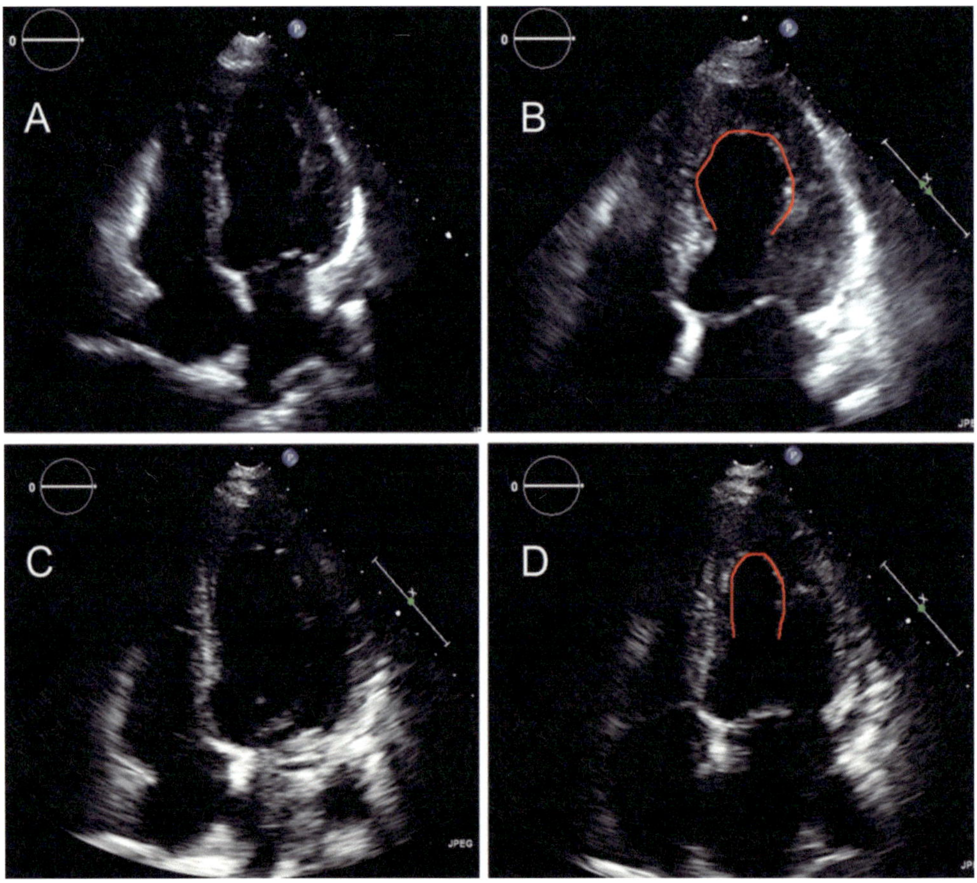

Figure 8. Diastolic and systolic frame of the LV in acute phase of takotsubo cardiomyopathy (panels A and B, respectively) and during recovery (panels C and D, respectively). Apical systolic expansion is noted during acute illness (panel B). Apical endocardial border is highlighted in red. Normalization of apical systolic morphology and function is noted upon recovery (panel D).

5.3. PeriPartum Cardiomyopathy (PPCM)

The diagnosis of PPCM rests on the echocardiographic identification of new left ventricular systolic dysfunction during a limited period surrounding childbirth. Other causes of cardiomyopathy should be excluded [54]. Features are typically that of dilated cardiomyopathy, though LV cavity dimensions may be normal. Echocardiogram is used to monitor the effectiveness of treatment. In one study of PPCM recovery of LV function was reported in 54% of study population [55]. This was more likely to happen in women with EF of > 30% at diagnosis [55]. However, even in those with recovery of resting LV function by echo, contractile reserve on dobutamine echo is reduced [56].The condition is likely to recur during subsequent pregnancy even following recovery of LV function. The condition is associated with a worse prognosis where recovery of LV function is incomplete or did not occur after the index pregnancy [57]. Patients with LVEF of < 25% at diagnosis or in whom LV function has not normalized should be counseled against subsequent pregnancy [58]. Early and serial echocardiogram may be considered during subsequent pregnancies in all patients with prior history of PPCM.

5.4. Tachycardia Induced Cardiomyopathy (TIC)

There are no diagnostic features of TIC on echocardiogram. Non-specific dilated cardiomyopathy may ensue from chronic tachyarrhythmia of either supraventricular or ventricular origin [59-60]. Treatment of tachyarrhythmia is associated with recovery of LV systolic function, though some degree of adverse LV remodeling may persist [61]. Diastolic dysfunction by echo is encountered which may not reverse after normalization of LV systolic function [62].

5.5. Ischemic cardiomyopathy

On standard echocardiogram findings that constitute ischemic cardiomyopathy include regional wall motion abnormalities, wall thinning with aneurysmal dilatation of the infarcted myocardial segment, left ventricular (LV) cavity dilatation and decline in LV systolic performance that is out of proportion to the degree of underlying CAD (Figure-9).

Beyond recognition of an underlying ischemic process, an issue that frequently merits clarification is that of hibernating viable myocardium and non-viable infarcted myocardium [63]. This is particularly difficult to distinguish when infarcted myocardial segments have normal or relatively normal thickness or when global LV contractile dysfunction as that seen in DCM is encountered. For this low-dose dobutamine echocardiography test is useful. Augmented contractility with dobutamine typically seen as a biphasic response is noted with hibernating myocardium. Newer methods of assessing longitudinal fiber contraction during dobutamine echo by long axis pulsed wave Doppler and M-mode is considered to be superior, particularly in patients with LBBB [64].

5.6. Valvular cardiomyopathy

It is defined as ventricular dysfunction that is out of proportion to the abnormal loading conditions of the heart [11]. Left ventricle is affected by regurgitant lesions of the mitral and

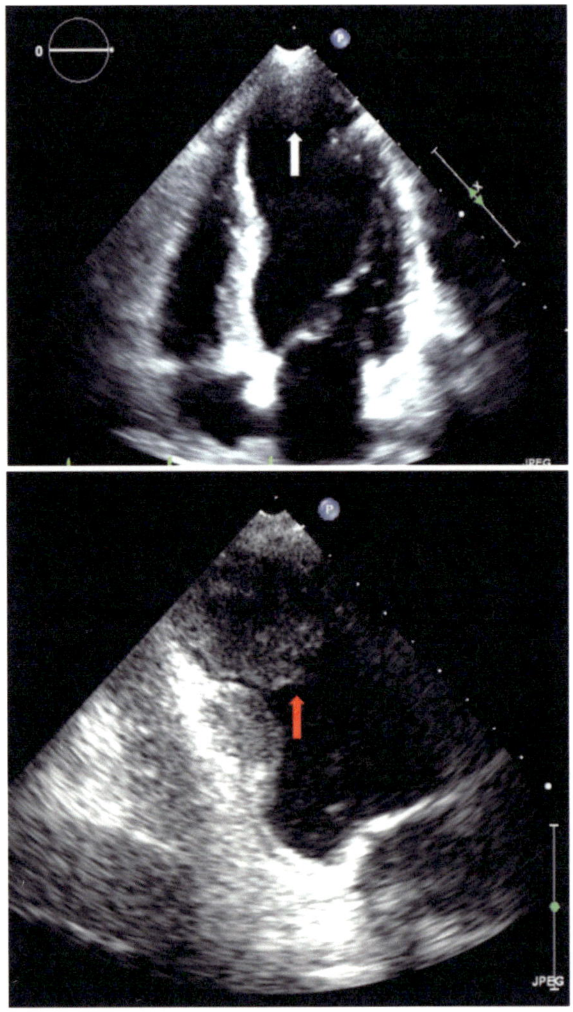

Figure 9. Apical LV aneurysm (white arrow) is seen in a patient with ischemic cardiomyopathy. In another patient apical LV aneurysm is associated with a large LV mural thrombus (red arrow).

aortic valves and by increased afterload of aortic stenosis. Primary valve abnormality can be readily identified though findings can be blunted in the failing heart.

5.6.1. Aortic stenosis

Increased afterload of aortic stenosis results in concentric left ventricular (LV) hypertrophy. LV cavity size is normal and systolic function preserved. With progressive disease LV dilatation and impaired systolic function ensues. In patients with severe systolic dysfunction assessment of aortic stenosis by Doppler can be challenging due to low flow velocity. Inotropic augmentation of contractility and flow with dobutamine can be used in such cases [65].

5.6.2. Aortic regurgitation

LV cavity enlargement is present, which can be marked. Systolic function is initially preserved but declines with advanced disease. Increase in LV end-diastolic pressure may blunt the color Doppler signal of aortic regurgitation. Serial estimation of LV cavity dimension and volume is necessary for aortic valve replacement prior to irreversible contractile dysfunction. LVEF of ≤ 50%, LV end-diastolic dimension of ≥ 70 mm and LV end-systolic dimension of ≥ 50 mm are echo criteria for surgical intervention in asymptomatic individuals [66]. Abnormal longitudinal and circumferential strain is noted in the preclinical phase [67]. Incremental value of these strain parameters for therapeutic intervention is not well established.

5.6.3. Mitral regurgitation

LV volume overload is well tolerated with preserved LV systolic function early in the disease. Progressive decline in LV systolic function can be underestimated when using LV ejection fraction as a marker of systolic performance. Left atrial enlargement is followed by LV cavity enlargement. Progressive increase in left atrial pressure may decrease the color Doppler signal of mitral regurgitation in advanced cases. LV end-systolic dimension of ≥ 45 mm or LVEF of ≤ 60% is used to time surgical intervention [68].

5.7. Hypertensive heart disease and cardiomyopathy

There is an increase in LV mass consequent to concentric hypertrophy of LV. Systolic function is preserved. Variable degree of diastolic function is noted. In patients with severe LV hypertrophy echocardiographic differentiation from other disease states with LV hypertrophy is challenging. Restrictive filling pattern is seen in severe disease. Progressive disease is associated with LV cavity dilatation and decline in LV systolic function similar to that seen in dilated cardiomyopathy.

5.8. Metabolic cardiomyopathy

5.8.1. Amyloid heart disease

Cardiac amyloidosis is an infiltrative disorder of the heart which on echo is seen as thick-walled left and right ventricles with normal left ventricular cavity dimension and systolic function. Advanced disease is associated with decline in left ventricular systolic function. Increased echogenicity from thickening of heart valves, biatrial enlargement and thickened interatrial septum are other morphologic features of established disease. Pericardial effusion is seen in more than half of patients [69] (Figure-10). Increased granular appearance of the heart in earlier description of cardiac amyloidosis is not distinct on modern echo hardware and image processing [70]. Assessment of transmitral flow and mitral annular velocities by Doppler reveals impaired diastolic function. Restrictive diastolic filling pattern is noted in advanced cases. Unlike in restrictive filling pattern, reduced mitral A- velocity may be seen with normal mitral E-deceleration time. This finding suggests atrial myopathy and reduced contractility from amyloid infiltration [71]. Some overlapping clinical and echocardiographic features of hypertrophic cardiomyopathy are seen in 5% of cases. In contrast to a hypertrophied ventricle, low voltage in precordial leads is seen on ECG, and systolic anterior motion of mitral valve which is a frequent observation in hypertrophic cardiomyopathy on echo, is uncommon in patients with cardiac amyloidosis. By novel echo techniques longitudinal strain and strain rate show systolic dysfunction despite preserved radial contraction as determined by fractional shortening. The value of strain parameters in early diagnosis and in prognosis is being evaluated [72]. Furthermore, strain measurement by 2D speckle tracking shows variation in longitudinal strain from base to apex with relative preservation of apical strain. This finding can be helpful in distinguishing cardiac amyloidosis from hypertrophic cardiomyopathy and hypertrophy associated with increased afterload state of aortic stenosis [73].

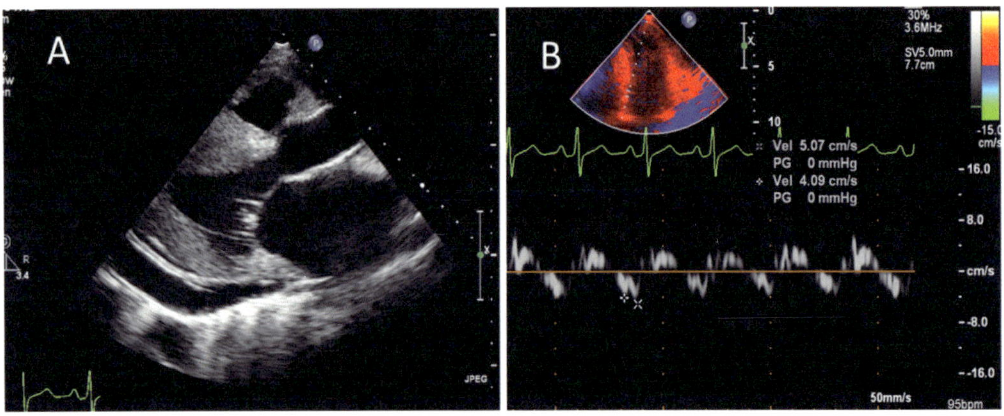

Figure 10. Severe concentric left ventricular wall thickening and small pericardial effusion is present in this patient with cardiac amyloidosis (panel A). Impaired mitral annular velocity is indicative of abnormal diastolic function (reduced mitral annular velocities with reversal of E' to A' ratio) (panel B).

5.8.2. Hemochromatosis

There are no specific morphologic features on echocardiogram. Dilated cardiomyopathy is seen in advanced stages of hemochromatosis [74]. Non-invasive diagnosis of cardiac involvement is dependent on demonstration of myocardial iron deposit on cardiac MRI [75]. In cases with established cardiac involvement, assessment of myocardial kinetics by Doppler and tissue strain may reveal functional impairment prior to development of overt cardiomyopathy. The value of these new techniques in determining prognosis and in serial follow up of patients following therapeutic intervention has been the subject of recent studies.

5.9. Toxic cardiomyopathy: Alcohol and anthracyclines

Echo findings are non-specific. Dilated cardiomyopathy from cardiotoxicity of alcohol cannot be distinguished from idiopathic dilated cardiomyopathy. Impairment of left ventricle systolic function is a concern for both anthracycline and some non-anthracycline based chemotherapeutic regimens. Dose dependent cardiotoxicity from anthracyclines is reversible if detected early and upon institution of effective heart failure therapy [76]. Serial assessment of left ventricle systolic function, preferably by echo, is routine in such cases. Impaired tissue kinetics by measures of myocardial strain and strain rate is noted prior to gross impairment of left ventricle systolic function. This may have a role in influencing management [77].

6. Conclusion

Value of echocardiography in the diagnosis, prognosis and monitoring of therapy in patients with cardiomyopathy is discussed in the preceding review. 3DE, Doppler and speckle strain and left ventricular torsion may have a role in preclinical disease states. Incorporation of these diagnostic methods in routine clinical assessment of patients with cardiomyopathy is dependent on emerging data on the usefulness and reproducibility of these techniques.

Author details

Gohar Jamil[1], Ahmed Abbas[1], Abdullah Shehab[2] and Anwer Qureshi[1*]

*Address all correspondence to: aqureshi@tawamhospital.ae

1 Division of Cardiology, Tawam Hospital, Al Ain, United Arab Emirates

2 Faculty of Medicine and Health Sciences, United Arab Emirates University, Al Ain, United Arab Emirates

References

[1] Jenkins, C, Bricknell, K, Hanekom, L, & Marwick, T. H. Reproducibility and accuracy of echocardiographic measurements of left ventricular parameters using real-time three-dimensional echocardiography, J Am Coll Cardiol , 44-2004.

[2] Sonne, C, Sugeng, L, Takeuchi, M, et al. Real-Time 3-Dimensional Echocardiographic Assessment of Left Ventricular Dyssynchrony: Pitfalls in Patients with Dilated Cardiomyopathy. J Am Coll Cardiol Img. (2009). , 2(7), 802-812.

[3] Nagueh, S. F, Middleton, K. J, Kopelen, H. A, Zoghbi, W. A, & Quinones, M. A. Doppler tissue imaging: a noninvasive technique for evaluation of left ventricular relaxation and estimation of filling pressures. *J Am Coll Cardiol*. (1997). , 30, 1527-1533.

[4] Ommen, S. R, Nishimura, R. A, Appleton, C. P, Miller, F. A, Oh, J. K, Redfield, M. M, & Tajik, A. J. Clinical utility of Doppler echocardiography and tissue Doppler imag-

ing in the estimation of left ventricular filling pressures: a comparative simultaneous Doppler-catheterization study. Circulation. (2000)., 102, 1788-1794.

[5] Carolyn, Y, Ho, C. Y, & Solomon, S. D. A Clinician's Guide to Tissue Doppler Imaging. Circulation. (2006). ee398., 396.

[6] Cardim, N, Oliveira, A. G, Longo, S, Ferreira, T, Pereira, A, Reis, R. P, & Correia, J. M. Doppler tissue imaging: regional myocardial function in hypertrophic cardiomyopathy and in athlete's heart. J Am Soc Echocardiogr. (2003)., 16, 223-232.

[7] Yu, C. M, Fung, J. W, Zhang, Q, Chan, C. K, Chan, Y. S, Lin, H, Kum, L. C, Kong, S. L, Zhang, Y, & Sanderson, J. E. Tissue Doppler imaging is superior to strain rate imaging and postsystolic shortening on the prediction of reverse remodeling in both ischemic and nonischemic heart failure after cardiac resynchronization therapy. Circulation. (2004)., 110, 66-73.

[8] Castro, PL, Greenberg, NL, Drinko, J, & Garcia, . . Potential pitfalls of strain rate imaging: angle dependency. Biomed Sci Instrum 2000; 36:197-202.

[9] Geyer, H, Caracciolo, G, Abe, H, et al. Assessment of myocardial mechanics using speckle tracking echocardiography: fundamentals and clinical applications. J Am Soc Echocardiogr (2010)., 23, 351-369.

[10] Rüssel, I. K, Götte, M. J, Bronzwaer, J. G, Knaapen, P, Paulus, W. J, & Van Rossum, A. C. Left ventricular torsion: an expanding role in the analysis of myocardial dysfunction. JACC Cardiovasc Imaging. (2009). May;, 2(5), 648-55.

[11] Richardson, P, Mckenna, W, Bristow, M, Maisch, B, Mautner, B, Connell, O, Olsen, J, Thiene, E, & Goodwin, G. J. Report of the 1995 World Health Organization/International Society and Federation of Cardiology Task Force on the definition and classification of cardiomyopathies. Circulation (1996)., 93, 841-842.

[12] Maron, B. J, Towbin, J. A, Thiene, M. D, Antzelevitch, G, Corrado, C, Arnett, D, Moss, D, Seidman, A. J, & Young, C. E, M. D. JB. Contemporary Definitions and Classification of the Cardiomyopathies. An American Heart Association Scientific Statement from the Council on Clinical Cardiology, Heart Failure and Transplantation Committee; Quality of Care and Outcomes Research and Functional Genomics and Translational Biology Interdisciplinary Working Groups; and Council on Epidemiology and Prevention. Circulation.(2006)., 113, 1807-1816.

[13] Maron, B. J, & Epstein, S. E. Hypertrophic cardiomyopathy. Recent observations regarding the specificity of three hallmarks of the disease: asymmetric septal hypertrophy, septal disorganization and systolic anterior motion of the anterior mitral leaflet, Am J Cardiol , 45-1980.

[14] Weyman, A. E. Principles and Practice of Echocardiography2nd edition (1994). Lea and Febiger New York, NY

[15] Wigle, E. D, Rakowski, H, Kimball, B. P, & Williams, W. G. Hypertrophic cardiomyopathy. Clinical spectrum and treatment. Circulation (1995). , 92, 1680-92.

[16] Kato, T. S, Noda, A, Izawa, H, et al. Discrimination of nonobstructive hypertrophic cardiomyopathy from hypertensive left ventricular hypertrophy on the basis of strain rate imaging by tissue Doppler ultrasonography. Circulation (2004). , 110, 3808-14.

[17] Harris, K. M, Spirito, P, Maron, M. S, et al. Prevalence, clinical profile, and significance of left ventricular remodeling in the end-stage phase of hypertrophic cardiomyopathy. Circulation (2006). , 114, 216-25.

[18] Maron, B. J, Spirito, P, Green, K. J, Wesley, Y. E, Bonow, R. O, & Arce, J. Noninvasive assessment of left ventricular diastolic function by pulsed Doppler echocardiography in patients with hypertrophic cardiomyopathy. J Am Coll Cardiol (1987). , 10, 733-42.

[19] Nagueh, S. F, Middleton, K. J, Kopelen, H. A, Zoghbi, W. A, & Quinones, M. A. Doppler tissue imaging: a noninvasive technique for evaluation of left ventricular relaxation and estimation of filling pressures. J Am Coll Cardiol (1997). , 30, 1527-33.

[20] Maron, B. J, Gottdiener, J. S, & Perry, L. W. Specificity of systolic anterior motion of anterior mitral leaflet for hypertrophic cardiomyopathy. Prevalence in large population of patients with other cardiac diseases. Br Heart J (1981). , 45, 206-212.

[21] Nagueh, S. F, & Mahmarian, J. J. Noninvasive cardiac imaging in patients with hypertrophic cardiomyopathy, J Am Coll Cardiol (2006). , 48, 2410-2422.

[22] Nagueh, S. F, Bachinski, L. L, Meyer, D, et al. Tissue Doppler imaging consistentlydetects myocardial abnormalities in patients with hypertrophic cardiomyopathy and provides a novel means for an early diagnosis before and independently of hypertrophy. Circulation (2001). , 104, 128-30.

[23] Vinereanu, D, Florescu, N, Sculthorpe, N, Tweddel, A. C, Stephens, M. R, & Fraser, A. G. Differentiation between pathologic and physiologic left ventricular hypertrophy by tissue Doppler assessment of long-axis function in patients with hypertrophic cardiomyopathy or systemic hypertension and in athletes. Am J Cardiol (2001). , 88, 53-8.

[24] Marcus, F. I, Fontaine, G. H, Guiraudon, G, et al. Right ventricular dysplasia: a report of 24 adult cases, Circulation (1982). , 65, 384-398.

[25] Basso, C, Thiene, G, Corrado, D, Angelini, A, & Nava, A. Valente M; Arrhythmogenic right ventricular cardiomyopathy. Dysplasia, dystrophy, or myocarditis? Circulation (1996). , 94, 983-991.

[26] Marcus, F. I, Mckenna, W. J, Sherrill, D, et al. Diagnosis of arrhythmogenic right ventricular cardiomyopathy/dysplasia: proposed modification of the task force criteria, Circulation (2010). , 121, 1533-1541.

[27] Yoerger, D. M, Marcus, F, Sherrill, D, et al. Multidisciplinary Study of Right Ventricular Dysplasia Investigators. Echocardiographic findings in patients meeting task force criteria for arrhythmogenic right ventricular dysplasia: new insights from the Multidisciplinary Study of Right Ventricular Dysplasia, J Am Coll Cardiol (2005). , 45, 860-865.

[28] Sedmera, D, Pexieder, T, Vuillemin, M, Thompson, R. P, & Anderson, R. H. Developmental patterning of the myocardium. *Anat Rec* (2000). , 258, 319-337.

[29] Chin, T. K, Perloff, J. K, Williams, R. G, Jue, K, & Mohrmann, R. Isolated noncompaction of left ventricular myocardium. A study of eight cases. Circulation (1990). , 82, 507-513.

[30] Dusek, J, Ostadal, B, & Duskova, M. Postnatal persistence of Postnatal persistence of spongy myocardium with embryonic blood supply. Arch Pathol (1975). , 99, 312-317.

[31] Jenni, R, Oechslin, E, & Schneider, J. Attenhofer Jost C, Kaufmann PA. Echocardiographic and pathoanatomical characteristics of isolated left ventricular non-compaction: a step towards classification as a distinct cardiomyopathy. Heart (2001). , 86, 666-671.

[32] Petersen, S. E, Selvanayagam, J. B, Wiesmann, F, Robson, M. D, Francis, J. M, Anderson, R. H, Watkins, H, & Neubauer, S. Left ventricular non-compaction: insights fromcardiovascular magnetic resonance imaging J Am Coll Cardiol (2005). , 46, 101-105.

[33] Baker, G. H, Pereira, N. L, Hlavacek, A. M, & Chessa, K. Shirali G: Transthoracic Real-Time Three-Dimensional Echocardiography in the Diagnosis and Description of Noncompaction of Ventricular Myocardium. Echocardiography (2006).

[34] Glazier, J. J, & Connell, J. B O. Dilated and toxic cardiomyopathy; Cardiology: Mosby, (2001).

[35] Codd, M. B, Sugrue, D. D, Gersh, B. J, & Melton, L. J. Epidemiology of idiopathic dilated and hypertrophic cardiomyopathy. A population-based study in Olmsted County, Minnesota, 1975-1984. *Circulation.* (1989). , 80, 564-572.

[36] Michels, V. V, Moll, P. P, Miller, F. A, et al. The frequency of familial dilated cardiomyopathy in a series of patients with idiopathic dilated cardiomyopathy. N Engl J Med.(1992). , 326, 77-82.

[37] Yiu, S. F, Enriquez-sarano, M, Tribouilloy, C, Seward, J. B, & Tajik, A. J. Determinants of the degree of functional mitral regurgitation in patients with systolic left ventricular dysfunction: a quantitative clinical study. Circulation (2000). , 102, 1400-6.

[38] Robbins, J. D, Maniar, P. B, Cotts, W, Parker, M. A, Bonow, R. O, & Gheorghiade, M. Prevalence and severity of mitral regurgitation in chronic systolic heart failure. Am J Cardiol (2003). , 91, 360-2.

[39] Lewis, J. F, Webber, J. D, Sutton, L. L, Chesoni, S, & Curry, C. L. Discordance in degree of right and left ventricular dilatation in patients with dilated cardiomyopathy: recognition and clinical implications. J Am Coll Cardiol.(1993). , 21, 649-54.

[40] Kaul, S, Tei, C, Hopkins, J. M, & Shah, P. M. (1984). Assessment of right ventricular function using two-dimensional echocardiography. Am Heart J , 107, 526-531.

[41] Ghio, S, Recusani, F, Klersy, C, Sebastiani, R, Lauisa, M. L, Campana, C, et al. Prognostic usefulness of the tricuspid annular plane systolic excursion in patients with congestive heart failure secondary to idiopathic or ischemic dilated cardiomyopathy. Am J Cardiol (2000). , 85, 837-42.

[42] Chua, S, Levine, R. A, Yosefy, C, Handschumacher, M. D, Chu, J, Qureshi, A, Neary, J, Ton-nu, T. T, Fu, M, Wu, C. J, & Hung, J. (2009). Assessment of right ventricular function by real-time three-dimensional echocardiography improves accuracy and decreases interobserver variability compared with conventional two-dimensional views. Eur J Echocardiogr , 10, 619-624.

[43] Ammash, N. M, Seward, J. B, Bailey, K. R, Edwards, W. D, & Tajik, A. J. Clinical profile and outcome of idiopathic restrictive cardiomyopathy. Circulation (2000). , 101, 2490-6.

[44] Petros Nihoyannopoulos and David Dawson Restrictive Cardiomyopathies Eur J Echocardiogr (2009) 10(8): iii23-iii33.

[45] Appleton, C. P, Hatle, L. K, & Popp, R. L. Relation of transmitral flow velocity patterns to left ventricular diastolic function: new insights from a combined hemodynamic and Doppler echocardiographic study. J Am Coll Cardiol. (1988). , 12, 426-440.

[46] Ha, J. W, Ommen, S. R, Tajik, A. J, Barnes, M. E, Ammash, N. M, Gertz, M. A, & Seward, J. B. Oh JKDifferentiation of constrictive pericarditis from restrictive cardiomyopathy using mitral annular velocity by tissue Doppler echocardiography. Am J Cardiol. (2004). August 1; , 94(3), 316-319.

[47] Rajagopaian, N, Garcia, M. J, Rodriguez, L, et al. Comparison of new Doppler echocardiographic methods to differentiate constrictive pericardial heart disease and restrictive cardiomyopathy. Am J Cardiol , 87, 86-94.

[48] Disparate patterns of left ventricular mechanics differentiate constrictive pericarditis-from restrictive cardiomyopathySengupta PP, Krishnamoorthy VK, Abhayaratna WP, Korinek J, Belohlavek M, Sundt TM 3rd, Chandrasekaran K, Mookadam F, Seward JB, Tajik AJ, Khandheria BK. JACC Cardiovasc Imaging. (2008). Jan; , 1(1), 29-38.

[49] Dote, K, Sato, H, Tateishi, H, Uchida, T, & Ishihara, M. Myocardial stunning due to simultaneous multivessel coronary spasms: a review of 5 cases. J Cardiol (1991). , 21, 203-214.

[50] Good, C. W, Hubbard, C. R, Harrison, T. A, & Qureshi, A. Echocardiographic Guidance in Treatment of Cardiogenic Shock Complicating Transient Left Ventricular Apical Ballooning Syndrome: J Am Coll Cardiol Img (2009). March 2; (3):372-374.

[51] Elesber AA, Prasad A, Bybee KA, Valeti U, Motiei A, Lerman A, Chandrasekaran K, Rihal CS, Transient Cardiac Apical Ballooning Syndrome: Prevalence and Clinical Implications of Right Ventricular Involvement. J Am Coll Cardiol, 2006; 47:1082-1083.

[52] Haghi, D, Athanasiadis, A, Papavassiliu, T, Suselbeck, T, Fluechter, S, Mahrholdt, H, Borggrefe, M, & Sechtem, U. Right ventricular involvement in Takotsubo Cardiomyopathy. Eur Heart J (2006). , 27, 2433-2439.

[53] Mrdovic, I, Kostic, J, Perunicic, J, Asanin, A, Vasiljevic, Z, & Ostojic, M. Right Ventricular Takotsubo Cardiomyopathy. J Am Coll Cardiol, (2010). , 55(16), 1751-1751.

[54] Pearson, G. D, Veille, J. C, & Rahimtoola, S. Peripartum cardiomyopathy: National Heart, Lung, and Blood Institute and Office of Rare Diseases (National Institutes of-Health) workshop recommendations and review. JAMA , 283(9), 1183-8.

[55] Elkayam, U, Akhter, M. W, & Singh, H. Pregnancy-associated cardiomyopathy: clinical characteristics and a comparison between early and late presentation. Circulation (2050). , 111(16), 2050-5.

[56] Lampert, M, Weinert, L, Hibbard, J, Korcarz, C, Lindheimer, M, & Lang, R. M. Contractile reserve in patients with peripartum cardiomyopathy and recovered left ventricular function. Am J Obstet Gynecol (1997). , 176, 189-195.

[57] Elkayam, U, Tummala, P. P, Rao, K, Akhter, M. W, Karaalp, I. S, Wani, O. R, Hameed, A, Gviazda, I, & Shotan, A. Maternal and fetal outcomes of subsequent pregnancies in women with peripartum cardiomyopathy. N Engl J Med (2001). , 344, 1567-1571.

[58] Sliwa, K, Hilfiker-kleiner, D, Petrie, M. C, Mebazaa, A, Pieske, B, Buchmann, E, Regitz-zagrosek, V, Schaufelberger, M, Tavazzi, L, Van Veldhuisen, D. J, Watkins, H, Shah, A. J, Seferovic, P. M, Elkayam, U, Pankuweit, S, Papp, Z, Mouquet, F, & Mcmurray, J. J. Current state of knowledge on aetiology, diagnosis, management, and therapy of peripartum cardiomyopathy: a position statement from the Heart Failure Association of the European Society of Cardiology Working Group on peripartum cardiomyopathy. Eur J Heart Fail (2010). , 12, 767-778.

[59] Mclaran, C. J, Bersh, B. J, Sugrue, D. D, Hammill, S. C, & Seward, J. B. Holes DR: Tachycardia-induced myocardial dysfunction-A reversible phenomenon? Br Heart J (1985). , 53, 323-327.

[60] Packer, D. L, Bardy, G. H, Worley, S. J, Smith, M. S, Cobb, F. R, Coleman, R. E, & Gallagher, J. J. German LD: Tachycardia induced cardiomyopathy: A reversible form of left Ventricular dysfunction. Am J Cardiol (1986). , 57, 563-570.

[61] Dandamudi, G, Rampurwala, A. Y, Mahenthiran, J, Miller, J. M, & Das, M. K. Persistent left ventricular dilatation in tachycardia-induced cardiomyopathy patients after

appropriate treatment and normalization of ejection fraction. Heart Rhythm. (2008). , 5(8), 1111-4.

[62] Tomita, M, Spinale, F. G, Crawford, F. A, & Zile, M. R. Changes in left ventricular volume, mass and function during development and regression of supraventricular tachycardia induced cardiomyopathy: disparity between recovery of systolic vs. diastolic function. Circulation. *1991635644*, 83

[63] Carluccio, E, Biagioli, P, Alunni, G, Murrone, A, Giombolini, C, Ragni, M, Marino, P. N, Reboldi, G, & Ambrosio, G. Patients with hibernating myocardium show altered left ventricular volumes and shape, which revert following revascularization: Evidence that dysynergy may directly induce cardiac remodeling. J Am Coll of Cardiol. (2006). , 47, 969-977.

[64] Duncan, A. M, Francis, D. P, Gibson, D. G, & Henein, M. Y. Differentiation of ischemic from nonischemic cardiomyopathy during dobutamine stress by left ventricular long-axis function: additional effect of left bundle-branch block. Circulation. (2003). , 108, 1214-1220.

[65] Monin, J. L, Quéré, J. P, Monchi, M, Petit, H, Baleynaud, S, Chauvel, C, Pop, C, Ohlmann, P, Lelguen, C, Dehant, P, Tribouilloy, C, & Guéret, P. Low-gradient aortic stenosis, operativerisk stratification and predictors for long-term outcome: a multicenter study using dobutamine stress hemodynamics. Circulation (2003). , 108, 319-324.

[66] Vahanian, A, Baumgartner, H, Bax, J, Butchart, E, Dion, R, Filippatos, G, et al. Guidelines on the management of valvular heart disease: Task Force on the Management of Valvular Heart Disease of the European Society of Cardiology. Eur Heart J (2007). , 28, 230-68.

[67] Marciniak, A, Sutherland, G. R, Marciniak, M, Claus, P, Bijnens, B, & Jahangiri, M. Myocardial deformation abnormalities in patients with aortic regurgitation: a strain rate imaging study. Eur J Echocardiogr (2009). , 10, 112-9.

[68] Guidelines on the management of valvular heart disease (version 2012): The Joint Task Force on the Management of Valvular Heart Disease of the European Society of Cardiology (ESC) and the European Association for Cardio-Thoracic Surgery (EACTS) Eur Heart J (2012) 33(19): 2451-2496.

[69] Siqueira-filho, A. G. Cunha CLP, Tajik AJ, et al. M-mode and two-dimensional echocardiographic features in cardiac amyloidosis. Circulation. (1981). , 63, 188-196.

[70] Falk, R. H. Diagnosis and management of the cardiac amyloidosis. Circulation (2047). , 112(13), 2047-60.

[71] Murphy, L, & Falk, R. H. Left atrial kinetic energy in AL amyloidosis: can it detect early dysfunction? Am J Cardiol. (2000). , 86, 244-246.

[72] Koyama, J, Ray-sequin, P. A, & Falk, R. H. Longitudinal myocardial function assessed bytissue velocity, strain, and strain rate tissue Doppler echocardiography in patients with AL (primary) cardiac amyloidosis. Circulation. (2003). , 107, 2446-2452.

[73] Phelan, D, Collier, P, Thavendiranathan, P, Popovic, Z. B, Hanna, M, Plana, J. C, Marwick, T. H, & Thomas, J. D. Relative apical sparing of longitudinal strain using two-dimensional speckle-tracking echocardiography is both sensitive and specific for the diagnosis of cardiac amyloidosis. Heart. (2012). , 98, 1442-1448.

[74] Olson, L. J, Baldus, W. P, & Tajik, A. J. Echocardiographic features of idiopathic hemochromatosis. Am J Cardiol. (1987). Oct 1; , 60(10), 885-9.

[75] Anderson, L. J, Holden, S, Davis, B, et al. Cardiovascular T2* magnetic resonance for the early diagnosis of myocardial iron overload. Eur Heart J (2001). , 22, 2171-9.

[76] Cardinale, D, Colombo, A, Lamantia, G, Colombo, N, Civelli, M, Giacomi, G. D, Rubino, M, Veglia, F, Fiorentini, C, & Cipolla, C. M. Anthracycline-Induced Cardiomyopathy Clinical Relevance and Response to Pharmacologic Therapy. J Am Coll Cardiol. (2010). , 55(3), 213-220.

[77] Migrino, R. Q, Aggarwal, D, Konorev, E, Brahmbhatt, T, Bright, M, & Kalyanaraman, B. Early detection of doxorubicin cardiomyopathy using two-dimensional strain chocardiography. Ultrasound Med Biol. (2008). Feb; Epub 2007 Oct 23., 34(2), 208-14.

Chapter 2

Left Ventricular Twist in Cardiomyopathy

B.M. van Dalen and M.L. Geleijnse

Additional information is available at the end of the chapter

http://dx.doi.org/10.5772/55281

1. Introduction

Merely 50 years ago, Inge Edler and Helmut Hertz were the first to use an ultrasound transducer, borrowed from a local shipyard where it was used for the detection of cracks in metal plates, to record the motion of cardiac structures. Ever since then, the clinical use of echocardiography has steadily increased. Echocardiography is an attractive imaging modality for several reasons. It is highly available, relatively inexpensive, it does not involve ionising radiation, and images are displayed in realtime allowing prompt diagnosis. However, despite a staggering technical progress in echocardiography, regional myocardial function was, until recently, still assessed by visual analysis of wall motion, a relatively inaccurate and poorly reproducible manner.

During the last 10 years, tissue Doppler imaging has been developed to quantify regional myocardial function [1]. Initially formatted as a one-dimensional method for measurement of regional longitudinal myocardial velocity profiles, tissue Doppler imaging has been further developed to allow measurements of one-dimensional regional strain [2]. This index measures local deformation as opposed to (passive and active) motion and thereby better reflects regional myocardial function. However, tissue Doppler imaging is inextricably limited by the angle-dependency of the technique. Because of this limitation, it is not clinically feasible to measure myocardial deformation in directions not parallel to the direction of the Doppler beam, such as left ventricular rotation. Although some have tried to override this limitation by applying complex algorithms [3], measurement of left ventricular rotation by echocardiography has only recently become clinically feasible by the development of speckle tracking echocardiography.

1.1. Left ventricular twist

In the 16th century, Leonardo daVinci already described the rotational motion of the left ventricle [4,5] and in 1669, Richard Lower observed that myocardial contraction could be compared with 'the wringing of a linen cloth to squeeze out the water' [6]. The mechanistic basis for this wringing motion or twist lies in the complex spiral architecture of the left ventricle as revealed by the anatomical studies of Streeter et al. [7] and Greenbaum et al. [8] The left ventricle consists of obliquely oriented muscle fibres that vary from a smaller-radius, right-handed helix at the subendocardium to a larger-radius, left-handed helix at the subepicardium. The functional consequence of this three-dimensional helical structure is a cyclic systolic twisting deformation, resulting from clockwise basal rotation and counterclockwise apical rotation (as seen from the apex). Left ventricular twist plays a pivotal role in the mechanical efficiency of the heart, making it possible that only 15% fibre shortening results in a 60% reduction in left ventricular volume [9]. Moreover, diastolic untwisting of the left ventricle plays a crucial role in diastolic suction [10]. In the last decades, left ventricular twist has mainly been studied with tagged magnetic resonance imaging (MRI). However, lack of availability, limited temporal resolution, and the time-consuming and complex data analysis have precluded its use in routine clinical practice. More recently, it became possible to study left ventricular twist with tissue Doppler techniques and two-dimensional speckle tracking echocardiography. As mentioned before, this latter technique offers the opportunity to track myocardial deformation independently of both cardiac translation and the insonation angle.

1.2. Assessment of left ventricular twist

Ever since the description of the rotational motion of the left ventricle by Leonardo da Vinci [4,5] in the 16th century, left ventricular twist has intrigued clinicians and researchers in their quest to understand the performance of the human heart. In the early 1960s, Harrison et al. [11] developed a method to measure external ventricular wall dimensions during the cardiac cycle. Silver tantalum clips were sutured into the human epicardium during cardiac surgery and these markers were viewed by calibrated cineradiographs. Ingels et al. [12] further developed this technique and studies of left ventricular twist continued throughout the 1980s. Unfortunately, progress was limited due to the invasive nature of the technique with its inherent limitations; the surgical implantation of the clips frequently led to local inflammation, hemorrhage and fibrosis, possibly affecting left ventricular twist. In addition, implantation of the clips could only be done in surgically accessible areas, which limited the left ventricular areas studied. In 1990, Buchalter et al. [13] described for the first time the non-invasive assessment of left ventricular twist with MRI. A tagging technique was employed to label specific areas of the myocardium prior to image acquisition. Tagging is achieved by selective radio-frequency excitation of narrow planes and appears as black lines on the image acquisition. Using dedicated software, displacement of these tagging lines can be monitored, allowing quantification of left ventricular deformation. However, the limited availability, the poor temporal resolution, and the time-consuming and complex data analysis have precluded its use in routine clinical practice.

More recently, assessment of left ventricular twist by speckle tracking echocardiography has become available. The fundamental principle of deformation imaging by speckle tracking echocardiography is simple. A certain segment of myocardial tissue is shown in an ultrasound image as a pattern of gray values caused by the interference of ultrasound reflected by the tissue. Such a pattern, resulting from the spatial distribution of the gray values, is commonly referred to as a speckle pattern. If the position of the myocardial segment within the ultrasound image changes, one can presume that the position of the speckle pattern will change accordingly. Since each region of the myocardium has its own rather unique speckle pattern, the speckle pattern can serve as a fingerprint of the region of interest of the myocardium. Furthermore, given a sufficiently high frame rate, it can be assumed that particular speckle patterns are preserved between subsequent image frames [14]. Thus, tracking of the speckle pattern during the cardiac cycle allows one to follow the motion of this myocardial segment within the two-dimensional ultrasound image. Several studies have shown [15,16] that twist data derived from commercially available speckle tracking software correlated well with tagged MRI. To be able to evaluate serial studies of left ventricular twist by speckle tracking echocardiography in the same patient, the technique needs to be reproducible as well. Van Dalen et al. [17] studied the feasibility and variability of left ventricular twist measurement and found that the method is feasible in approximately two thirds of subjects and has good intraobserver, interobserver and temporal reproducibility, allowing to study changes over time in left ventricular twist in an individual patient.

In this chapter, the important physiological role of left ventricular twist and untwist will be explained. Furthermore, cardiomyopathies may show striking alterations of left ventricular twist. The pathophysiological background and potential clinical role of these changes is discussed.

2. Physiology of left ventricular twist

According to the Hippocratic treatise "On the Heart", the heart is shaped like a pyramid, has a deep crimson colour, and is an extremely strong muscle. From the top of the heart, rivers that irrigate the "mortal habitation" flow into the body. If these rivers dry up, then the person dies [18]. Leonardo da Vinci's investigations of the heart and circulation began nearly 18 centuries later, in the 1490s. Da Vinci made a number of advances in the understanding of the heart and blood flow. For example, he showed that the heart is indeed a muscle, that it has four chambers an he linked the pulse in the wrist with left ventricular contraction. Furthermore, as mentioned before, Da Vinci was the first to describe the rotational motion of the left ventricle [4,5]. However, it lasted until the late 1960s before left ventricular twist was described in more detail by Streeter et al. [7] following a study of post-mortem canine hearts. Using a rapid method of fixation, they were able to analyze these hearts in either systole, begin diastole or end-diastole. Fibre angle, representing the angle between the myofibres as projected onto the circumferential-longitudinal plane and the circumferential axis, was introduced for quantification of fibre orientation. This angle changed continuously from the subendocardium to the subepicardium, typically ranging from +60 degrees at the subendocardium to –60 degrees at the subepicardium. Left ventricular twist is supposed to originate from the dynamic interaction between these oppositely wound subepicardial and subendocardial myocardial fibre helices, whereby the direction of left ventricular twist is governed by the subepicardial fibres, mainly owing to their longer arm of movement [19]. Left ventricular twist plays a pivotal role in the mechanical efficiency of the heart, making it possible that only 15% fibre shortening results in a 60% reduction in left ventricular volume [20]. Furthermore, mathematical models have shown that the counterdirectional arrangement of muscle fibres in the heart is energetically efficient and important for equal redistribution of stresses and strain in the heart [21]. However, controversy remains present. The group of Buckberg published in 2005 a comprehensive compendium, "Rethinking the cardiac helix; a structure function journey", of the Liverpool meeting: "New concepts of cardiac anatomy & physiology" [22]. Buckberg et al. believe that, based on anatomical studies by Torrent-Guasp [23] the heart is a helix that contains an apex, and that sequential contraction of the basal, descending, and ascending loop of the helix leads to the physiological pattern of myocardial contraction [24]. Although interesting, other anatomical studies have failed to reproduce the findings of Torrent-Guasp, and during the past few years this latter theory seems to gradually lose appreciation as compared to the theory of dynamic interaction between oppositely wound subepicardial and subendocardial myocardial fibres [25]. Taber et al. [19] used a theoretical model to underscore the importance of the arrangement of myocardial fibres for left ventricular function. Peak systolic twist approximately doubled with a change in de epicardial / endocardial fibre angles from +90 degrees / –90 degrees to +60 degrees / –60 degrees. The importance of fibre orientation for left ventricular twist was highlighted in clinical context as well [26]. Left ventricular sphericity index was found to have an independent positive linear relation with peak systolic twist in dilated cardiomyopathy patients. Even in dilated cardiomyopathy patient with similar left ventricular ejection fraction, left ventricular sphericity index remained positively correlated to left ventricular twist. Interestingly, in normal hearts the left ventricular sphericity index had a parabolic relation with apical peak systolic rotation and peak systolic twist. A left ventricular sphericity index of about 2.1 was associated with the highest peak systolic twist, lower and higher sphericity indices were associated with less peak systolic twist. The findings of this study seem to support the hypothesis by Taber et al. that alterations in fibre-orientation influence left ventricular peak systolic twist. Furthermore, the curvature of the left ventricular wall is related to wall tension. Since deformation of myocardial fibres is known to be inversely related to wall tension, changes in cardiac shape may also lead to changes in left ventricular twist by means of alterations in wall tension [21].

In 1995, Moon et al. [27] investigated the effects of load and inotropic state on left ventricular twist. They studied 6 cardiac transplant recipients 1 year after heart transplantation. At the time of surgery 12 radiopaque midwall left ventricular myocardial markers were implanted. The authors claimed that pressure and volume loading did not affect left ventricular twist. However, in more recent tagged MRI studies by MacGowan et al. [28] and Dong et al. [29] it has been shown that afterload changes do affect left ventricular twist. Dong et al. also investigated the influence of preload and contractility. An isolated increase in preload resulted in an increase in left ventricular twist. From a multiple linear regression analysis, they concluded that the effect of preload on left ventricular twist was about two-thirds as great as that of afterload. Since left ventricular twist is critically dependent on the arrangement of fibres in the myocardium, the dependence of left ventricular twist on pre- and afterload-induced changes in left ventricular volumes is intuitive. Dong et al. also observed that dobutamine increased left ventricular twist, even at identical pre- and afterload, indicating that there is a direct inotropic effect on left ventricular twist that is not mediated through changes in volume, but through changes in force.

Finally, several groups investigated the influence of aging on left ventricular twist [30-32]. Nakai et al. [30] and Takeuchi et al. [31] reported increased left ventricular twist with aging. Because left venticular peak systolic twist is calculated as the maximal value of *instantaneous* left ventricular apical rotation minus left ventricular basal rotation, any difference between the timing of left ventricular basal and apical peak systolic rotation (defined as rotational deformation delay) will result in less left ventricular peak systolic twist. In a study by Van Dalen et al. [32] it was shown that the increase of left ventricular twist with aging results not only from an increase in apical peak systolic rotation but also from a decrease in rotational deformation delay. The function of subendocardial fibres declines with age, even in normal hearts [33,34]. Loss of the opposed action of subendocardial fibres will allow the subepicardial fibres to cause more pronounced left ventricular apical rotation and thereby left ventricular twist. Time-to-peak left ventricular basal rotation remained relatively unchanged with aging, whereas left ventricular apical peak rotation occurred later in systole with advancing age, approaching time-to-peak basal rotation and thereby decreasing rotational deformation delay. Although the increase in time-to-peak left ventricular apical rotation may be caused by an increase in collagenous tissue in the conduction system with advancing age [34], this would implicate an increase in time-to-peak left ventricular basal rotation as well, leaving rotational deformation delay unchanged. The increase in time-to-peak left ventricular apical rotation with advancing age may also be explained by prolonged contraction duration, which was previously found in aged myocardium of animals [35,36]. This prolonged contraction duration results from a prolonged active state rather than changes in passive properties or myocardial catecholamine content [37]. Whether this is the true explanation of the increase in time-to-peak left ventricular apical rotation with advancing age, and why time-to-peak left ventricular basal rotation would not be influenced by this phenomenon, still needs to be clarified. Nevertheless, both increased left ventricular apical rotation and decreased rotational deformation delay seem to be characteristics of "physiological cardiac aging", and may contribute to the preservation of left ventricular ejection fraction in the elderly.

3. Physiology of left ventricular untwist

Untwisting starts after the peak of left ventricular twist, just before the end of systole. The twisting deformation of the left ventricle during systole results not only in ejection of blood but also in storage of potential energy. During the isovolumic relaxation period the twisted fibres behave like a compressed coil that springs open while abruptly releasing the potential energy. This process may be actively supported by still depolarized subendocardial fibres that are – in contrast to the systolic period – now not opposed by active contraction of the subepicardial fibres [38]. However, the effective force of contraction of myocardial fibres is expected to be minimal during this part of the cardiac cycle. Nevertheless, dissimilarities of apparent stiffness of the endocardium and epicardium caused by differences in breakdown of actin-myosin cross-bridges may be of influence. The group of Shapiro and Rademakers was one of the first to investigate the physiology of left ventricular untwisting in more detail with MRI [39]. They found, in an open-chest canine model, that left ventricular untwisting and filling are dissociated in time. In the normal resting heart about 40% of left ventricular untwisting occurs during isovolumic relaxation. Dobutamine enhanced the extent of left ventricular untwisting before mitral valve opening and further accentuated the dissociation between left ventricular untwisting and filling. The untwisting rate, the mean left ventricular untwisting velocity during the isovolumic relaxation phase, is proportional to the rate of isovolumic pressure decay [40]. In addition, left ventricular untwisting precedes and is a strong predictor of the intraventricular pressure gradient, a marker of diastolic suction during early left ventricular filling. This may be caused by a temporal dispersion between basal and apical de-rotation, the diastolic reversal of systolic rotation [41]. At the left ventricular apical level there is faster de-rotation, as compared to the basal level, which may be explained by the relatively increased systolic apical rotation, and thus stored potential energy. Interestingly, at the left ventricular basal level there is still a profound de-rotation from mitral valve opening until the peak of early left ventricular filling velocity. This may be explained by the temporal dispersion in basal and apical repolarization. Since the basal endocardial fibres are the latest to be repolarized (repolarization progresses from the apex to the base of the heart and from the epicardium to the endocardium, and takes approximately 150ms), an extra de-rotating force may still be present during this period at the basal level. Furthermore, there is a brief episode of re-rotation at the basal level from the peak to the end of the early left ventricular filling velocity that may partially be explained by the sudden omission of the de-rotational forces of the endocardial fibres, at the moment of complete cardiac repolarization. In contrast, during this period continuing de-rotation is seen at the left ventricular apical level. Since rotation is related to an increase and de-rotation to a decrease in left ventricular pressure, this phenomenon may facilitate blood flow all the way to the apex. Thus, left ventricular untwisting provides a temporal link between two crucial diastolic phenomena, relaxation and diastolic suction.

In adolescents and young adults, there may be a marked contribution of active left ventricular relaxation to left ventricular filling, resulting in an accentuated early diastolic filling velocity with a short deceleration time, resembling restrictive left ventricular filling at Doppler echocardiography ('pseudo-restrictive' left ventricular filling pattern). Very rapid left ventricular untwisting plays a pivotal role in this physiological rapid early diastolic filling [42]. In contrast, in dilated cardiomyopathy patients, untwisting is delayed and this impairment to utilize suction may impair left ventricular filling [42].

Marked changes in left ventricular diastolic function are known to occur in healthy elderly [43,44]. As described before, with advancing age left ventricular twist increases, probably due to both a decrease in rotational deformation delay and subendocardial dysfunction leading to loss of the counteraction of the subendocardial fibre helix. The early diastolic release of

http://dx.doi.org/10.5772/55281

increased potential energy stored during this augmented systolic twisting deformation may be the cause of preserved peak diastolic untwisting velocity and untwisting rate with aging. A strong age-independent relation between left ventricular peak systolic twist and peak diastolic untwisting velocity and untwisting rate supports this hypothesis. Nevertheless, although peak diastolic untwisting velocity and untwisting rate do not change significantly with advancing age, both parameters are significantly impaired when normalized for the increased extent of left ventricular twist. This results in a progressive delay in relative left ventricular untwisting and in the time-to-peak diastolic untwisting velocity with aging. This may reflect the increased stiffness known to occur in aging. In addition, the same subendocardial dysfunction that is supposed to lead to increased left ventricular twist with aging, may also lead to loss of the active part of untwisting normally caused by in early diastole still depolarized subendocardial fibres. Relatively reduced and delayed left ventricular untwisting may help to explain the increased duration of isovolumic relaxation in the elderly. Because left ventricular untwisting generates the left ventricular pressure gradient that helps filling the left ventricle [10], impediment of left ventricular untwisting may lead to delayed generation of this pressure gradient, and thereby to delayed opening of the mitral valve.

4. Left ventricular twist in cardiac disease

4.1. Subendocardial dysfunction

As mentioned before, left ventricular twist originates from the dynamic interaction between oppositely wound subepicardial and subendocardial myocardial fibres. The direction of left ventricular twist is governed by the subepicardial fibres, mainly owing to their longer arm of movement. Subendocardial ischemia with loss of contraction of the counteracting subendocardial fibres will lead to increased left ventricular twist. Therefore, left ventricular twist, and in particular changes within one patient, may provide an easily assessable marker of subendocardial ischemia. Increased left ventricular twist has been described in aging healthy subjects (as discussed previously), and in patients with hypertrophic cardiomyopathy (HCM), aortic stenosis (AS), or diabetes.

In HCM patients, left ventricular twist is increased [45,46]. Actually, in particular left ventricular basal rotation is augmented [46]. The increased basal rotation may be explained by loss of counteraction of the subendocardial fibre helix, caused by endocardial ischemia due to microvascular dysfunction [47,48]. Also, larger radius differences between the subepicardium and subendocardium in hypertrophic muscle may increase the dominant action of the subepicardial fibres and increase basal rotation. Interestingly, left ventricular apical rotation and twist are dependent on the pattern of left ventricular hypertrophy. In patients with a sigmoidal septal curvature, left ventricular apical rotation and twist are increased as compared to patients with a reverse septal curvature. This may be partly explained by the degree of subendocardial ischemia, since patients with a sigmoidal septal curvature more often have left ventricular outflow tract obstruction. The extravascular compressive forces caused by gradients due to the outflow obstruction may lead to more extensive microvascular dysfunction and subendocardial ischemia.

AS patients are consistently found to have increased left ventricular twist, mainly due to increased left ventricular apical rotation [49-51]. Furthermore, left ventricular apical rotation and twist correlate positively to the severity of AS. This underlines the potential role of subendocardial ischemia as the cause of increased left ventricular apical rotation and twist in AS since the severity of subendocardial ischemia is known to be related to the severity of AS [52]. In addition, left ventricular apical rotation and twist are highest in AS patients with symptoms (angina) or electrocardiographic signs (strain) compatible with subendocardial ischemia [53]. However, deformation of myocardial fibres is known to be inversely related to wall tension. Since increased afterload in AS leads to increased endocardial wall tension, increased left ventricular twist in AS may also be caused by decreased endocardial deformation as a result of increased endocardial wall tension, independently of ischemia.

Increased left ventricular twist was also described in diabetics with a normal left ventricular ejection fraction [54-56]. Several potential mechanisms for the supposed loss of counteraction of the subendocardial fibres have been mentioned, including metabolic disturbances triggered by hyperglycemia, increased free fatty acid oxidation, altered calcium homeostasis, myocyte death, fibrosis, small-vessel diseases, and cardiac autonomic neuropathy.

In all the above mentioned examples, increased left ventricular twist may serve as a compensatory mechanism to balance loss of left ventricular myocardial contraction in other directions, which with subendocardial dysfunction is usually a loss of contraction in the longitudinal direction, and thereby preserve left ventricular ejection fraction.

4.2. Diastolic dysfunction

The need for objective evidence of left ventricular diastolic dysfunction has led to an extensive search for accurate, noninvasive, load-independent methods to quantify its severity. Takeuchi et al. [57] examined whether left ventricular hypertrophy adversely affects left ventricular untwisting in hypertension patients. Patients with moderate to severe left ventricular hypertrophy had reduced and delayed left ventricular untwisting as compared to patients without left ventricular hypertrophy, which may contribute to the left ventricular relaxation abnormality seen in these patients.

In both HCM [58] and AS [51], the untwisting rate, the mean untwisting velocity during the isovolumic relaxation phase, is decreased and untwisting is delayed. Subendocardial ischemia may lead to loss of active untwisting normally caused by the subendocardial fibres during early diastole. In addition, the impaired compliance of the left ventricles of these patients will prevent optimal transformation of the potential energy stored in systolic left ventricular twisting into kinetic energy. However, *peak* diastolic untwisting velocity is decreased in HCM patients, whereas it is increased in AS patients. In AS patients, systolic left ventricular twist is clearly increased as compared to controls. The increased potential energy stored in this more twisted left ventricular will be released after all, which may lead to increased, but delayed, peak diastolic untwisting velocity, that may serve as a compensatory mechanism to help left ventricular filling. Conversely, in HCM patients systolic twist is only moderately increased, which may thwart this phenomenon. This hypothesis is supported by the fact that increased peak diastolic untwisting velocity hace been found in a subgroup of HCM patients with mild diastolic dysfunction, who had increased systolic twist. It has been suggested that increased untwisting might be a compensatory mechanism, preventing the need to increase left atrial pressure.

4.3. Noncompaction cardiomyopathy

Noncompaction cardiomyopathy (NCCM) is a myocardial disorder characterized by excessive and prominent trabeculations associated with deep recesses that communicate with the ventricular cavity but not the coronary circulation [59]. Although NCCM was included in the 2006 World Health Organization classification of cardiomyopathies [60], it remains subject to controversy owing to lack of consensus on its aetiology, pathogenesis, diagnosis, and management [61]. The final stage of the development of myocardial architecture is characterized by the formation of compact myocardium and development of oppositely wound epicardial and endocardial myocardial fibre helices [62,63]. Since NCCM is probably caused by intrauterine arrest of this final stage of cardiac embryogenesis [64], it may be anticipated that left ventricular twist characteristics are altered, beyond that seen in patients with impaired left ventricular function and normal compaction. This has been confirmed in a clinical study. NCCM patients were found to show left ventricular rigid body rotation, that is predominantly instantaneous rotation at the basal and apical level in the same direction, with near absent left ventricular twist. In a subsequent, larger study left ventricular rigid body rotation was confirmed to be an objective, quantitative, and reproducible criterion with a good predictive value for the diagnosis of NCCM as established by expert opinion [65]. Interestingly, all familial NCCM patients showed rigid body rotation. Since the diagnosis of NCCM seems most certain in patients with familial NCCM, this finding underscores the excellent sensitivity of solid body rotation for NCCM. Of additional interest was the finding that NCCM patients who were first-degree relatives from one family had identical left ventricular rotation patterns, suggesting a genetic-functional relationship in NCCM.

4.4. Cardiac resynchronization therapy

Although a significant reduction of left ventricular twist was observed in patients with advanced heart failure, left ventricular twist did not improve after resynchronization therapy, despite significant gains in left ventricular global and short-axis function in responders. In fact, non-responders showed further reduction of left ventricular twist [66]. However, in a more recent study, subendocardial and subepicardial left ventricular twist were investigated separately, which did lead to identification of prognostic value of left ventricular twist in the population undergoing resynchronization [67]. At 6-month follow-up, 53% of the patients showed favorable outcomes after resynchronization therapy. In a multivariate logistic regression analysis, only the immediate improvement of subepicardial left ventricular twist was independently related to favorable outcomes. Furthermore, the immediate improvement of subepicardial left ventricular twist had incremental value over established parameters.

Several reasons may explain this finding. First, subepicardial left ventricular twist may reflect the positive effects of cardiac resynchronization therapy better than subendocardial left ventricular twist, because the subepicardial layer is the major determinant of left ventricular twist. Second, left ventricular pacing in cardiac resynchronization therapy is applied from the epicardial surface, which may be more closely related to mechanical changes in the subepicardial than the subendocardial left ventricular layer.

4.5. Ischemic heart disease

Sun et al. [68] subjected 7 pigs to myocardial infarction by occlusion of the left anterior descending coronary artery. After 8 weeks, left ventricular twist was decreased significantly in the left anterior descending coronary artery territory areas, whereas there was no change in twist in adjacent and remote left ventricular areas. Therefore, the authors proposed that left ventricular twist may be suitable for noninvasive quantification of left ventricular regional function in ischemic heart disease. Kroeker et al. [69], using an optical device coupled to the left ventricular apex in 16 open-chest dogs, also found a decrease of left ventricular apical rotation with ischemia caused by occlusion of the left anterior descending coronary artery. Interestingly, in the first 10 seconds of occlusion, there was a paradoxical increase in left ventricular apical rotation, which was attributed to isolated subendocardial ischemia leading to loss of the counteractive action of the subendocardial helix of myofibres.

In clinical studies in patients with a prior anterior myocardial infarction it was found that, although left ventricular basal rotation was preserved, left ventricular apical rotation was decreased, leading to decreased left ventricular twist [70]. In patients with a left ventricular aneurysm, left ventricular apical rotation was nonexistent or even inverted, leading to severely decreased left ventricular twist.

4.6. Congenital heart disease

In the majority of left ventricular twist studies in congenital heart disease, investigators focused on patients with a congenital transposition of the great arteries. In patients operated with atrial switch, the systemic right ventricle shows absence of twist, whereas the subpulmonary left ventricle shows reduced twist [71,72]. Furthermore, there are regional differences of apical rotation of the subpulmonary left ventricular, whereas apical rotation is homogeneous in a normal left ventricle [73,74]. In a theoretical model of situs inversus totalis, and in 8 patients with this condition [75,76] it was shown that, although gross anatomy is mirror imaged, this is not the case for left ventricular systolic deformation. Both the left ventricular base and apex rotated in a counterclockwise direction, whereas the midventricular section exhibited hardly any rotation. These findings may be explained by the arrangement of myofibres in these patients. Anatomical studies have revealed that in situs inversus totalis arrangement of myofibres is normal in the apical regions leading to normal counterclockwise rotation, whereas at the basal level a partly mirror-imaged pattern of the normal transmural change in fibre angle is seen.

5. Conclusion

Even though left ventricular twist is indispensable for proper left ventricular function, little is known about it in "the cardiology community". Mainly due to the development of speckle tracking echocardiography, allowing accurate, reproducible and rapid bedside assessment of left ventricular twist, interest in this important mechanical aspect of left ventricular deformation has been rapidly increasing.

Although the vital physiological role of left ventricular twist is indisputable, the clinical relevance of assessment of left ventricular twist in cardiomyopathies still needs to be confirmed. Nonetheless, left ventricular twist evaluation has already provided significant pathophysiological insight in a broad variety of cardiomyopathies. It has become clear that increased left ventricular twist in for example HCM, AS, and diabetics, but also in a healthy ageing population, may serve as a compensatory mechanism to preserve ejection fraction. Furthermore, demonstration of left ventricular rigid body rotation in NCCM may provide a unique way to objectively confirm this difficult diagnosis. Diastolic left ventricular untwisting represents the elastic recoil caused by the release of restoring forces that have been generated during the preceding systolic left ventricular twist and has an important contribution in left ventricular filling through suction generation. Measurement of left ventricular untwisting may become an important element of diastolic function evaluation in cardiomyopathies in the future.

Author details

B.M. van Dalen and M.L. Geleijnse

Erasmus University Medical Center Rotterdam, The Netherlands

References

[1] Sutherland GR, Hatle L, Claus P, D'hooge J, Bijnens BH. Doppler Myocardial Imaging 2006;Hasselt, Belgium: BSWK, bvba:1-4.

[2] Heimdal A, Stoylen A, Torp H, Skjaerpe T. Real-time strain rate imaging of the left ventricle by ultrasound. J Am Soc Echocardiogr 1998;11(11):1013-9.

[3] Notomi Y, Setser RM, Shiota T, Martin-Miklovic MG, Weaver JA, Popovic ZB, et al. Assessment of left ventricular torsional deformation by Doppler tissue imaging: validation study with tagged magnetic resonance imaging. Circulation 2005;111(9): 1141-7.

[4] Da Vinci L. Quoted by Evans L. Starling's Principles of Human Physiology. 1936;London, UK: J.A. Churchill:706.

[5] Keele KD. Leonardo da Vinci's elements of the science of man. 1983;New York, USA: Academic Press.

[6] Lower R. Tractus de Corde. In Gunter RT, ed. Early Science in Oxford. 1968;Oxford, London, UK: Sawsons, Pall Mall:1669.

[7] Streeter DD, Jr., Spotnitz HM, Patel DP, Ross J, Jr., Sonnenblick EH. Fiber orientation in the canine left ventricle during diastole and systole. Circ Res 1969;24(3):339-47.

[8] Greenbaum RA, Ho SY, Gibson DG, Becker AE, Anderson RH. Left ventricular fibre architecture in man. Br Heart J 1981;45(3):248-63.

[9] Sallin EA. Fiber orientation and ejection fraction in the human left ventricle. Biophys J 1969;9(7):954-64.

[10] Notomi Y, Martin-Miklovic MG, Oryszak SJ, Shiota T, Deserranno D, Popovic ZB, et al. Enhanced ventricular untwisting during exercise: a mechanistic manifestation of elastic recoil described by Doppler tissue imaging. Circulation 2006;113(21):2524-33.

[11] Harrison DC, Goldblatt A, Braunwald E, Glick G, Mason DT. Studies on Cardiac Dimensions in Intact, Unanesthetized Man. I. Description of Techniques and Their Validation. Ii. Effects of Respiration. Iii. Effects of Muscular Exercise. Circ Res 1963;13:448-67.

[12] Ingels NB, Jr., Daughters GT, 2nd, Stinson EB, Alderman EL. Measurement of midwall myocardial dynamics in intact man by radiography of surgically implanted markers. Circulation 1975;52(5):859-67.

[13] Buchalter MB, Weiss JL, Rogers WJ, Zerhouni EA, Weisfeldt ML, Beyar R, et al. Noninvasive quantification of left ventricular rotational deformation in normal humans using magnetic resonance imaging myocardial tagging. Circulation 1990;81(4): 1236-44.

[14] Ramamurthy BS, Trahey GE. Potential and limitations of angle-independent flow detection algorithms using radio-frequency and detected echo signals. Ultrason Imaging 1991;13(3):252-68.

[15] Notomi Y, Lysyansky P, Setser RM, Shiota T, Popovic ZB, Martin-Miklovic MG, et al. Measurement of ventricular torsion by two-dimensional ultrasound speckle tracking imaging. J Am Coll Cardiol 2005;45(12):2034-41.

[16] Helle-Valle T, Crosby J, Edvardsen T, Lyseggen E, Amundsen BH, Smith HJ, et al. New noninvasive method for assessment of left ventricular rotation: speckle tracking echocardiography. Circulation 2005;112(20):3149-56.

[17] van Dalen BM, Soliman OI, Vletter WB, Kauer F, van der Zwaan HB, Ten Cate FJ, et al. Feasibility and reproducibility of left ventricular rotation parameters measured by speckle tracking echocardiography. Eur J Echocardiogr 2009;10(5):669-76.

[18] Lloyd GER. Hippocratic Writings.London: Penguin Books; 1978:347-353.

[19] Taber LA, Yang M, Podszus WW. Mechanics of ventricular torsion. J Biomech 1996;29(6):745-52.

[20] Sallin EA. Fiber orientation and ejection fraction in the human left ventricle. Biophys J 1969;9(7):954-64.

[21] Vendelin M, Bovendeerd PH, Engelbrecht J, Arts T. Optimizing ventricular fibers: uniform strain or stress, but not ATP consumption, leads to high efficiency. Am J Physiol Heart Circ Physiol 2002;283(3):H1072-81.

[22] Buckberg GD. Rethinking the cardiac helix--a structure/function journey: overview. Eur J Cardiothorac Surg 2006;29 Suppl 1:S2-149.

[23] Torrent-Guasp F, Buckberg GD, Clemente C, Cox JL, Coghlan HC, Gharib M. The structure and function of the helical heart and its buttress wrapping. I. The normal macroscopic structure of the heart. Semin Thorac Cardiovasc Surg 2001;13(4):301-19.

[24] Buckberg GD. Basic science review: the helix and the heart. J Thorac Cardiovasc Surg 2002;124(5):863-83.

[25] Sengupta PP, Khandheria BK, Narula J. Twist and untwist mechanics of the left ventricle. Heart Fail Clin 2008;4(3):315-24.

[26] van Dalen BM, Kauer F, Vletter WB, Soliman OI, van der Zwaan HB, Ten Cate FJ, et al. Influence of cardiac shape on left ventricular twist. J Appl Physiol. 2010 Jan;108(1): 146-51.

[27] Moon MR, Ingels NB, Jr., Daughters GT, 2nd, Stinson EB, Hansen DE, Miller DC. Alterations in left ventricular twist mechanics with inotropic stimulation and volume loading in human subjects. Circulation 1994;89(1):142-50.

[28] MacGowan GA, Burkhoff D, Rogers WJ, Saleft ventricularador D, Azhari H, Hees PS, et al. Effects of afterload on regional left ventricular torsion. Cardiovasc Res 1996;31(6):917-25.

[29] Dong SJ, Hees PS, Huang WM, Buffer SA, Jr., Weiss JL, Shapiro EP. Independent effects of preload, afterload, and contractility on left ventricular torsion. Am J Physiol 1999;277(3 Pt 2):H1053-60.

[30] Nakai H, Takeuchi M, Nishikage T, Kokumai M, Otani S, Lang RM. Effect of aging on twist-displacement loop by 2-dimensional speckle tracking imaging. J Am Soc Echocardiogr 2006;19(7):880-5.

[31] Takeuchi M, Nakai H, Kokumai M, Nishikage T, Otani S, Lang RM. Age-related changes in left ventricular twist assessed by two-dimensional speckle-tracking imaging. J Am Soc Echocardiogr 2006;19(9):1077-84.

[32] van Dalen BM, Soliman OI, Vletter WB, Ten Cate FJ, Geleijnse ML. Age-related changes in the biomechanics of left ventricular twist measured by speckle tracking echocardiography. Am J Physiol Heart Circ Physiol 2008;295(4):H1705-11.

[33] Lumens J, Delhaas T, Arts T, Cowan BR, Young AA. Impaired subendocardial contractile myofiber function in asymptomatic aged humans, as detected using MRI. Am J Physiol Heart Circ Physiol 2006;291(4):H1573-9.

[34] Nikitin NP, Witte KK, Thackray SD, de Sileft ventriculara R, Clark AL, Cleland JG. Longitudinal ventricular function: normal values of atrioventricular annular and myocardial velocities measured with quantitative two-dimensional color Doppler tissue imaging. J Am Soc Echocardiogr 2003;16(9):906-21.

[35] Lakatta EG, Sollott SJ. Perspectives on mammalian cardiovascular aging: humans to molecules. Comp Biochem Physiol A Mol Integr Physiol 2002;132(4):699-721.

[36] Lakatta EG, Gerstenblith G, Angell CS, Shock NW, Weisfeldt ML. Prolonged contraction duration in aged myocardium. J Clin Invest 1975;55(1):61-8.

[37] Weisfeldt ML, Loeven WA, Shock NW. Resting and active mechanical properties of trabeculae carneae from aged male rats. Am J Physiol 1971;220(6):1921-7.

[38] Ashikaga H, Criscione JC, Omens JH, Covell JW, Ingels NB, Jr. Transmural left ventricular mechanics underlying torsional recoil during relaxation. Am J Physiol Heart Circ Physiol 2004;286(2):H640-7.

[39] Rademakers FE, Buchalter MB, Rogers WJ, Zerhouni EA, Weisfeldt ML, Weiss JL, et al. Dissociation between left ventricular untwisting and filling. Accentuation by catecholamines. Circulation 1992;85(4):1572-81.

[40] Notomi Y, Popovic ZB, Yamada H, Wallick DW, Martin MG, Oryszak SJ, et al. Ventricular untwisting: a temporal link between left ventricular relaxation and suction. Am J Physiol Heart Circ Physiol 2008;294(1):H505-13.

[41] van Dalen BM, Soliman OI, Vletter WB, ten Cate FJ, Geleijnse ML. Insights into left ventricular function from the time course of regional and global rotation by speckle tracking echocardiography. Echocardiography 2009;26(4):371-7.

[42] van Dalen BM, Soliman OI, Vletter WB, ten Cate FJ, Geleijnse ML. Left ventricular untwisting in restrictive and pseudorestrictive left ventricular filling: novel insights into diastology. Echocardiography. 2010 Mar;27(3):269-74.

[43] Mantero A, Gentile F, Gualtierotti C, Azzollini M, Barbier P, Beretta L, et al. Left ventricular diastolic parameters in 288 normal subjects from 20 to 80 years old. Eur Heart J 1995;16(1):94-105.

[44] Prasad A, Popovic ZB, Arbab-Zadeh A, Fu Q, Palmer D, Dijk E, et al. The effects of aging and physical activity on Doppler measures of diastolic function. Am J Cardiol 2007;99(12):1629-36.

[45] Young AA, Kramer CM, Ferrari VA, Axel L, Reichek N. Three-dimensional left ventricular deformation in hypertrophic cardiomyopathy. Circulation 1994;90(2):854-67.

[46] van Dalen BM, Kauer F, Soliman OI, Vletter WB, Michels M, ten Cate FJ, et al. Influence of the pattern of hypertrophy on left ventricular twist in hypertrophic cardiomyopathy. Heart 2009;95(8):657-61.

[47] Cecchi F, Olivotto I, Gistri R, Lorenzoni R, Chiriatti G, Camici PG. Coronary microvascular dysfunction and prognosis in hypertrophic cardiomyopathy. N Engl J Med 2003;349(11):1027-35.

[48] Soliman OI, Geleijnse ML, Michels M, Dijkmans PA, Nemes A, van Dalen BM, et al. Effect of successful alcohol septal ablation on microvascular function in patients with obstructive hypertrophic cardiomyopathy. Am J Cardiol 2008;101(9):1321-7.

[49] Nagel E, Stuber M, Burkhard B, Fischer SE, Scheidegger MB, Boesiger P, et al. Cardiac rotation and relaxation in patients with aortic valeft ventriculare stenosis. Eur Heart J 2000;21(7):582-9.

[50] Stuber M, Scheidegger MB, Fischer SE, Nagel E, Steinemann F, Hess OM, et al. Alterations in the local myocardial motion pattern in patients suffering from pressure overload due to aortic stenosis. Circulation 1999;100(4):361-8.

[51] van Dalen BM, Tzikas A, Soliman OI, Kauer F, Heuvelman HJ, Vletter WB, et al. Left ventricular twist and untwist in aortic stenosis. Int J Cardiol. 2011 May 5;148(3): 319-24.

[52] Smucker ML, Tedesco CL, Manning SB, Owen RM, Feldman MD. Demonstration of an imbalance between coronary perfusion and excessive load as a mechanism of ischemia during stress in patients with aortic stenosis. Circulation 1988;78(3):573-82.

[53] van Dalen BM, Tzikas A, Soliman OI, Kauer F, Heuvelman HJ, Vletter WB, et al. Assessment of subendocardial contractile function in aortic stenosis: a Study using Speckle Tracking Echocardiography. Echocardiography 2013 (in press).

[54] Fonseca CG, Dissanayake AM, Doughty RN, Whalley GA, Gamble GD, Cowan BR, et al. Threedimensional assessment of left ventricular systolic strain in patients with type 2 diabetes mellitus, diastolic dysfunction, and normal ejection fraction. Am J Cardiol 2004;94(11):1391-5.

[55] Chung J, Abraszewski P, Yu X, Liu W, Krainik AJ, Ashford M, et al. Paradoxical increase in ventricular torsion and systolic torsion rate in type I diabetic patients under tight glycemic control. J Am Coll Cardiol 2006;47(2):384-90.

[56] Ma H, Xie M, Wang J, Lu Q, Wang X, Lu X, et al. Ultrasound speckle tracking imaging contributes to early diagnosis of impaired left ventricular systolic function in pa-

tients with type 2 diabetes mellitus. J Huazhong Univ Sci Technolog Med Sci 2008;28(6):719-23.

[57] Takeuchi M, Borden WB, Nakai H, Nishikage T, Kokumai M, Nagakura T, et al. Reduced and delayed untwisting of the left ventricle in patients with hypertension and left ventricular hypertrophy: a study using two-dimensional speckle tracking imaging. Eur Heart J 2007;28(22):2756-62.

[58] van Dalen BM, Kauer F, Michels M, Soliman OI, Vletter WB, van der Zwaan HB, et al. Delayed left ventricular untwisting in hypertrophic cardiomyopathy. J Am Soc Echocardiogr. 2009 Dec;22(12):1320-6.

[59] Ritter M, Oechslin E, Sutsch G, Attenhofer C, Schneider J, Jenni R. Isolated noncompaction of the myocardium in adults. Mayo Clin Proc 1997;72(1):26-31.

[60] Maron BJ, Towbin JA, Thiene G, Antzelevitch C, Corrado D, Arnett D, et al. Contemporary definitions and classification of the cardiomyopathies: an American Heart Association Scientific Statement from the Council on Clinical Cardiology, Heart Failure and Transplantation Committee; Quality of Care and Outcomes Research and Functional Genomics and Translational Biology Interdisciplinary Working Groups; and Council on Epidemiology and Prevention. Circulation 2006;113(14):1807-16.

[61] Sen-Chowdhry S, McKenna WJ. Left ventricular noncompaction and cardiomyopathy: cause, contributor, or epiphenomenon? Curr Opin Cardiol 2008;23(3):171-5.

[62] Greenbaum RA, Ho SY, Gibson DG, Becker AE, Anderson RH. Left ventricular fibre architecture in man. Br Heart J 1981;45(3):248-63.

[63] Sanchez-Quintana D, Garcia-Martinez V, Climent V, Hurle JM. Morphological changes in the normal pattern of ventricular myoarchitecture in the developing human heart. Anat Rec 1995;243(4):483-95.

[64] Jenni R, Oechslin EN, van der Loo B. Isolated ventricular non-compaction of the myocardium in adults. Heart 2007;93(1):11-5.

[65] van Dalen BM, Caliskan K, Soliman OI, Kauer F, van der Zwaan HB, Vletter WB, van Vark LC, Ten Cate FJ, Geleijnse ML. Diagnostic value of rigid body rotation in noncompaction cardiomyopathy. J Am Soc Echocardiogr. 2011;24(5):548-55.

[66] Zhang Q, Fung JW, Yip GW, Chan JY, Lee AP, Lam YY, et al. Improvement of left ventricular myocardial short-axis, but not long-axis function or torsion after cardiac resynchronisation therapy: an assessment by two-dimensional speckle tracking. Heart 2008;94(11):1464-71.

[67] Bertini M, Delgado V, Nucifora G, Marsan NA, Ng AC, Shanks M, et al. Effect of cardiac resynchronization therapy on subendo- and subepicardial left ventricular twist mechanics and relation to favorable outcome. Am J Cardiol. 2010;106(5):682-7.

[68] Sun JP, Niu J, Chou D, Chuang HH, Wang K, Drinko J, et al. Alterations of regional myocardial function in a swine model of myocardial infarction assessed by echocardiographic 2-dimensional strain imaging. J Am Soc Echocardiogr 2007;20(5):498-504.

[69] Kroeker CA, Tyberg JV, Beyar R. Effects of ischemia on left ventricular apex rotation. An experimental study in anesthetized dogs. Circulation 1995;92(12):3539-48.

[70] Nagel E, Stuber M, Lakatos M, Scheidegger MB, Boesiger P, Hess OM. Cardiac rotation and relaxation after anterolateral myocardial infarction. Coron Artery Dis 2000;11(3):261-7.

[71] Pettersen E, Helle-Valle T, Edvardsen T, Lindberg H, Smith HJ, Smevik B, et al. Contraction pattern of the systemic right ventricle shift from longitudinal to circumferential shortening and absent global ventricular torsion. J Am Coll Cardiol 2007;49(25): 2450-6.

[72] Pettersen E, Lindberg H, Smith HJ, Smevik B, Edvardsen T, Smiseth OA, et al. Left ventricular function in patients with transposition of the great arteries operated with atrial switch. Pediatr Cardiol 2008;29(3):597-603.

[73] Fogel MA, Gupta K, Baxter BC, Weinberg PM, Haselgrove J, Hoffman EA. Biomechanics of the deconditioned left ventricle. Am J Physiol 1996;271(3 Pt 2):H1193-206.

[74] Fogel MA, Weinberg PM, Fellows KE, Hoffman EA. A study in ventricular-ventricular interaction. Single right ventricles compared with systemic right ventricles in a dual-chamber circulation. Circulation 1995;92(2):219-30.

[75] Delhaas T, Kroon W, Decaluwe W, Rubbens M, Bovendeerd P, Arts T. Structure and torsion of thenormal and situs inversus totalis cardiac left ventricle. I. Experimental data in humans. Am J Physiol Heart Circ Physiol 2008;295(1):H197-201.

[76] Kroon W, Delhaas T, Bovendeerd P, Arts T. Structure and torsion in the normal and situs inversus totalis cardiac left ventricle. II. Modeling cardiac adaptation to mechanical load. Am J Physiol Heart Circ Physiol 2008;295(1):H202-10.

Chapter 3

Contractile Reserve in Dilated Cardiomyopathy

Takahiro Okumura and Toyoaki Murohara

Additional information is available at the end of the chapter

http://dx.doi.org/10.5772/55413

1. Introduction

Dilated cardiomyopathy (DCM) is one of the most common types of cardiomyopathy worldwide. It is characterized by progressive chamber dilatation and myocardial systolic dysfunction and diagnosed by finding left ventricular (LV) enlargement and impaired systolic LV function (LV ejection fraction less than 50% or fractional shortening of less than 25-30%). Angiotensin-converting enzyme inhibitors and ß-blockers are the best and popular therapeutic interventions for DCM that promotes amelioration of systolic LV dysfunction among 20-45% DCM patients [1 - 5]; nonetheless, the 5-year mortality rate of DCM remains 10-35% under these medical therapy [6 - 8].

The predictive assessment of LV function is clinically important in medical management of DCM, particularly when considering the indication for heart transplantation. In most patients with heart failure, symptoms are not present at rest but become limiting with exercise. Nevertheless, the major measures for LV function of DCM, such as echocardiography, are generally performed under the static condition. In addition, LV contractile function at rest is not reliable for an assessment of the reversibility of LV contraction, that is contractile reserve [3, 4]. Therefore, it is important to evaluate LV functional response under dynamic conditions by use of pharmacological as well as exercise stress [9].

This article reviews the current status of myocardial contractile reserve with our findings, including procedures for evaluating contractile reserve, clinical implications, and molecular biological significance.

2. Contractile reserve in DCM

2.1. Myocardial contractile reserve

Myocardial contractile reserve measured by stress testing has been defined as a difference LV function at rest and under load. To date, the assessment of myocardial contractile reserve limitedly applied to evaluate the myocardial viability exclusively in patients with LV dysfunction and coronary artery disease. Nowadays, glowing evidences suggest the clinical importance to evaluating the contractile reserve in non-ischemic DCM [9, 10]. In particular to the case of DCM, the assessment of myocardial contractile reserve is mainly focused to evaluate the presence of residual LV contractile reserve.

2.2. Pathophysiological implications

Determinant factors of myocardial contractile reserve include the Frank-Starling mechanism, the force-frequency effect, and adrenergic stimulation [11, 12]. In DCM patients, myocardial contractile reserve to adrenergic stimulation is impaired [9].

Myocardial contractile reserve by stress testing provide important prognostic information in DCM [13]. Previous studies reported that patients exhibiting load-induced enhancement of systolic LV function had better clinical outcomes [10, 14 - 17] and LV contractile reserve is a useful marker to predict future LV functional improvement in the treatment of beta blocker or after cardiac resynchrnonization therapy [18 - 21].

In addition, myocardial contractile reserve is associated with other prognostic biomarkers and molecule expressions in cardiomyocyte. Firstly, LV inotropic reserve is associated with exercise capacity [14]. The contractile reserve correlates with peak oxygen consumption (peak VO_2) in cardiopulmonary exercise testing [22, 23]. Moreover, patients with greater increase in myocardial contractile reserve achieved a greater peak VO_2 [23]. Secondly, impaired LV contractile reserve was reported to be associated with cardiac sympathetic dysfunction measured by myocardial iodine-123-metaiodobenzylgluanidine (^{123}I-MIBG) scintigraphy [24]. Finally, we reported that reduced adrenergic myocardial contractile reserve related to myocardial expression of contractile regulatory protein mRNAs, such as beta$_1$-adrenergic receptor, sarcoplasmic reticulum Ca^{2+}-adrenergic triphosphatase, and phospholamban [25].

Moreover, the assessment of LV response using a stress testing may also help in the screening or monitoring the presence of latent myocardial dysfunction in patients with the initial phase of cardiomyopathy overt normal resting echocardiographic parameters who had exposure to cardiotoxic agents [26].

3. How to evaluate contractile reserve?

Myocardial contractile reserve is usually defined as a difference between LV function at rest and under load. LV function has been evaluated by a variety of modalities, such as echocardiography, cardiac pool scintigraphy, and cardiac catheterization. Exercise and inotropic stress have been used as stress protocols for the assessment of contractile reserve. Both stresses provoke a generalized increase of regional wall motion with an increment of ejection fraction [27]. Although regional LV wall dysfunction is commonly caused by coronary artery ischemia, regional wall motion abnormality is sometimes shown in non-ischemic cardiomyopathy [28].

The selection of evaluation method and stress modality mainly depends on the patient's exercise capacity, the purpose of the examination, and medical contraindications.

3.1. Exercise stress

Exercise stress is a very useful and the best physiological stressor. Therefore, exercise testing should be performed in patients who are physically allowed [27]. Images can be obtained by use of pre- and within one minute of post- treadmill, upright or supine cycle exercise. However, the weakness of stress echocardiography is that it depends on image quality and its use by the occasional user may be attached with loss of accuracy.

3.2. Dobutamine stress

Pharmacologic stress testing is preferred for patients unable to exercise. Use of low dose dobutamine seems to be the best stress method for the assessment of myocardial contractile reserve, unless there is a contraindication [29]. The protocol of dobutamine infusions vary from investigators, but the patient usually undergo the stress testing using standardised incremental infusions of 5, 10, and 20 μg/kg/min [30]. The safety dose has been documented as high as 40 μg/kg/min and serious complications occurs in about 0.3 %.

3.3. Interpretension

In stress echocardiography, global LV function at rest is assessed by calculation of ejection fraction or wall motion score index on the resting images. After collecting stress images, both data are compared for the development of global function. As for the evaluation of regional function, regional wall motion scoring is generally used. Generally, the critical level to define the presence of contractile reserve is defined as an increase of more than 5% in the global LV ejection fraction [31].

Some studies have evaluated the adrenergic contractile reserve by measurement of increase in the maximal first derivative of LV pressure (LV dP/dt_{max}) using a cardiac catheter in patients with non-ischemic LV dysfunction [15, 32].

3.4. Stress testing protocol in our studies

Our protocol for the evaluation of myocardial contractile reserve consists of low-dose dobutamine infusion and cardiac catheterization (Figure 1). Although a lot of investigations which reported dobutamine stress testing were measured by echocardiography, we more accurately evaluate LV response using catheterization with a high-fidelity micromanometer.

Initially, routine diagnostic left and right heart catheterization are performed. A 6-F fluid-filled pigtail catheter with a high-fidelity micromanometer (CA-61000-PLB Pressure-tip Catheter, CD Leycom, Zoetermeer, The Netherlands) is placed in the LV cavity for measurement of LV pressure. We evaluate LV dP/dt_{max} as an index of LV contractility [33]. After collection of baseline hemodynamic data, dobutamine is infused intravenously at incremental doses of 5, 10, and 15 μg/kg/min and hemodynamic measurements are made at the end of each 5-minute infusion period. In addition, we calculate ΔLV dP/dt_{max} as an index of myocardial contractile reserve [25]. ΔLV dP/dt_{max} is defined as the percentage increase in LV dP/dt_{max} induced by dobutamine, and this index is defined on the basis of the formula.

$$\Delta LV\ dP/dt_{max}(x) = [LV\ dP/dt_{max}(x) - LV\ dP/dt_{max}(\text{baseline})] \,/\, LV\ dP/dt_{max}(\text{baseline})$$

where x = the dose of dobutamine (μg/kg/min)

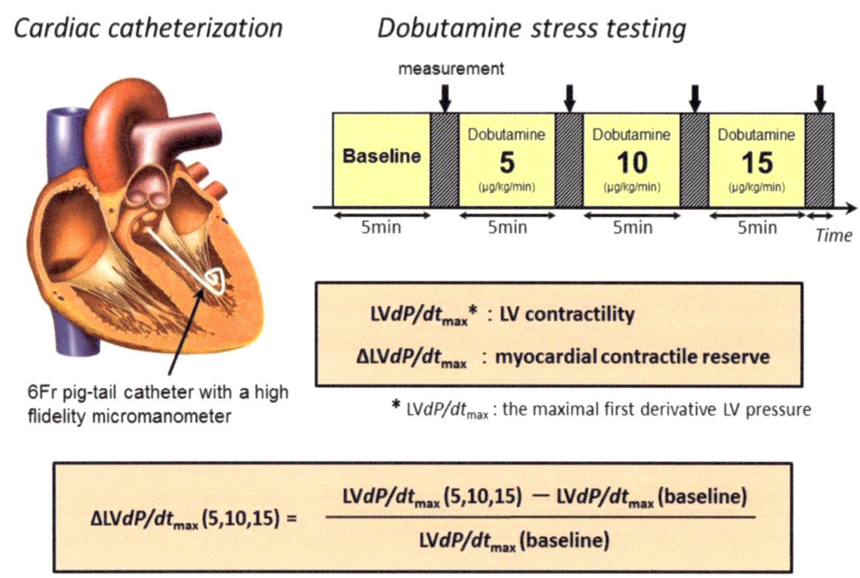

Figure 1. Protocol for evaluating myocardial contractile reserve in DCM

4. Clinical implications of myocardial contractile reserve

4.1. Exercise capacity and contractile reserve

The presence of LV inotropic response during dobutamine stress testing is associated with a better performance [14]. Patients with markedly reduced myocardial contractility at rest, but with good residual contractile reserve, have a favorable exercise capacity. On the other hand, patients with mildly abnormal myocardial contractility at rest, but reduced contractile reserve have a poor capacity [34].

http://dx.doi.org/10.5772/55413

Recently, we reported the association between myocardial contractile reserve and exercise capacity in 38 idiopathic DCM patients [23]. Peak VO_2 was significantly correlated with ΔLV dP/dt_{max}, but not with LV dP/dt_{max} at baseline. In addition, the correlation became more pronounced as the dose of dobutamine was increased (Figure 2). Multivariate regression analysis revealed that ΔLV dP/dt_{max} was independently correlated with peak VO_2 ($p=0.011$). There was no correlation between minute ventilation/carbon dioxide production (VE/VCO_2) slope and ΔLV dP/dt_{max}.

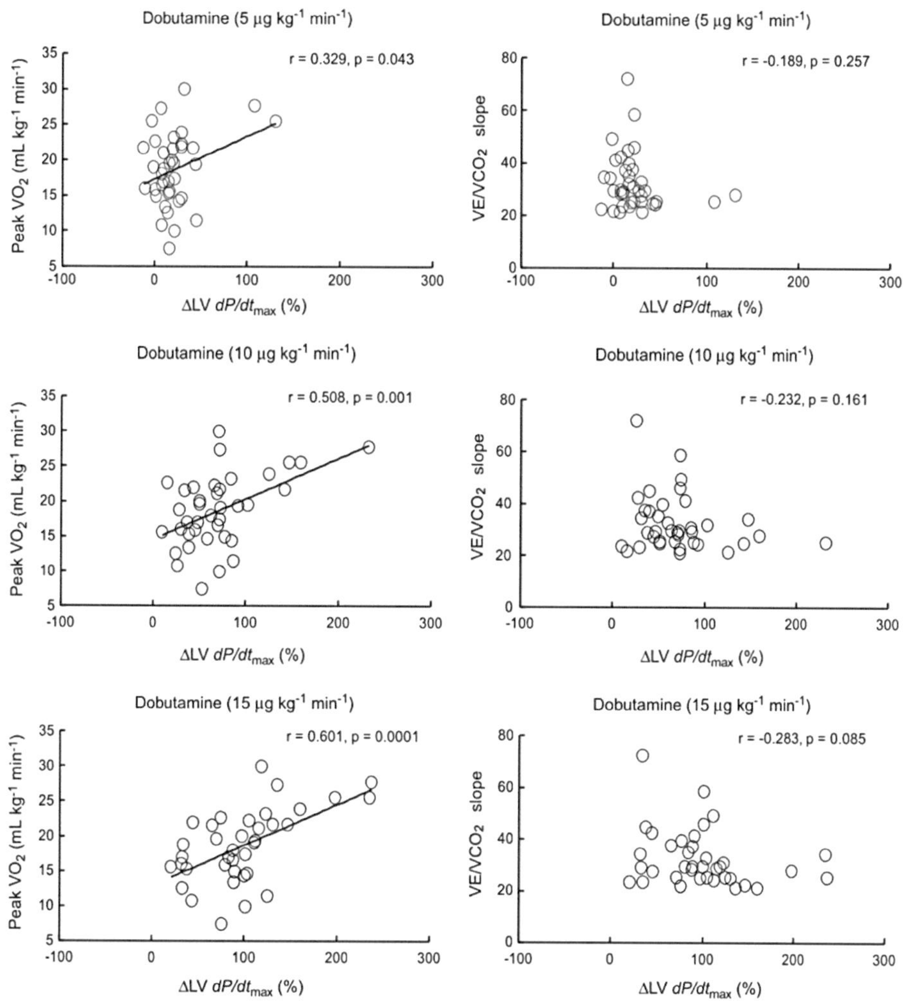

ΔLV dP/dt_{max} was significantly correlated with peak VO_2, and the correlation became more pronounced as the dose of dobutamine was increased. In contrast, no significant inverse correlation between ΔLV dP/dt_{max} and VE/VCO_2 slope was apparent, even at the maximum dose of dobutamine. ΔLV dP/dt_{max} is the percentage increase in LV dP/dt_{max} induced by dobutamine. [23]

Figure 2. Correlation between myocardial contractile reserve and peak VO_2, VE/VCO_2 slope.

Paraskevaidis, et al. reported the utility of evaluating the presence of myocardial contractile reserve in patients with intermediate values of peak VO_2 (10-14 mL/kg/min) [35]. They concluded that contractile reserve may yield the greatest incremental prognostic value in gray zone candidates for cardiac transplantation and provide further information for the risk stratification.

These results suggested that myocardial contractile reserve can be used as an adjunct or an alternative to predict peak VO_2 in patients with heart failure, especially when the patients fall into the gray zone of peak VO_2 or when the patients have a difficulty in ambulation.

4.2. Cardiac sympathetic function and contractile reserve

In 2005, we reported the correlation of impaired contractile reserve with cardiac sympathetic dysfunction in 24 DCM patients [24]. A significant correlation was observed between the delayed ^{123}I-MIBG heart-mediastinum ratio (HMR) and the percentage change in LV dP/dt_{max} from the baseline to the peak heart rate (Figure 3). The delayed ^{123}I-MIBG HMR was significantly lower in patients with a worsening change in LV dP/dt_{max} ($p=0.004$). As for the expression of mRNA, there is no significant difference in abundance for sarcoplasmic reticulum Ca^{2+}-ATPase (SERCA2). However, SERCA2/glyceraldehyde-3-phosphate dehydrogenase (GAPDH) ratio was significantly lower in low HMR group, indicating that reduced expression of SERCA2 is associated with impaired cardiac sympathetic activity.

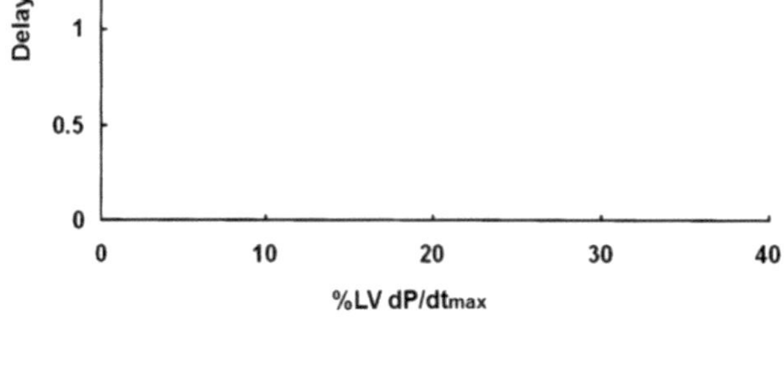

Figure 3. Relationship between the delayed ^{123}I-MIBG HMR and the percentage change in LV dP/dt_{max} from the baseline to the peak or critical heart rate. (modified from [24])

This result indicated that the myocardial ^{123}I-MIBG scintigraphy may reflect myocardial contractile reserve, and may be useful in non-invasively predicting residual contractile reserve.

http://dx.doi.org/10.5772/55413

4.3. Prognosis and contractile reserve

LV contractility has been considered to be the most powerful predictor of prognosis in DCM. Around 2000, an array of studies reported the association between LV contractile reserve and prognosis, and the presence of contractile reserve came to be considered as the most powerful prognostic predictor [10, 14 - 17].

We investigated the contractile reserve during dobutamine infusion in relation to the prognosis in 52 patients with mildly symptomatic DCM. In the ΔLV $dP/dt_{max}(10)$ <60% group, cardiac events were significantly higher than in the ΔLV $dP/dt_{max}(10)$ ≥60% group. Peak VO_2 <18 (mL/kg/min) (HR:3.18, p=0.029) and ΔLV $dP/dt_{max}(10)$ <60% (HR:3.25, p=0.026) were comparable predictors of cardiac events (Figure 4). This result indicated that evaluating the myocardial contractile reserve in dobutamine stress testing and peak VO_2 in cardiopulmonary exercise testing may be complementary approaches to predict a prognosis of non-ischemic DCM.

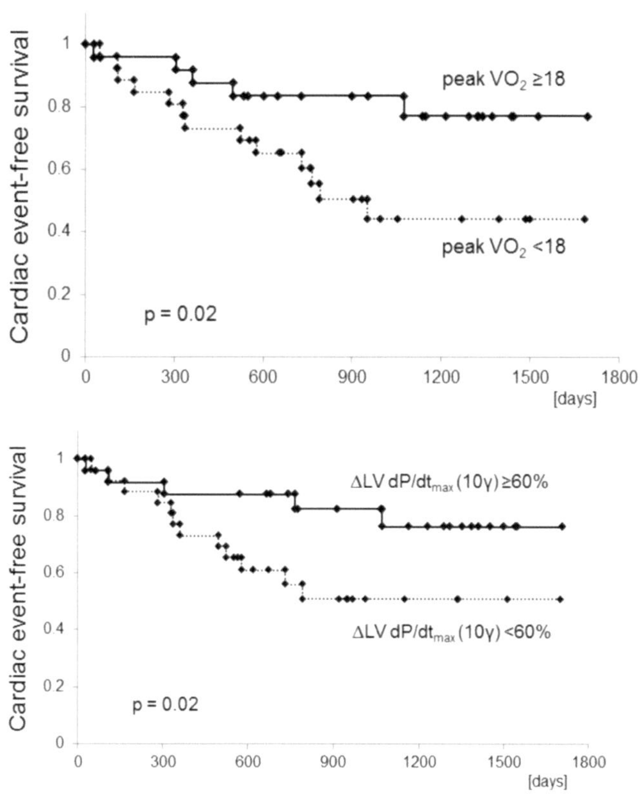

In the peak VO_2 <18 (mL/kg/min) group, cardiac events were significantly higher than in the peak VO_2 ≥18 group. In addition, cardiac events were significantly higher in the ΔLV $dP/dt_{max}(10)$ <60% group than in the ΔLV $dP/dt_{max}(10)$ ≥60% group. Peak VO_2 <18 (HR:3.18, p=0.029) and ΔLV $dP/dt_{max}(10)$ <60% (HR:3.25, p=0.026) were comparable predictors of cardiac events.

Figure 4. Kaplan-Meier analysis of cardiac event-free survival in 52 DCM patients.

Kasama S, et al. evaluated the LV response using dobutamine gated blood pool scintigraphy in 22 DCM patients [20]. In the good response group to 15 μg/kg/min dobutamine (the presence of contractile reserve; echocardiographic LV ejection fraction >5% improvement), LV systolic function was significantly improved after 1 year of ß-blocker therapy. Cardiac sympathetic nerve activity and New York Heart Association functional class also improved with cardiac reverse remodeling. In addition, they investigated contractile reserve using ^{99m}Tc-tetrofosmin quantitative gated single photon emission computed tomography (SPECT) and the similar findings were shown [21].

4.4. Molecular biological significance and contractile reserve

Recently, we reported that dobutamine stress testing is a useful diagnostic tool for evaluating adrenergic myocardial contractile reserve. This residual contractile reserve is related to alterd myocardial expression of $ß_1$-adrenergic receptor, SERCA2a, and phospholamban genes in DCM [25]. In this study, 46 asymptomatic or mildly-symptomatic DCM patients were enrolled and classified into 3 groups based on baseline LV ejection fraction and ΔLV dP/dt_{max} (Figure 5). The amounts of $ß_1$-adrenergic receptor, SERCA2a, and phospholamban mRNA were significantly smaller in group IIa and IIb than in group I (Table 1). This result indicated that impaired contractile reserve by dobutamine stress testing may be associated with molecular remodeling caused by the overactivation of sympathetic nerve system.

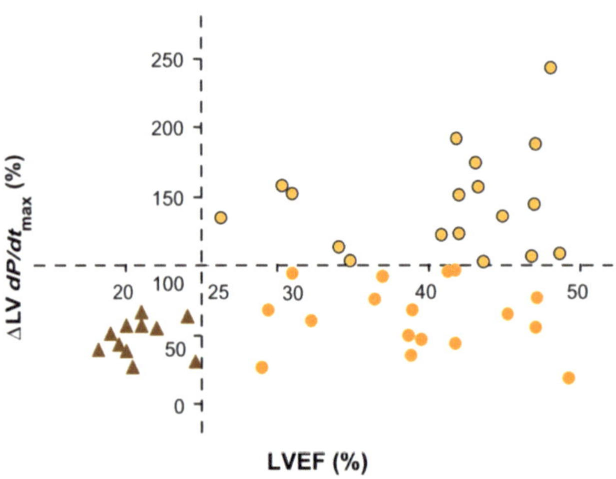

Patients were classified into 3 groups: group I (orange with black circles), ΔLV dP/dt_{max} >100% (LV ejection fraction [LVEF] >25%); group IIa (orange circles), ΔLV dP/dt_{max} ≤100% and LVEF >25%; and group IIb (brown triangles), ΔLV dP/dt_{max} ≤100% and LVEF ≤25%. [25]

Figure 5. Relation between baseline LV ejection fraction and LV dP/dt_{max}

mRNA	Group I	Group IIa	Group IIb
$Beta_1$-AR	1.39 ± 0.68	0.71 ± 0.19*	0.66 ± 0.29*
$Beta_2$-AR	1.29 ± 0.92	0.95 ± 0.18	0.91 ± 0.40
GRK2	1.54 ± 0.63	1.53 ± 0.26	1.59 ± 0.58
G_5 alpha	1.18 ± 0.40	0.94 ± 0.17	1.04 ± 0.34
G_{i2} alpha	0.78 ± 0.35	0.77 ± 0.15	0.85 ± 0.25
SERCA2a	0.60 ± 0.29	0.36 ± 0.08*	0.37 ± 0.12*
Phospholamban	0.82 ± 0.28	0.56 ± 0.12*	0.36 ± 0.16*
Ryanodine receptor-2	0.74 ± 0.42	0.56 ± 0.17	0.69 ± 0.23
Calsequestrin	1.34 ± 0.58	1.16 ± 0.25	1.30 ± 0.44
Na^+/Ca^{2+} exchanger	1.69 ± 0.76	1.14 ± 0.14	1.46 ± 0.84

Data are means ± SD. *p <0.05 vs. group I.
AR = adrenergic receptor; GRK2 = G protein-coupled receptor kinase 2; mRNA = messenger ribonucleic acid; SERCA2a = sarcoplasmic reticulum Ca^{2+} adenosine triphosphatase 2a.

Data are means ± SD. * p<0.05 vs. group I.

AR= adrenergic receptor, GRK2+ G protein-coupled receptor kinase 2; mRNA = messenger ribonucleic acid; SERCA 2a = sarcoplasmic reticulum Ca^{2+} adenosine triphosphate 2a.

Table 1. Relative Abundance of Contractile Regulatory Protein mRNAs in Endomyocardial Biopsy Specimens Relative to the Corresponding Amount of Glyceraldehyde-3-Phosphate Dehydrogenase mRNA [25]

4.5. Latest findings about contractile reserve

At present, it is reported that the patients with non-ischemic DCM have an impairment of coronary microcirculation and their coronary flow reserve is diminished [36, 37]. Skalidis EI, et al. investigated the association between LV contractile reserve and coronary flow reserve [38]. They studied 14 patients with idiopathic DCM and 11 control subjects. A significant correlation between coronary flow reserve and the corresponding contractile reserve in the vascular territory was reported. Interstingly, Otasevic P, et al. reported the relation of myocardial histomorphometric features in endomyocardial biopsy specimens and LV contractile reserve assessed by dobutamine stress echocardiography [39]. It was revealed that myocyte diameter and interstitial fibrosis strongly correlated with change in the wall motion score index, followed by the change in LV ejection fraction. Recently, Yamada S, et al. invetigated the association between myocardial blood volume and LV contractile reserve in 21 DCM patients using myocardial contrast echocardiography [40]. Myocardial blood volume was not correlated with any parameters of resting LV function, but significantly correlated with percent increase in LV ejection fraction during dobutamine stress testing. They speculated in their paper that myocardial histomorphometric features in DCM conceivably cause the reduction in myocardial blood volume, being related to the depressed contractile reserve.

5. Conclusions and future perspectives

As present, stress testing, especially by dobutamine infusion, is considered to be useful for detecting residual contractile reserve in DCM. Myocardial contractile reserve is usually detected by echocardiography, but sometimes evaluated by other modalities for accuracy, such as quantitative gated SPECT, cardiac pool scintigraphy, and LV pressure analysis. A lot of previous studies revealed that the presence of residual contractile reserve is associated with a good prognosis and impaired contractile reserve is affected by multiple factors including, but not limited to, exercise intolerance, cardiac sympathetic dysfunction, reduced myocardial blood flow and histopathological changes. In addition, the possibility is suggested that myocardial contractile reserve would predict a reversibility of LV dysfunction after initiation of cardioprotective therapy. Evaluating residual contractile reserve may have key information to predict response to interventional therapy. Therefore, further studies are required in order to detect non-responders with no available future reverse remodeling.

Acknowledgements

The authors express gratitude to Yasuko Kureishi Bando and Takahisa Kondo for careful reading of the manuscript. We would also like to thank the patients who participated in our researches.

Author details

Takahiro Okumura* and Toyoaki Murohara

Department of Cardiology, Nagoya University Graduate School of Medicine, Japan

References

[1] Steimle AE, Stevenson LW, Fonarow GC et al. Prediction of improvement in recent onset cardiomyopathy after referral for heart transplantation. *Journal of the American College of Cardiology* 1994; 23: 553-9.

[2] Cicoira M, Zanolla L, Latina L et al. Frequency, prognosis and predictors of improvement of systolic left ventricular function in patients with 'classical' clinical diagnosis of idiopathic dilated cardiomyopathy. *European journal of heart failure* 2001; 3: 323-30.

[3] Metra M, Nodari S, Parrinello G et al. Marked improvement in left ventricular ejection fraction during long-term beta-blockade in patients with chronic heart failure: clinical correlates and prognostic significance. *American heart journal* 2003; 145: 292-9.

http://dx.doi.org/10.5772/55413

[4] Kawai K, Takaoka H, Hata K et al. Prevalence, predictors, and prognosis of reversal of maladaptive remodeling with intensive medical therapy in idiopathic dilated cardiomyopathy. *The American journal of cardiology* 1999; 84: 671-6.

[5] Francis GS, Johnson TH, Ziesche S et al. Marked spontaneous improvement in ejection fraction in patients with congestive heart failure. *The American journal of medicine* 1990; 89: 303-7.

[6] Di Lenarda A, Secoli G, Perkan A et al. Changing mortality in dilated cardiomyopathy. The Heart Muscle Disease Study Group. *British heart journal* 1994; 72: S46-51.

[7] Sugrue DD, Rodeheffer RJ, Codd MB et al. The clinical course of idiopathic dilated cardiomyopathy. A population-based study. *Annals of internal medicine* 1992; 117: 117-23.

[8] Azuma A, Matsuo A, Nakamura T et al. Improved survival of idiopathic dilated cardiomyopathy in the 1990s. *Japanese circulation journal* 1999; 63: 333-8.

[9] Ramahi TM, Longo MD, Cadariu AR et al. Dobutamine-induced augmentation of left ventricular ejection fraction predicts survival of heart failure patients with severe non-ischaemic cardiomyopathy. *European heart journal* 2001; 22: 849-56.

[10] Naqvi TZ, Goel RK, Forrester JS, Siegel RJ. Myocardial contractile reserve on dobutamine echocardiography predicts late spontaneous improvement in cardiac function in patients with recent onset idiopathic dilated cardiomyopathy. *Journal of the American College of Cardiology* 1999; 34: 1537-44.

[11] Holubarsch C, Ludemann J, Wiessner S et al. Shortening versus isometric contractions in isolated human failing and non-failing left ventricular myocardium: dependency of external work and force on muscle length, heart rate and inotropic stimulation. *Cardiovascular research* 1998; 37: 46-57.

[12] Ross J, Jr., Miura T, Kambayashi M et al. Adrenergic control of the force-frequency relation. *Circulation* 1995; 92: 2327-32.

[13] Picono E. Stress Echocardiography, 4th ed. New York: Springer; 2003.

[14] Scrutinio D, Napoli V, Passantino A et al. Low-dose dobutamine responsiveness in idiopathic dilated cardiomyopathy: relation to exercise capacity and clinical outcome. *European heart journal* 2000; 21: 927-34.

[15] Dubois-Rande JL, Merlet P, Roudot F et al. Beta-adrenergic contractile reserve as a predictor of clinical outcome in patients with idiopathic dilated cardiomyopathy. *American heart journal* 1992; 124: 679-85.

[16] Pratali L, Picano E, Otasevic P et al. Prognostic significance of the dobutamine echocardiography test in idiopathic dilated cardiomyopathy. *The American journal of cardiology* 2001; 88: 1374-8.

[17] Drozdz J, Krzeminska-Pakula M, Plewka M et al. Prognostic value of low-dose dobutamine echocardiography in patients with idiopathic dilated cardiomyopathy. *Chest* 2002; 121: 1216-22.

[18] Mastumura Y,et al. Low-dose dobutamine stress echocardiography predicts the improvement of left ventricular systolic function and long-term prognosis in patients with idiopathic dilated cardiomyopathy, *Journal of Medical Ultrasonics* 2006; 33: 17-22.

[19] Ypenburg C, Sieders A, Bleeker GB et al. Myocardial contractile reserve predicts improvement in left ventricular function after cardiac resynchronization therapy. *American heart journal* 2007; 154: 1160-5.

[20] Kasama S, Toyama T, Hoshizaki H et al. Dobutamine gated blood pool scintigraphy predicts the improvement of cardiac sympathetic nerve activity, cardiac function, and symptoms after treatment in patients with dilated cardiomyopathy. *Chest* 2002; 122: 542-8.

[21] Kasama S, Toyama T, Kumakura H et al. Dobutamine stress 99mTc-tetrofosmin quantitative gated SPECT predicts improvement of cardiac function after carvedilol treatment in patients with dilated cardiomyopathy. *Journal of nuclear medicine : official publication, Society of Nuclear Medicine* 2004; 45: 1878-84.

[22] Neskovic AN, Otasevic P. Stress-echocardiography in idiopathic dilated cardiomyopathy: instructions for use. *Cardiovascular ultrasound* 2005; 3: 3.

[23] Okumura T, Hirashiki A, Yamada S et al. Association between cardiopulmonary exercise and dobutamine stress testing in ambulatory patients with idiopathic dilated cardiomyopathy: A comparison with peak VO(2) and VE/VCO(2) slope. *International journal of cardiology* 2011 (epub).

[24] Ohshima S, Isobe S, Izawa H et al. Cardiac sympathetic dysfunction correlates with abnormal myocardial contractile reserve in dilated cardiomyopathy patients. *Journal of the American College of Cardiology* 2005; 46: 2061-8.

[25] Kobayashi M, Izawa H, Cheng XW et al. Dobutamine stress testing as a diagnostic tool for evaluation of myocardial contractile reserve in asymptomatic or mildly symptomatic patients with dilated cardiomyopathy. *JACC Cardiovascular imaging* 2008; 1: 718-26.

[26] Bountioukos M, Doorduijn JK, Roelandt JR et al. Repetitive dobutamine stress echocardiography for the prediction of anthracycline cardiotoxicity. *European journal of echocardiography : the journal of the Working Group on Echocardiography of the European Society of Cardiology* 2003; 4: 300-5.

[27] Marwick TH. Stress echocardiography. *Heart* 2003; 89: 113-8.

[28] Armstrong WF. Echocardiography in coronary artery disease. *Progress in cardiovascular diseases* 1988; 30: 267-88.

[29] Allman KC, Shaw LJ, Hachamovitch R, Udelson JE. Myocardial viability testing and impact of revascularization on prognosis in patients with coronary artery disease and left ventricular dysfunction: a meta-analysis. *Journal of the American College of Cardiology* 2002; 39: 1151-8.

[30] Becher H, Chambers J, Fox K et al. BSE procedure guidelines for the clinical application of stress echocardiography, recommendations for performance and interpretation of stress echocardiography: a report of the British Society of Echocardiography Policy Committee. *Heart* 2004; 90 Suppl 6: vi23-30.

[31] Werner GS, Schaefer C, Dirks R et al. Prognostic value of Doppler echocardiographic assessment of left ventricular filling in idiopathic dilated cardiomyopathy. *The American journal of cardiology* 1994; 73: 792-8.

[32] Fowler MB, Laser JA, Hopkins GL et al. Assessment of the beta-adrenergic receptor pathway in the intact failing human heart: progressive receptor down-regulation and subsensitivity to agonist response. *Circulation* 1986; 74: 1290-302.

[33] Somura F, Izawa H, Iwase M et al. Reduced myocardial sarcoplasmic reticulum Ca^{2+}-ATPase mRNA expression and biphasic force-frequency relations in patients with hypertrophic cardiomyopathy. *Circulation* 2001; 104: 658-63.

[34] Nagaoka H, Isobe N, Kubota S et al. Myocardial contractile reserve as prognostic determinant in patients with idiopathic dilated cardiomyopathy without overt heart failure. *Chest* 1997; 111: 344-50.

[35] Paraskevaidis IA, Adamopoulos S, Kremastinos DT. Dobutamine echocardiographic study in patients with nonischemic dilated cardiomyopathy and prognostically borderline values of peak exercise oxygen consumption: 18-month follow-up study. *Journal of the American College of Cardiology* 2001; 37: 1685-91.

[36] Treasure CB, VitaJ A, Cox DA, et al. Endothelium-dependent dilation of the coronary microvasculature is impaired in dilated cardiomyopathy. *Circulation* 1990; 81: 772-9.

[37] Rigo F, Ciampi Q, Ossena G, et al. Prognostic value of left and right coronary flow reserve assessment in nonischemic dilated cardiomyopathy by transthoracic Doppler echocardiography. *Journal of Cardiac Failure* 2011 Jan; 17 (1): 39-46.

[38] Skalidis EI, Parthenakis FI, Patrianakos AP, et al. Regional coronary flow and contractile reserve in patients with idiopathic dilated cardiomyopathy. *Journal of American College of Cardiology* 2004; 44: 2027-32.

[39] Otasevic P, Popovic ZB, Vasiljevic JD, et al. Relation of myocardial histomorphometric features and left ventricular contractile reserve assessed by high-dose dobutamine stress echocardiography in patients with idiopathic dilated cardiomyopathy. *The European Journal of Heart Failure* 2005; 7: 49-56.

[40] Yamada S, Iwano H, Komuro K, et al. Relation between myocardial blood volume and left ventricular contractile reserve in patients with dilated cardiomyopathy. *Journal of Medical Ultrasonics* 2010; 37 (4): 491-497.

Section 2

Pathophysiology and Molecular Mechanisms

Chapter 4

Cardiomyopathies: When the Goliaths of Heart Muscle Hurt

Maegen A. Ackermann and
Aikaterini Kontrogianni-Konstantopoulos

Additional information is available at the end of the chapter

http://dx.doi.org/10.5772/55609

1. Introduction

Cardiomyopathy, a primary cause of human death, is defined as a disease of the myocardium, which results in insufficient pumping of the heart. It is classified into four major forms; hypertrophic cardiomyopathy (HCM), dilated cardiomyopathy (DCM), restrictive cardiomyopathy (RMC), and arrhythmogenic right ventricular cardiomyopathy (ARVC) [1]. These are characterized by extensive remodeling of the myocardium initially manifested as hypertrophy, evidenced by an increase in the thickness of the left ventricular wall and interventricular septum due to interstitial fibrosis and enlarged myocyte size. Following hypertrophy the heart muscle reverts to a dilated state, characterized by a profound expansion of the intraventricular volume and a modest increase in ventricular wall thickness [2]. These changes, initially compensatory, eventually become maladaptive.

During the past ~20 years, several mutations in genes encoding sarcomeric proteins have been causally linked to cardiomyopathies [1]. Among the long list of affected proteins are three members of the family of giant sarcomeric proteins of striated muscles: titin, nebulette, a member of the nebulin subfamily, and obscurin, each encoded by single genes namely *TTN*, *NEBL*, and *OBSCN*, respectively [3]-[10]. This chapter will briefly describe the molecular structure of these genes, assisting the reader to excellent detailed reviews when appropriate, and further provide a comprehensive and up-to-date listing of the mutations that have been identified and directly linked to the development of cardiomyopathy.

2. Titin

Titin, the largest member of the superfamily of giant sarcomeric proteins, is a 3-4 MDa protein encoded by the single *TTN* gene. The 363 exons that make up *TTN* undergo extensive alternative splicing resulting in the expression of several large variants of the protein [11]. A single titin molecule spans a half sarcomere, with its NH_2-terminus anchored to the Z-disc and its COOH-terminus extending into the M-band [11]-[14]. Titin possesses a modular structure, composed mainly of immunoglobulin (Ig) and fibronectin type III (FN-III) domains. Specifically, its Z-disc portion is composed of Ig domains along with ~45-residue long repeats unique to that region (Z-repeats) and possesses binding sites for several sarcomeric proteins (Figure 1) [7]. The portion of titin that spans the I-band is composed mainly of Ig domains intersected by titin specific N2A and N2B regions along with several ~30-residue long PEVK repeats (Figure 2). Titin's I-band region holds binding sites for actin and thin filament proteins, as well as docking sites for many signaling molecules [7]. Within its A-band portion, titin is organized in repeats containing numerous FN-III domains interspersed by Ig domains, which provide repetitive binding sites for myosin and thick filament associated proteins (Figure 3) [7]. The portion of titin that extends into the M-band begins with a Ser/Thr kinase domain followed by additional Ig domains and M-band specific insertions (Figure 4) [7]. Through this region, titin interacts with many other structural proteins to form a scaffold at the M-band.

Within the sarcomere, titin, through its PEVK domain, functions as a "molecular spring," contributing to the biomechanical properties and structural integrity of striated muscle cells during the contractile cycle [15], [16]. In addition, it acts as a "molecular blueprint" coordinating the assembly of structural, regulatory, and contractile proteins [17]. Given the elastic nature and scaffolding role of titin, it is not surprising that mutations along the length of *TTN* are intimately associated with the development of cardiomyopathy.

To date, at least 107 mutations in *TTN* have been causally linked to HCM, DCM, and ARVC. Many of these mutations occur within essential binding sites along its length, with a high incidence of mutations occurring within the region that spans the A-band, disrupting the ability of titin to bind to myosin thick filaments. The remaining mutations are present within the extensible region of titin affecting its ability to respond to the constant stretching of the sarcomere during repeating cycles of contraction and relaxation. Notably, 84 of these mutations, found exclusively in the I- and A-band regions of titin, alter the length of the protein. Thus, mutations within *TTN* compromise the structural integrity of sarcomeres and lead to impaired contractile activity of cardiac muscle cells.

2.1. Cardiomyopathy linked mutations within titin's Z-disc region

The extreme NH_2-terminus of titin is only mildly affected by cardiomyopathy-causing mutations; only 4 missense mutations and 3 insertion/deletion (indel) polymorphisms have been identified within the Z-disc portion of titin. A missense mutation identified in codon 54 leads to conversion of a valine residue to methionine (V54M) in the region encoding the first Ig domain of titin [18]. The V54M mutation is located in the telethonin-binding domain of titin and functional analysis revealed a decrease of titin's ability to interact with telethonin in the

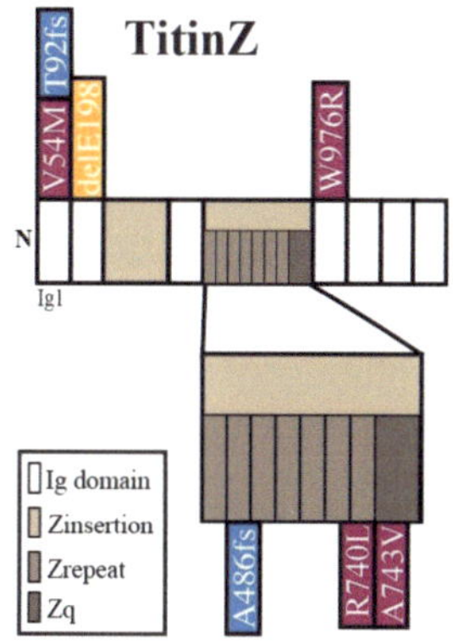

Figure 1. Schematic representation of the Z-disc region of titin, illustrating its motifs and cardiomyopathy associated mutations. Insertions or deletions predicted to cause frame shifts (fs) and single amino acid deletions (del) are noted in blue and yellow, respectively. Missense mutations are shown with a magenta background. Mutations in the *TTN* gene within this region are shown relative to the domains in which they are found.

presence of this mutation [18]. Sequencing of the DNA encoding the Z-disc region of titin in patients with HCM revealed a G to T transversion in codon 740 that is located within the 7th Z-repeat of titin and results in the replacement of an arginine residue with leucine (R740L) [19]. The mutation was not found in DNA from corresponding controls, suggesting it is not a polymorphism. Yeast two-hybrid assays showed that the mutation increased binding to α-actinin by ~40% [19]. Interestingly the opposite biochemical effect was observed in a father and daughter with DCM where a point mutation in codon 743 resulting in an alanine to valine (A743V) conversion in the Zq region of titin was identified [18]. The A743V mutation, which is also localized within the α-actinin binding site on titin, significantly decreases the binding capacity of titin for α-actinin [18]. Additionally, a kindred with autosomal dominant DCM was analyzed and shown to have a point mutation in exon 18 encoding Ig4 that results in the conversion of a tryptophan residue to arginine (W976R), but the functional consequence of this mutation is currently unknown [20]. Recently, Golbus et al identified 3 indels within the Z-disc portion of titin in a large population of individuals exhibiting cardiac disease [5]. Due to the nature of this extensive study, phenotypic data regarding the subjects is unavailable, however they have been linked to either DCM or HCM.

2.2. Cardiomyopathy linked mutations within the region of titin that spans the I-band region

To date, several mutations within the region of titin that spans the I-band have been linked to DCM and HCM. In particular, three mutations within titin's N2B region at the beginning of its I-band portion have been identified. A missense mutation in the N2B region of titin (S3753Y) was identified in two siblings with familial HCM [18], and shown to increase binding to four-and-a-half-LIM domain protein 2 (FLH2) by ~26% in a yeast two-hybrid assay [21]. In addition, in patients exhibiting a DCM phenotype a transversion of C to T in codon 4007 was found to result in the conversion of a glutamine residue to an early termination codon (Q4007X), and another missense mutation in codon 4417 was identified to replace a serine residue with an asparagine (S4417N) [18]. The premature stop codon (Q4007X) occurs just prior to the binding site for FHL2 while the S4417N mutation decreases the binding capacity of titin for FHL2, as determined by yeast two-hybrid studies [21]. Within titin's PEVK region 3 missense mutations have been identified in DCM and HCM patients (G3470D, R8500H, and R8604Q) [22], [23]. Mutations R8500H and R8604Q were shown to increase the binding capacity of titin for cardiac ankyrin repeat protein (CARP) as determined by coimmunoprecipitation assays [22]. The pathogenicity of the G3470D is still unknown, however. Moreover, using population based studies of DCM and HCM patients, Golbus et al recently identified 9 indels within the portion of titin that spans the I-band [5].

In a large study, using next generation sequencing, Herman et al analyzed 203 and 231 patients with DCM and HCM, respectively and the corresponding control subjects for mutations in the *TTN* gene [6]. The frequency of *TTN* polymorphisms was significantly higher in DCM than HCM patients or normal subjects. Interestingly, of the mutations identified, all were shown to cause alterations in full-length titin, many of which caused early termination. Two of these truncations occurred as a result of missense mutations within the N2B region and also within Ig94 following the PEVK region. In addition, several splice site donor/acceptor mutations were found to cause truncations within the PEVK region and Ig85. The study also revealed 3 deletion and 2 insertion mutations affecting the I-band region of titin. Specifically, frameshift mutations within Ig11, 45, 61, and 85 alter the length of the protein, while a large duplication of exons 72-124 corresponding to Ig50 through the PEVK region increased *TTN*'s already large size by ~28kb. The functional significance of these mutations, which alter the length of full-length titin, is currently unknown.

Studies linking *TTN* to the development of DCM and HCM date back about a decade, however, it is only recently that *TTN* has been linked to ARVC. A recent study using DNA screening of patients diagnosed with ARVC revealed 3 missense mutations along the I-band region of titin [9]. The study identified a threonine to isoleucine transversion within codon 2896 (T2896I) located in Ig16 as well as two mutations within the PEVK region (Y8031C and H8848Y). Proteomic techniques revealed that the T2896I mutation reduces the structural stability of Ig16 and increases its propensity for degradation [9]. The pathogenicity of the other two mutations has not yet been determined.

2.3. Cardiomyopathy linked mutations within titin's A-band region

The region of titin spanning the A-band can be considered a "hot spot" for cardiomyopathy-linked changes with an overwhelming 63 identified mutations. In the early 2000's, Gerull et al analyzed two siblings with autosomal dominant DCM and identified a unique mutation in titin [20]. A 2-bp insertion mutation in exon 326, caused a frameshift at K20995 within Ig115 resulting in a premature stop codon leading to proteolytic degradation of titin, probably near or within the PEVK domain, as determined by antibody labeling [20]. A few years later, the same group discovered a frameshift mutation at A27460 within FN-III107, also resulting in a premature stop codon, and proteolytic degradation of titin [24].

Recently, two additional insertions within FN-III domains present at the A-band have been identified in patients with DCM. The first causes a frame shift at S19628 and the second a frameshift at G26124 resulting in early termination within domains FN-III 42 and 97, respec-

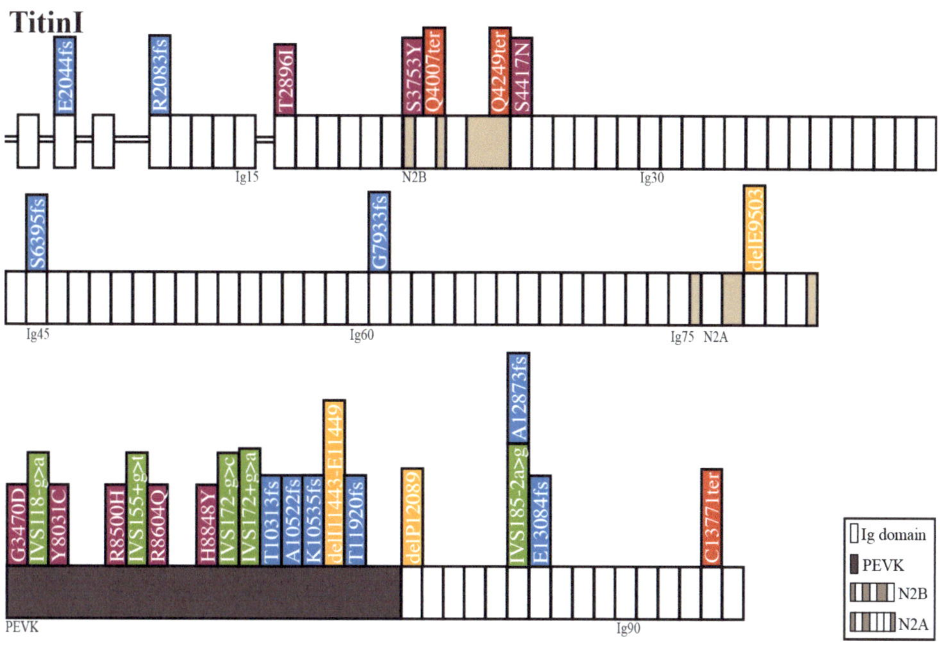

Figure 2. Schematic representation of the I-band region of titin, illustrating its motifs and cardiomyopathy associated mutations. Mutations in the *TTN* gene within this region are shown relative to the domains in which they are found. Insertions or deletions predicted to cause frame shifts (fs) and single amino acid deletions (del) are noted in blue and yellow, respectively. Missense mutations are shown with a magenta background. A red background indicates nonsense mutations resulting in premature stop codons (ter). Splice site donor/acceptor mutations are shown in green.

tively [10]. In addition to the several length altering mutations noted within the I-band region of titin by Herman et al, many more have been found within the region spanning the A-band [6]. An astonishing 23 missense mutations have been identified to cause early termination within several of the Ig and FN-III domains throughout the A-band. Another 11 spice site donor/acceptor mutations were found to cause truncations throughout the A-band. In addition, 13 deletion, 4 insertion, and 2 insertion/deletion mutations have been shown to cause frameshifts in the coding region of titin, resulting in altered full-length titin protein. The functional significance of these mutations is not yet known, however. Moreover, Golbus et al recently identified 3 indels within the portion of titin that spans the A-band in a large population of individuals exhibiting cardiac disease [5]. Due to the nature of this extensive study phenotypic data regarding the subjects in unavailable, however they have been linked to either DCM or HCM.

In addition, 4 missense mutations affecting patients with ARVC have been identified within the A-band region of titin. DNA screening of patients exhibiting signs of ARVC revealed 4 missense mutations affecting both FN-III and Ig domains along the A-band region of titin (I16949T, A18579T, A19309S, P30847L) [9]. The molecular effects of these mutations have not yet been determined.

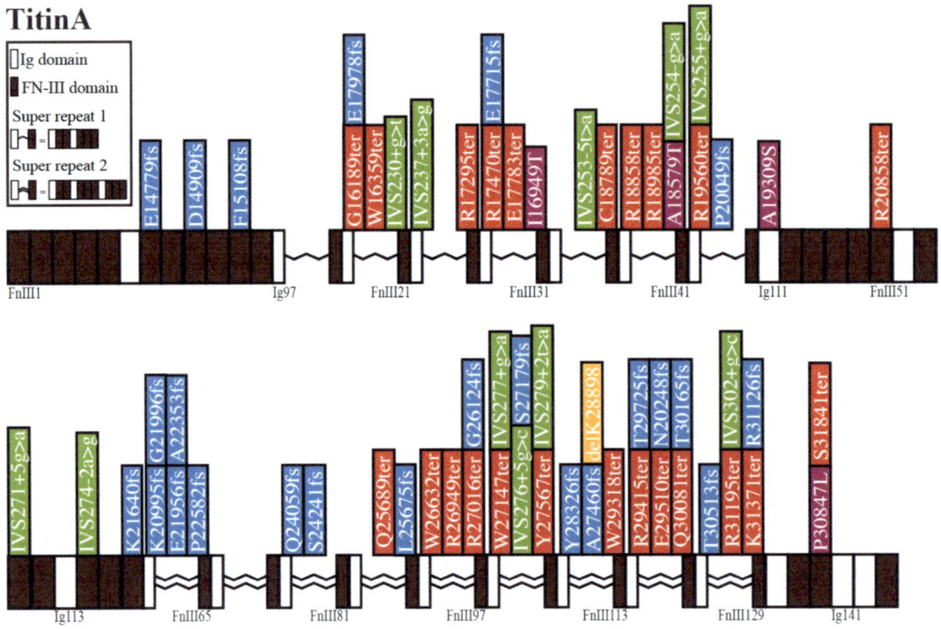

Figure 3. Schematic representation of the A-band region of titin, illustrating its motifs and cardiomyopathy-associated mutations. Mutations in the *TTN* gene within this region are shown relative to the domains in which they are found. Insertions or deletions predicted to cause frame shifts (fs) and single amino acid deletions (del) are noted in blue and yellow, respectively. A red background indicates nonsense mutations resulting in premature stop codons (ter). Splice site donor/acceptor mutations are shown in green. Missense mutations are shown with a magenta background.

2.4. Cardiomyopathy linked mutations within the region of titin that extends into the M-band

Similar to the NH_2-terminus of titin, the COOH-terminus remains relatively unaffected by cardiomyopathy causing mutations. A total of 6 mutations have been described within the portion of titin that extends into the M-band. Sequencing of DNA from patients with DCM and ARVC has identified 2 missense mutations localized to the M-band region of titin. Specifically, in two related individuals exhibiting late-onset DCM, an arginine to glutamine conversion at amino acid 32069 was identified (R32069Q) [21]. In addition, a patient diagnosed with ARVC possessed a methionine to threonine transition at codon 33291 (M33291T) [9]. These mutations localize to Ig146 and Ig152, respectively, however, their pathogenicity has not yet been determined. A recent study using population based analysis of DCM and HCM patients, identified 2 indels within the M-band portion of titin [5]. Phenotypic data regarding the subjects, as well as the mechanistic affects of the mutations are unavailable. Interestingly, 2 deletion mutations within the M-band region of titin were identified in 2 non-related families exhibiting early onset myopathy, affecting skeletal muscle, with fatal cardiomyopathy. Sequence analysis indicated a deletion mutation of 1 bp in exon 360 (Mex3) and an 8 bp deletion in exon 358 (Mex1) [25]. Both deletions left the titin kinase domain intact but resulted in premature stop codons at Ig domains 147 and 150 and a loss of the COOH-terminal 447 and

808 amino acids, respectively. Genetic analysis showed the defects in the *TTN* gene to be homozygous, leaving the heterozygote parents clinically unaffected. These mutations (1bp deletion in exon 360 and an 8bp deletion in exon 358) in the *TTN* gene are the first to be identified that produce both skeletal and cardiac muscle defects.

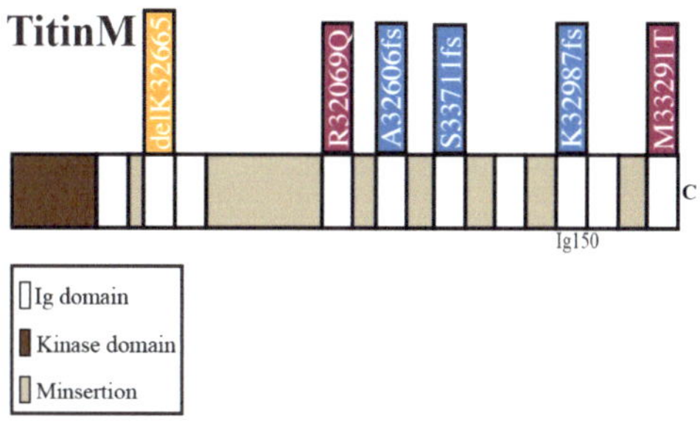

Figure 4. Schematic representation of the M-band region of titin, illustrating its motifs and cardiomyopathy-associated mutations. Mutations in the *TTN* gene within this region are shown relative to the domains in which they can be found. Insertions or deletions predicted to cause frame shifts (fs) and single amino acid deletions (del) are noted in blue and yellow, respectively. Missense mutations are shown with a magenta background.

Although titin has been implicated in cardiomyopathies for over a decade, only recently has its direct role begun to be expounded. Many of the follow-up results on identified cardiomyopathy linked mutations of *TTN* indicate that these mutations can alter titin's binding capacity to its ligands, however, it remains to be proven that this is sufficient to cause DCM and HCM. Further study of the functional consequences of the *TTN* mutations, especially those causing truncated variants, using *in vivo* animal models is still necessary to elucidate titin's role in cardiomyopathies.

3. Nebulin

Nebulin is a giant (~500-800 kDa) sarcomeric protein of striated muscles [26]. Similar to titin, nebulin is oriented longitudinally across the sarcomere, spanning the length of the thin filament [27]. Its NH_2-terminus extends to the pointed ends of thin filaments in the sarcomeric I-band, and its COOH-terminus resides within the Z-disc [28]. The nebulin gene, *NEB*, contains 183 exons and is the product of extensive gene duplication, resulting in a protein of highly repetitive domain structure [29]. Nebulin is mostly composed of tandem nebulin-repeats with the central motifs organized as super-repeats. In addition, nebulin contains a glutamine rich region at its NH_2-terminus, as well as a serine rich region and a Src Homology 3 (SH3) domain at its COOH-terminus. The organization of the nebulin repeats complements the periodicity of actin filaments [28]. Consistent with this, alternative splicing of the *NEB* gene generates proteins of different sizes, which correspond to thin filaments of various lengths [30], [31]. In addition to its role in stabilizing thin filaments, nebulin has also been implicated as a regulator of thin filament length [32], [33].

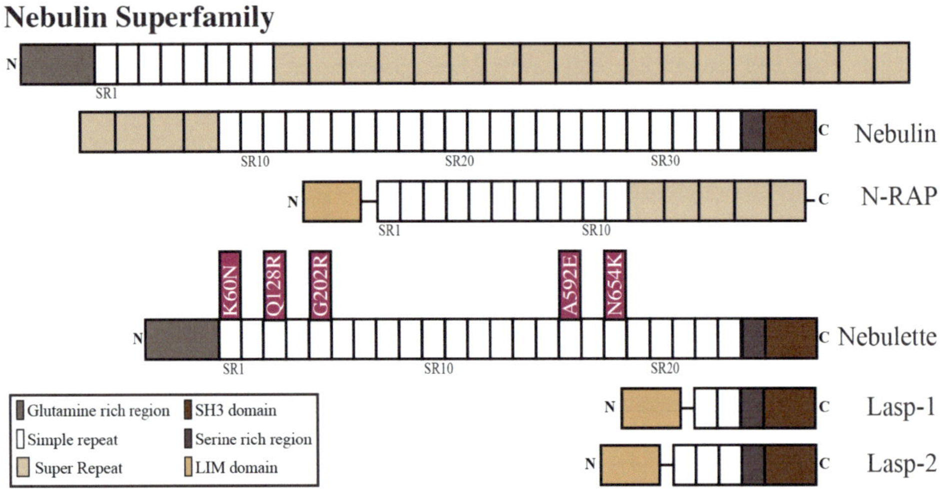

Figure 5. Schematic representation of the nebulin superfamily members, illustrating their motifs and cardiomyopathy associated mutations. Mutations in the *NEBL* gene are shown relative to the domains in which they are found. Missense mutations are shown with a magenta background.

In addition to being a member of the family of large sarcomeric proteins of striated muscle, nebulin is also a member of a family of actin-binding cytoskeletal proteins, which includes N-RAP, nebulette, LASP-1, and LASP-2 (Figure 5). The unifying domain of nebulin family members is the actin binding nebulin-repeat, of ~35 amino acids in length, each containing an SDxxYK motif [34]. For the remainder of the chapter, we will focus on nebulette as it is the only member of the nebulin family that has been linked to cardiomyopathies. Cardiac specific nebulette is functionally similar to nebulin whereby it aids in the stabilization of actin filaments [26]. Nebulette localizes to the Z-disc [35], where it interacts with the thin filament proteins troponin and tropomyosin [36]. Mutations in the nebulettte gene, *NEBL,* which cause disruption of the stabilization of the Z-disc, have been linked to the development of cardiomyopathy [4], [8].

Nebulette's involvement in cardiomyopathies was first identified in the early 2000's when Arimura et al screened *NEBL* paired normal subjects and patients with idiopathic dilated cardiomyopathy (IDC) for mutations in the nebulette gene [4]. The study identified several polymorphisms in *NEBL* with one variant showing a high frequency in patients with non-familial IDC. Patients carrying this variant possess a missense mutation, N654K, in the 18th nebulin repeat of nebulette. The mechanism by which this mutation causes disruptions in the heart is unknown, however due to its location this mutation likely disrupts nebulette's incorporation into the Z-disc. Notably, this observation has brought about a new role for nebulette as a genetic marker for patients with non-familial IDC.

Recently, more direct evidence for the involvement of nebulette in the development of heart disease was demonstrated in several patients diagnosed with DCM [8]. Linkage analysis revealed four sequence variations in the *NEBL* gene in regions encoding nebulin-repeats along the length of the molecule. Specifically, variants K60N, Q128R, and G202R are located in nebulin-repeats that bind to F-actin and the tropomyosin-troponin complex, while A592E is located in the region that is incorporated into the Z-disc. Variants K60N and G202R found in nebulin-repeats 1 and 5, respectively, were identified in adult patients developing clinical manifestations of DCM. On the contrary variant Q128R, located in nebulin-repeat 3, was identified in a newborn patient diagnosed with DCM and endocardial fibroelastosis. The remaining variant, A592E, located in nebulin-repeat 16 was also found in a newborn displaying clinical features of DCM. *In vivo* studies using cardiac specific nebulette mutant mice were able to recapitulate human cardiac disease phenotypes and begun to unravel the mechanisms by which these mutations affect cardiac function [8]. Specifically, variants K60N and Q128R were embryonic lethal with hearts exhibiting structural abnormalities. Additionally, mutant mice carrying G202R or A592E variants resulted in left ventricular dilation and impaired cardiac function. These functional defects were coupled with improper localization of mutant nebulette resulting in dramatic structural alterations in I-band and Z-disc proteins. Taken together these studies suggest that nebulette is required for normal maintenance of the sarcomere and stability of the Z-disc and identifies *NEBL* as a contributor to the development of ICD and DCM.

4. Obscurin

Obscurin is the third giant protein of the contractile apparatus of striated muscles. Similar to titin and nebulin the obscurin gene, *OBSCN*, gives rise to a large (~720 kDa; obscurin A) multidomain protein composed mainly of Ig and FN-III domains [7]. In addition, obscurin possesses several signaling motifs within its COOH-terminal half, including an IQ motif, an SH3 domain, as well as tandem Rho Guanine Nucleotide Exchange Factor (RhoGEF) and Pleckstrin Homology (PH) motifs. Similar to *TTN* and *NEB*, *OBSCN* is also subjected to alternative splicing giving rise to several isoforms of differing sizes (Figure 6) [37]. Specifically, the *OBSCN* gene gives rise to another large isoform, referred to as obscurin-B, which has a molecular mass of ~870 kDa. Obscurin B contains two serine/threonine kinase domains, which replace the non-modular COOH-terminus of obscurin A. The kinase domains may be expressed independently as smaller isoforms, containing one or both kinase domains (sMLCK or tMLCK, respectively). Unlike its counterparts, obscurins surround the sarcomere at the level of the Z-disc and M-band, where they are appropriately positioned to interact with several ligands and participate in their assembly and integration into the sarcomere and internal membrane systems [7]. Despite its large size, it is only recently that we learn of *OBSCN*'s linkage to cardiomyopthies.

Although the role of *OBSCN* in cardiomyopthies is still unclear, several studies have documented an upregulation of obscurins during cardiac hypertrophic responses to pressure overload and myopathic responses to mutations in titin [38]-[40]. In addition, up-regulation of different *OBSCN* gene products, including full length obscurin and several of the smaller MLCK variants was reported to occur in mice with myocardial hypertrophy induced by aortic constriction [38]. This increase in expression was mainly observed in obscurin isoforms that contained the RhoGEF and kinase signaling motifs, and occurred early in the hypertrophic response and also during hypertrophic growth. Concurrent with this, targeted loss of the obscurin RhoGEF domain resulted in myocytes lacking intercalated discs and in more severe cases in failure of the contractile filaments to organize into mature sarcomeres [41]. It is likely that upregulation of obscurins, is associated with the increase in contractile structures observed during hypertrophy, however, the mechanism by which this occurs remains unresolved.

More direct evidence for the involvement of *OBSCN* in the development of heart disease was demonstrated in a single patient with HCM [3]. Linkage analysis revealed a sequence variation in the *OBSCN* gene in the region encoding the site of interaction for the Z-disc region of titin (Ig58/59), specifically an R4344Q variant in the Ig58 domain of obscurin. *In vitro* studies showed that this variant resulted in decreased binding of obscurin to titin as well as mis-localization of obscurin to the Z-disc. Despite this single case, it suggests that, like titin and nebulette, mutations in the *OBSCN* gene lead to the development cardiomyopathies.

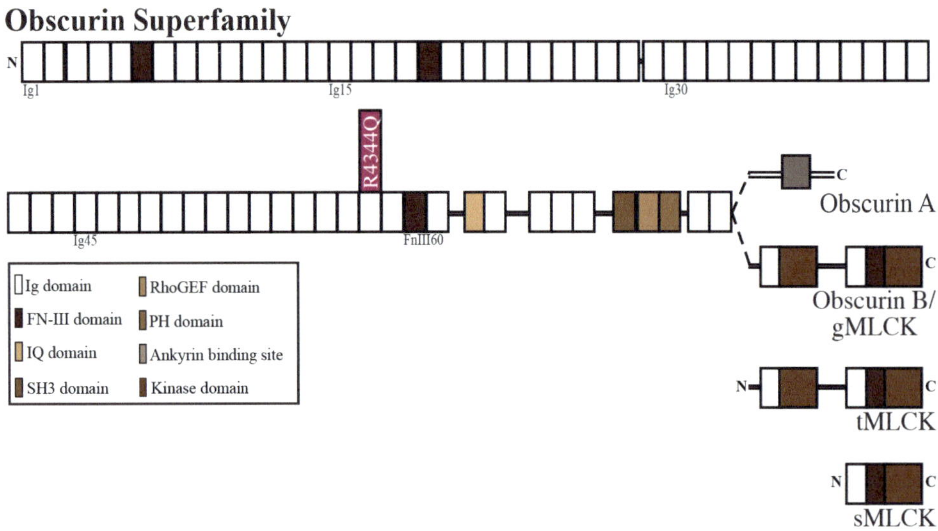

Figure 6. Schematic representation of the obscurin isoforms, illustrating their motifs and cardiomyopathy associated mutation. The missense mutation in the *OBSCN* gene is shown relative to the domain in which it is localized with a magenta background.

5. Concluding remarks

Over two decades ago the first HCM-causing mutation in a sarcomeric gene was identified in β-myosin heavy chain. Since then both HCM and DCM have come to be known as diseases of the sarcomere. In fact, sarcomeric dysfunction is the underlying cause of many genetically mediated HCM and DCM disorders and accounts for ~60% of HCM and ~10-20% of DCM reported cases [42]-[45]. To date, more than 1500 distinct mutations of sarcomeric proteins have been linked to cardiomyopathies [46], [47]. Given the many roles that have been described for

http://dx.doi.org/10.5772/55609

titin, nebulette, and obscurin in cardiac muscle, and the effects of the identified mutations in their localization, activity, and regulation, it is not surprising that many human diseases of heart muscle have been linked to these proteins. Notably, a striking 50 missense mutations within *TTN, NEBL,* and *OBSCN* (Table 1) with an additional 16 splice site donor/acceptor mutations (Table 2) and 47 deletion or insertion mutations within *TTN* (Table 3) have been associated with the development of different forms of cardiomyopathy. The severity of these diseases can vary from moderate to severe, depending on the nature of the mutation. The characterization of these mutations and their effects on cardiac pathophysiology is just beginning to be elucidated, however it is clear that this is just the tip of the iceberg. Understanding how these mutations alter sarcomeric structure and contractile activity could aid in improving clinical diagnosis and developing individualized therapies for cardiomyopathic patients.

Missense Mutations of Titin, Nebulette, and Obscurin					
Disease	**Mutation**	**Region on Protein**	**Sarcomeric Region**	**Effect**	**Reference**
			Mutations of TTN		
DCM	V54M*	Ig1	Z-disc	Reduced binding to telethonin	[18]
HCM	R740L*	Z-repeat 7	Z-disc	Increase binding to α-actinin	[19]
DCM	A743V*	Zq region	Z-disc	Reduce binding to α-actinin	[18]
DCM	W976R*	Ig4	Z-disc	Unknown	[20]
ARVC	T2896I*	Ig16	I-band	Unknown	[9]
HCM	S3753Y#	N2B	I-band	Increase binding to FLH2	[18]
DCM	Q4007X#	N2B	I-band	Truncation of titin	[18]
DCM	Q4249X^	N2B	I-band	Truncation of titin	[6]
DCM	S4417N#	Ig24	I-band	Decrease binding to FHL2	[18]
DCM	G3470D*	PEVK	I-band	Unknown	[23]
ARVC	Y8031C*	PEVK	I-band	Unknown	[9]
HCM	R8500H*	PEVK	I-band	Increase binding to CARP	[22]
HCM	R8604Q*	PEVK	I-band	Increase binding to CARP	[22]
ARVC	H8848Y*	PEVK	I-band	Unknown	[9]
DCM	C13771X^	Ig94	I-band	Truncation of titin	[6]
DCM	G16189X^	FNIII17	A-band	Truncation of titin	[6]
DCM	W16359X^	Ig100	A-band	Truncation of titin	[6]
DCM	R17295X^	FNIII25	A-band	Truncation of titin	[6]
DCM	R17470X^	Ig103	A-band	Truncation of titin	[6]
DCM	E17783X^	Ig104	A-band	Truncation of titin	[6]
ARVC	I16949T*	FNIII29	A-band	Unknown	[9]
DCM	C18789X^	FNIII36	A-band	Truncation of titin	[6]

Missense Mutations of Titin, Nebulette, and Obscurin					
Disease	**Mutation**	**Region on Protein**	**Sarcomeric Region**	**Effect**	**Reference**
DCM	R18858X^	Ig107	A-band	Truncation of titin	[6]
DCM	R18985X^	FNIII37	A-band	Truncation of titin	[6]
ARVC	A18579T*	FNIII41	A-band	Unknown	[9]
DCM	R19560X^	Ig109	A-band	Truncation of titin	[6]
ARVC	A19309S*	Ig111	A-band	Unknown	[9]
DCM	R20858X^	FNIII51	A-band	Truncation of titin	[6]
DCM	Q25689X^	Ig125	A-band	Truncation of titin	[6]
DCM	W26632X^	FNIII94	A-band	Truncation of titin	[6]
DCM	R26949X^	FNIII96	A-band	Truncation of titin	[6]
DCM	K27016X^	FNIII97	A-band	Truncation of titin	[6]
DCM	W27147X^	Ig129	A-band	Truncation of titin	[6]
DCM	Y27567X^	FNIII100	A-band	Truncation of titin	[6]
DCM	W29318X^	Ig134	A-band	Truncation of titin	[6]
DCM	R29415X^	FNIII114	A-band	Truncation of titin	[6]
DCM	E29510X^	FNIII115	A-band	Truncation of titin	[6]
DCM	Q30081X^	FNIII119	A-band	Truncation of titin	[6]
DCM	R31195X^	FNIII127	A-band	Truncation of titin	[6]
DCM	K31371X^	FNIII129	A-band	Truncation of titin	[6]
ARVC	P30847L*	FNIII131	A-band	Unknown	[9]
DCM	S31841X^	FNIII131	A-band	Truncation of titin	[6]
DCM	R32069Q*	Ig146	A-band	Unknown	[21]
ARVC	M33291T*	Ig152	A-band	Unknown	[9]
Mutations of NEBL					
DCM	K60N	Repeat 1		Sarcomeric structural abnormalities	[8]
DCM	Q128R	Repeat 3		Sarcomeric structural abnormalities	[8]
DCM	G202R	Repeat 5		Disruption of I-band and Z-disc proteins	[8]
DCM	A592E	Repeat 16		Disruption of I-band and Z-disc proteins	[8]
IDC	N654K	Repeat 18		Unknown	[4]
Mutations of OBSCN					
HCM	R4344Q	Ig58		Loss of titin Binding	[3]

Table 1. Listing of missense mutations found in *TTN, NEBL,* and *OBSCN* that have been causally linked to the development of cardiomyopathies. Sequences correspond to the following accession numbers: NM_133378.4*, NM_003319.4#, and NM_001256850.1^ for titin; NM_006393.2 for nebulette; and NM_052843.2 for obscurin. DCM: dilated cardiomyopathy, HCM: hypertrophic cardiomyopathy, ARVC: arrhythmogenic right ventricular cardiomyopathy, IDC: idiopathic dilated cardiomyopathy

Splice Site Donor/Acceptor Mutations of Titin					
Disease	**Mutation**	**Region on Protein**	**Sarcomeric Region**	**Effect**	**Reference**
		Mutations of TTN			
DCM	IVS118-g>a^	PEVK	I-band	Unknown	[6]
HCM	IVS155+g>t^	PEVK	I-band	Unknown	[6]
DCM	IVS172-g>c^	PEVK	I-band	Unknown	[6]
DCM	IVS172+g>a^	PEVK	I-band	Unknown	[6]
DCM	IVS185-2a>g^	Ig85	I-band	Unknown	[6]
DCM	IVS230+g>t^	FNIII19	A-band	Unknown	[6]
DCM	IVS237+3a>g^	FNIII22	A-band	Unknown	[6]
DCM	IVS253-5t>a^	Ig106	A-band	Unknown	[6]
DCM	IVS254-g>a^	FNIII41	A-band	Unknown	[6]
DCM	IVS255+g>a^	Ig109	A-band	Unknown	[6]
DCM	IVS271+5g>a^	FNIII53	A-band	Unknown	[6]
DCM	IVS274-2a>g^	FNIII55	A-band	Unknown	[6]
DCM	IVS276+5g>c^	FNIII99	A-band	Unknown	[6]
DCM	IVS277+g>a^	FNIII100	A-band	Unknown	[6]
DCM	IVS279+2t>a^	FNIII102	A-band	Unknown	[6]
DCM	IVS302+g>c^	FNIII128	A-band	Unknown	[6]

Table 2. Listing of splice site donor/acceptor mutations found in *TTN* that have been causally linked to the development of cardiomyopathies. Sequence correspond to accession number NM_001256850.1^ for titin. DCM: dilated cardiomyopathy, HCM: hypertrophic cardiomyopathy, IVS: intron

Deletion and Insertion Mutations of Titin						
Disease	**Mutation**	**Amino Acid**	**Region on Protein**	**Sarcomeric Region**	**Effect**	**Reference**
			Deletion Mutations			
DCM	6247 del g^	R2083fs	Ig11	I-band	Unknown	[6]
DCM	19183 del g^	S6395fs	Ig45	I-band	Unknown	[6]
HCM	23798-23810 del gtcaagatatctg^	G7933fs	Ig61	I-band	Unknown	[6]
DCM	44336 del a^	E14779fs	FNIII6	A-band	Unknown	[6]
DCM	44725 del t^	D14909fs	FNIII8	A-band	Unknown	[6]
DCM	45322 del t^	F15108fs	FNIII10	A-band	Unknown	[6]
DCM	53935 del c^	E17978fs	FNIII20	A-band	Unknown	[6]
HCM	60147 del c^	P20049fs	FNIII45	A-band	Unknown	[6]
DCM	64925 del t^	K21640fs	FNIII57	A-band	Unknown	[6]
DCM	65867 del a^	E21956fs	FNIII59	A-band	Unknown	[6]
DCM	67745 del t^	P22582fs	FNIII64	A-band	Unknown	[6]
DCM	81536-81537 del ct^	S27179fs	Ig129	A-band	Unknown	[6]
DCM	84977-84980 del atta^	Y28326fs	FNIII106	A-band	Unknown	[6]
DCM	82381 del g*	A27460	FNIII107	A-band	Truncation of titin	[24]
DCM	89180-89184 del ttaaa^	T29725fs	FNIII116	A-band	Unknown	[6]

Deletion and Insertion Mutations of Titin						
Disease	Mutation	Amino Acid	Region on Protein	Sarcomeric Region	Effect	Reference
DCM	91043 del a^	N30348fs	FNIII121	A-band	Unknown	[6]
DCM	93376-93377 del ag^	R31126fs	Ig139	A-band	Unknown	[6]
DCM	97824-97831 del agtgacca*	A32606fs	Ig147	M-band	Unknown	[6]
DCM	98964 del a*	K32987fs	Ig150	M-band	Unknown	[6]
Insertion Mutations						
DCM	38621 ins a^	A12873fs	Ig85	I-band	Unknown	[6]
DCM	28kb duplication of ex 72-124^		Ig50-PEVK	I-band	Unknown	[6]
DCM	53145 ins g^	E17715fs	FNIII28	A-band	Unknown	[6]
DCM	58880 insert a*	S19628fs	FNIII42	A-band	Truncation of titin	[10]
DCM	62986-62987 ins at ex. 326*	K20995fs	Ig115	A-band	Truncation of titin	[20]
DCM	72178 ins t^	Q24059fs	FNIII75	A-band	Unknown	[6]
DCM	78372 ins a*	G26124fs	FNIII97	A-band	Unknown	[10]
DCM	90493 ins cct^	T30165fs	FNIII120	A-band	Unknown	[6]
DCM	91537 ins a^	T30513fs	FNIII122	A-band	Unknown	[6]
Indel (Insertion/Deletion) Mutations						
	276 del g ins gt^	T92fs	Ig1	Z-disc	Unknown	[5]
	594-598 del actt ins a^	E198del	Ig2	Z-disc	Unknown	[5]
	1458 del c ins ct^	A486fs	Z-repeat 2	Z-disc	Unknown	[5]
	6131 del c ins ct^	E2044fs	3′ to Ig9	I-band	Unknown	[5]
	28509-28513 del ctct ins c^	E9503del	Ig77	I-band	Unknown	[5]
	30939 del gt ins g^	T10313fs	PEVK	I-band	Unknown	[5]
	31566 del a ins ag^	A10522fs	PEVK	I-band	Unknown	[5]
	31605 del tc ins t^	K10535fs	PEVK	I-band	Unknown	[5]
	34329-34347 del tttcctcttcaggagcaa ins t^	I11443-E11449del	PEVK	I-band	Unknown	[5]
	35760 del a ins ag^	T11920fs	PEVK	I-band	Unknown	[5]
	36267-36271 del cagg ins c^	P12089del	Ig80	I-band	Unknown	[5]
	39252-39254 del ttc ins t^	E13084fs	Ig86	I-band	Unknown	[5]
	65988 del gc ins g^	G21996fs	Ig115	A-band	Unknown	[5]
DCM	67057-67063 del gcatatg ins ta^	A22353fs	Ig116	A-band	Unknown	[6]
DCM	72723-72739 del a ins aga^	S24241fs	Ig121	A-band	Unknown	[6]
	77025 del a ins ag^	L25675fs	Ig125	A-band	Unknown	[5]
	86694-86697 del ttaa ins t^	K28898del	Ig133	A-band	Unknown	[5]
	97995-97998 del actt ins t^	K32665del	Ig144	M-band	Unknown	[5]
	101133 del ga ins g^	S33711fs	Ig148	M-band	Unknown	[5]

Table 3. Listing of deletion and insertion mutations found in TTN that have been causally linked to the development of cardiomyopathies. Sequences correspond to the following accession numbers: NM_133378.4* and NM_001256850.1^ for titin DCM: dilated cardiomyopathy, HCM: hypertrophic cardiomyopathy, del: deletion, ins: insertion, fs: frameshift

http://dx.doi.org/10.5772/55609

Acknowledgements

Our research has been supported by grants to A.K.K. through the National Institutes of Health (R21 HL106197) and the American Heart Association (GRNT 3780035) and to M.A.A from the National Institutes of Health (F32 AR058079).

Author details

Maegen A. Ackermann and Aikaterini Kontrogianni-Konstantopoulos

Department of Biochemistry and Molecular Biology, University of Maryland, School of Medicine, Baltimore, MD, USA

References

[1] Morimoto S. Sarcomeric proteins and inherited cardiomyopathies. Cardiovasc Res 2008;77:659-66.

[2] Ahmad F, Seidman JG, Seidman CE. The genetic basis for cardiac remodeling. Annu Rev Genomics Hum Genet 2005;6:185-216.

[3] Arimura T, Matsumoto Y, Okazaki O, et al. Structural analysis of obscurin gene in hypertrophic cardiomyopathy. Biochem Biophys Res Commun 2007;362:281-7.

[4] Arimura T, Nakamura T, Hiroi S, et al. Characterization of the human nebulette gene: a polymorphism in an actin-binding motif is associated with nonfamilial idiopathic dilated cardiomyopathy. Hum Genet 2000;107:440-51.

[5] Golbus JR, Puckelwartz MJ, Fahrenbach JP, Dellefave-Castillo LM, Wolfgeher D, McNally EM. Population-based variation in cardiomyopathy genes. Circ Cardiovasc Genet 2012;5:391-9.

[6] Herman DS, Lam L, Taylor MR, et al. Truncations of titin causing dilated cardiomyopathy. N Engl J Med 2012;366:619-28.

[7] Kontrogianni-Konstantopoulos A, Ackermann MA, Bowman AL, Yap SV, Bloch RJ. Muscle giants: molecular scaffolds in sarcomerogenesis. Physiol Rev 2009;89:1217-67.

[8] Purevjav E, Varela J, Morgado M, et al. Nebulette mutations are associated with dilated cardiomyopathy and endocardial fibroelastosis. J Am Coll Cardiol 2010;56:1493-502.

[9] Taylor M, Graw S, Sinagra G, et al. Genetic variation in titin in arrhythmogenic right ventricular cardiomyopathy-overlap syndromes. Circulation 2011;124:876-85.

[10] Yoskovitz G, Peled Y, Gramlich M, et al. A novel titin mutation in adult-onset familial dilated cardiomyopathy. Am J Cardiol 2012;109:1644-50.

[11] Bang ML, Centner T, Fornoff F, et al. The complete gene sequence of titin, expression of an unusual approximately 700-kDa titin isoform, and its interaction with obscurin identify a novel Z-line to I-band linking system. Circ Res 2001;89:1065-72.

[12] Gautel M, Mues A, Young P. Control of sarcomeric assembly: the flow of information on titin. Rev Physiol Biochem Pharmacol 1999;138:97-137.

[13] Labeit S, Barlow DP, Gautel M, et al. A regular pattern of two types of 100-residue motif in the sequence of titin. Nature 1990;345:273-6.

[14] Sanger JW, Sanger JM. Fishing out proteins that bind to titin. J Cell Biol 2001;154:21-4.

[15] Labeit S, Kolmerer B. Titins: giant proteins in charge of muscle ultrastructure and elasticity. Science 1995;270:293-6.

[16] Linke WA, Ivemeyer M, Olivieri N, Kolmerer B, Ruegg JC, Labeit S. Towards a molecular understanding of the elasticity of titin. J Mol Biol 1996;261:62-71.

[17] Wang K. Titin/connectin and nebulin: giant protein rulers of muscle structure and function. Adv Biophys 1996;33:123-34.

[18] Itoh-Satoh M, Hayashi T, Nishi H, et al. Titin mutations as the molecular basis for dilated cardiomyopathy. Biochem Biophys Res Commun 2002;291:385-93.

[19] Satoh M, Takahashi M, Sakamoto T, Hiroe M, Marumo F, Kimura A. Structural analysis of the titin gene in hypertrophic cardiomyopathy: identification of a novel disease gene. Biochem Biophys Res Commun 1999;262:411-7.

[20] Gerull B, Gramlich M, Atherton J, et al. Mutations of TTN, encoding the giant muscle filament titin, cause familial dilated cardiomyopathy. Nat Genet 2002;30:201-4.

[21] Matsumoto Y, Hayashi T, Inagaki N, et al. Functional analysis of titin/connectin N2-B mutations found in cardiomyopathy. J Muscle Res Cell Motil 2005;26:367-74.

[22] Arimura T, Bos JM, Sato A, et al. Cardiac ankyrin repeat protein gene (ANKRD1) mutations in hypertrophic cardiomyopathy. J Am Coll Cardiol 2009;54:334-42.

[23] Liu X, Rao L, Zhou B, et al. [Titin gene mutations in Chinese patients with dilated cardiomyopathy]. Zhonghua Xin Xue Guan Bing Za Zhi 2008;36:1066-9.

[24] Gerull B, Atherton J, Geupel A, et al. Identification of a novel frameshift mutation in the giant muscle filament titin in a large Australian family with dilated cardiomyopathy. J Mol Med (Berl) 2006;84:478-83.

[25] Carmignac V, Salih MA, Quijano-Roy S, et al. C-terminal titin deletions cause a novel early-onset myopathy with fatal cardiomyopathy. Ann Neurol 2007;61:340-51.

[26] Pappas CT, Bliss KT, Zieseniss A, Gregorio CC. The Nebulin family: an actin support group. Trends Cell Biol 2011;21:29-37.

[27] Wright J, Huang QQ, Wang K. Nebulin is a full-length template of actin filaments in the skeletal muscle sarcomere: an immunoelectron microscopic study of its orientation

and span with site-specific monoclonal antibodies. J Muscle Res Cell Motil 1993;14:476-83.

[28] Millevoi S, Trombitas K, Kolmerer B, et al. Characterization of nebulette and nebulin and emerging concepts of their roles for vertebrate Z-discs. J Mol Biol 1998;282:111-23.

[29] Donner K, Sandbacka M, Lehtokari VL, Wallgren-Pettersson C, Pelin K. Complete genomic structure of the human nebulin gene and identification of alternatively spliced transcripts. Eur J Hum Genet 2004;12:744-51.

[30] Clark KA, McElhinny AS, Beckerle MC, Gregorio CC. Striated muscle cytoarchitecture: an intricate web of form and function. Annu Rev Cell Dev Biol 2002;18:637-706.

[31] Kruger M, Wright J, Wang K. Nebulin as a length regulator of thin filaments of vertebrate skeletal muscles: correlation of thin filament length, nebulin size, and epitope profile. J Cell Biol 1991;115:97-107.

[32] McElhinny AS, Schwach C, Valichnac M, Mount-Patrick S, Gregorio CC. Nebulin regulates the assembly and lengths of the thin filaments in striated muscle. J Cell Biol 2005;170:947-57.

[33] Pappas CT, Krieg PA, Gregorio CC. Nebulin regulates actin filament lengths by a stabilization mechanism. J Cell Biol 2010;189:859-70.

[34] Labeit S, Gibson T, Lakey A, et al. Evidence that nebulin is a protein-ruler in muscle thin filaments. FEBS Lett 1991;282:313-6.

[35] Moncman CL, Wang K. Nebulette: a 107 kD nebulin-like protein in cardiac muscle. Cell Motil Cytoskeleton 1995;32:205-25.

[36] Bonzo JR, Norris AA, Esham M, Moncman CL. The nebulette repeat domain is necessary for proper maintenance of tropomyosin with the cardiac sarcomere. Exp Cell Res 2008;314:3519-30.

[37] Russell MW, Raeker MO, Korytkowski KA, Sonneman KJ. Identification, tissue expression and chromosomal localization of human Obscurin-MLCK, a member of the titin and Dbl families of myosin light chain kinases. Gene 2002;282:237-46.

[38] Borisov AB, Raeker MO, Kontrogianni-Konstantopoulos A, et al. Rapid response of cardiac obscurin gene cluster to aortic stenosis: differential activation of Rho-GEF and MLCK and involvement in hypertrophic growth. Biochem Biophys Res Commun 2003;310:910-8.

[39] Makarenko I, Opitz CA, Leake MC, et al. Passive stiffness changes caused by upregulation of compliant titin isoforms in human dilated cardiomyopathy hearts. Circ Res 2004;95:708-16.

[40] Wu Y, Bell SP, Trombitas K, et al. Changes in titin isoform expression in pacing-induced cardiac failure give rise to increased passive muscle stiffness. Circulation 2002;106:1384-9.

[41] Raeker MO, Bieniek AN, Ryan AS, Tsai HJ, Zahn KM, Russell MW. Targeted deletion of the zebrafish obscurin A RhoGEF domain affects heart, skeletal muscle and brain development. Dev Biol 2010;337:432-43.

[42] Hershberger RE, Norton N, Morales A, Li D, Siegfried JD, Gonzalez-Quintana J. Coding sequence rare variants identified in MYBPC3, MYH6, TPM1, TNNC1, and TNNI3 from 312 patients with familial or idiopathic dilated cardiomyopathy. Circ Cardiovasc Genet 2010;3:155-61.

[43] Hershberger RE, Parks SB, Kushner JD, et al. Coding sequence mutations identified in MYH7, TNNT2, SCN5A, CSRP3, LBD3, and TCAP from 313 patients with familial or idiopathic dilated cardiomyopathy. Clin Transl Sci 2008;1:21-6.

[44] Lakdawala NK, Funke BH, Baxter S, et al. Genetic testing for dilated cardiomyopathy in clinical practice. J Card Fail 2012;18:296-303.

[45] Morita H, Nagai R, Seidman JG, Seidman CE. Sarcomere gene mutations in hypertrophy and heart failure. J Cardiovasc Transl Res 2010;3:297-303.

[46] Maron BJ. A phenocopy of sarcomeric hypertrophic cardiomyopathy: LAMP2 cardiomyopathy (Danon disease) from China. Eur Heart J 2012;33:570-2.

[47] Seidman CE, Seidman JG. Identifying sarcomere gene mutations in hypertrophic cardiomyopathy: a personal history. Circ Res 2011;108:743-50.

Chapter 5

Na/K-ATPase Signaling and the Tradeoff Between Natriuresis and Cardiac Fibrosis

Joe Xie, Larry D. Dial and Joseph I. Shapiro

Additional information is available at the end of the chapter

http://dx.doi.org/10.5772/54722

1. Introduction

The care of patients with chronic renal insufficiency continues to be complicated by significant cardiovascular dysfunction causing substantial morbidity and mortality. These patients develop cardiovascular disease that is characterized by left ventricular dysfunction and left ventricular hypertrophy (LVH). It has been demonstrated that patients with chronic renal insufficiency develop elevated levels of cardiotonic steroids (CTS) such as marinobufagenin (MBG) in an effort to promote natriuresis and resolve the volume expansion associated with renal insufficiency and cardiac failure. In this review we will try to elucidate the mechanisms involved in the pathogenesis of uremic cardiomyopathy and the role of CTS in cardiac fibrosis.

2. Renal failure and cardiotonic steroids

Patients with renal insufficiency continue to demonstrate significantly high risk of cardiovascular disease with an associated mortality exceeding 50% cardiovascular causes including sudden cardiac death and heart failure [1]. While end stage renal disease confers a high risk of complications those patients with a more modest degree of renal insufficiency (stage 2 and stage 3) continue to have high risk of cardiac events including heart failure, arrhythmia, coronary events and sudden cardiac death all independent of traditional risk factors such as diabetes, hypertension and hyperlipidemia. The cardiac dysfunction most commonly manifest as diastolic dysfunction and left ventricular hypertrophy although systolic dysfunction can occur as a natural progression [2].

In the past there has been substantial interest and research related to digitalis-like substances (DLS) their accumulation in chronic renal failure and pathology associated with elevated circulating levels. Patients with chronic renal failure frequently developed antibodies to digoxin despite no administration of the drug [3, 4]. These DLS were later characterized as cardiotonic steroids and are significantly elevated due to decreased glomerular filtration and increased endogenous production. These endogenous ligands have been found to significantly alter renal sodium handling, inotropic activity and vascular tone [5, 6].

Cardiotonic steroids are known to play a key role in sodium excretion in response to volume expansion. Their effect is primarily mediated through binding to the Na/K-ATPase, a ubiquitous membrane ion transporter and a crucial protein in controlling the electrochemical gradient in cells. Recently, our understanding of the interaction between cardiotonic steroids and the Na/K-ATPase has undergone re-evaluation, and it has since been proposed that this binding leads to the generation of a signaling cascade, which not only produces the natriuretic response in dealing with volume expansion, but may also offer an explanation for the pro-fibrotic effects of cardiotonic steroids.

For many years, the understanding of renal physiology and the kidney's role in maintaining volume homeostasis revolved around the renin-angiotensin-aldosterone pathway, its effects on the glomerular filtration rate as well as contributions from the sympathetic nervous system. Standard therapies offered for congestive heart failure are mostly limited to modulation of this neurohumoral axis through drug therapy. However, this has been inadequate in explaining how volume expansion is handled by the body [7, 8]. In 1961, de Wardener introduced an entirely new concept in renal hemodynamics when he discovered that kidneys were still able to increase sodium excretion after saline infusion despite controlling glomerular filtration rate and aldosterone [9]. Thus, it was proposed that a "Third Factor" was also in play, named for its discovery after glomerular filtration rate (Factor-1) and aldosterone (Factor-2). Uncovering this "Third Factor" galvanized great interest over the next two decades, and significant contributions from Schrier, Kramer, Bricker, Gruber, and others resulted in our current understanding that the "Third Factor" was in fact a circulating endogenous digitalis-like substance, now commonly referred to as a cardiotonic steroid (CTS) [10-14]. CTS include plant-derived cardenolides such as ouabain and digoxin, and amphibian-derived bufadenolides such as marinobufagenin and proscillaridin A [15-18]. Ouabain and marinobufagenin were identified as endogenous hormones after they were detected in human plasma and urine [15-19]. Coincidentally, along with the fervent CTS research in renal physiology, many scientists were also interested in the role ouabain played as an ionotropic agent in myocardium. In 1963, Repke was the first to suggest the Na/K-ATPase was a receptor for these drugs [20]. Since then, extensive studies from many laboratories revealed that these compounds were specific ligands for the Na/K-ATPase, and in fact, produced their natriuretic and ionotropic effects through binding to the Na/K-ATPase [21].

2.1. Na/K-ATPase inhibition and CTS-regulated natriuresis

The Na/K-ATPase was discovered in 1957 by Jens Skou through his studies on crab nerves, and is a member of the P-type ATPase family responsible for the exchange of Na and K ions across cell membranes via the hydyolysis of ATP [22]. Its structure and function has since been extensively studied. It consists of a non-covalently linked alpha and beta subunit, of which multiple

http://dx.doi.org/10.5772/54722

isoforms in various combinations exist [23]. Four alpha isoforms and three beta isoforms have been identified and their expression is tissue-specific, as well as their sensitivity to CTS. The alpha-1 isoform appears to be the main functional receptor for CTS in the kidney [24-28].

When de Wardener first considered the possibility of a "Third Factor," ion pumping was the only function attributed to the Na/K-ATPase. Thus classically, the mechanism of CTS-induced natriuresis was understood as follows: volume expansion or a salt-heavy diet leads to an increase in circulating CTS, which in turn results in the inhibition of the Na/K-ATPase in the nephron, specifically, its ion pumping ability. Consequently, cytosolic Na+ begins to rise, and eventually this disruption in the Na+ gradient across the cell membrane decreases Na reabsorption in the renal proximal tubules (RPT) leading to increased sodium excretion. Systemically, increased levels of CTS also inhibit the Na/K-ATPase in vasculature, thereby altering intracellular Na gradients in vascular smooth muscle cells. This indirectly leads to the inhibition of the Na/Ca exchanger causing intracellular calcium in these smooth muscle cells to rise as well [29-31]. Chronically, this leads to an important trade-off. Despite its pivotal role in renal salt handling, this pathway has substantial consequences in the vasculature and has been implicated in the pathogenesis of hypertension [29-31] (Figure 1).

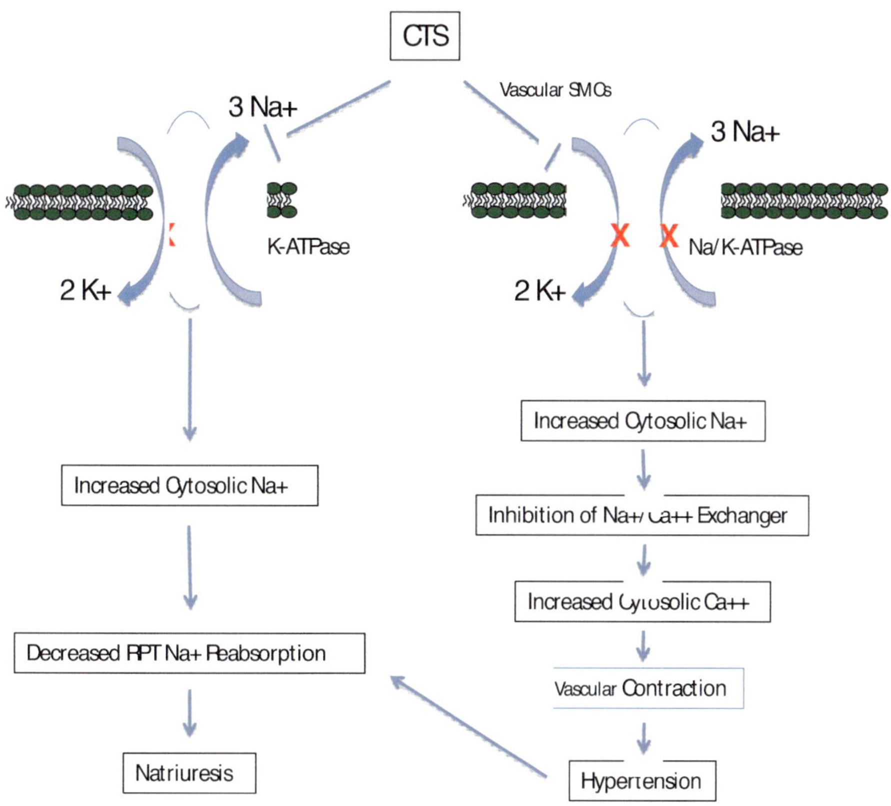

Figure 1. Ionic Mechanism for CTS Induced Hypertension

2.2. CTS and Na/K-ATPase-mediated signal transduction

In the late 1990's, Xie and colleagues suggested that the Na/K-ATPase had an additional signaling function in addition to its transportation of ions. He proposed that instead of only inhibiting the pumping activity of the Na/K-ATPase, CTS also bound to a non-pumping pool of Na/K-ATPase residing in caveolae [32]. This subset of Na/K-ATPase innately held Src, a non-receptor tyrosine kinase, in an inactive state. With the structural change induced by CTS binding, Src was subsequently released and activated. In turn, EGFR became transactivated and a number of additional downstream targets in the signaling cascade such as Ras/Raf/MAPK, PI3 kinase/Akt, phospholipase C/PKC, and the generation of ROS have been identified [33-40].

3. Uremic cardiomyopathy

It is well substantiated that cardiovascular mortality remains the leading cause of death in patients with end stage renal disease with the majority of the cases due to sudden cardiac death and coronary events [1]. While traditional risk factors associated with cardiac dysfunction exist in patients with renal failure the risk conferred can exceed twice that of normal patients [41]. The risk of cardiovascular disease is not limited to those with end stage renal failure but rather confers a gradual risk of increased cardiovascular and all-cause mortality as glomerular filtrate rate declines and albuminuria increases [42]. Systolic dysfunction in these patients have been less consistently demonstrated [43] but rather the development of LVH is more common and may be a predictor of higher mortality related to arrhythmia and sudden death in patients on dialysis [44]. The myocardial fibrosis initially described with uremia as early as 1943 by Rossle and later characterized by Ritz et al has a pivotal role in the development of uremic cardiomyopathy [45]. While traditional thought regarding cardiac fibrosis revolved around a reparative process related to myocardial necrosis; early fibrosis after subtotal nephrectomy without myocardial necrosis has been demonstrated suggesting the potential for a reactive process rather reparative. Mall and colleagues utilizing a uremic cardiomyopathy model in rats demonstrated that interstitial volume density increased with a resultant decrease in the capillary volume. Additionally, cytoplasmic and nuclear swelling occurred whereas the endothelial cells remained unchanged [46]. This reactive cardiac fibrosis can explain the alterations in left ventricular compliance in addition to the electrical conduction abnormalities causing arrythmogenic potential. The risk factors in patients with chronic renal failure believed to be involved in cardiac fibrosis and LVH include anemia, activation of the RAS aldosterone system, oxidative stress, hyperparathyroidism, hypertension and cardiotonic steroids.

4. Natriuresis versus fibrosis—A new trade-off model

The activation of Na/K-ATPase signaling by CTS also appears to be responsible for the coordinated inhibition of Na+ transporters in the nephron resulting in natriuresis. This concept is not without precedence. Dopamine, another known natriuretic hormone, increases sodium excretion through signal transduction by mediating the synchronized downregulation of basolateral Na/K-ATPase and apical Na/H antiporter isoform-3 (NHE3) after binding to D1 and D2 receptors in the nephron [47, 48]. Similarly, Liu and Shapiro as well as others noted that CTS at physiological concentrations activated the previously described signaling cascades, resulting in the endocytosis of both the basolateral Na/K-ATPase and apical NHE3 in cultured renal epithelial cells. As a result, this redistribution of membrane Na+ transporters in RPTs leads to a reduction in sodium reabsorption and increased sodium excretion [49-53].

Support for this theory has also been demonstrated in vivo. Lingrel first established that ouabain binding to the Na/K-ATPase is crucial in the natriuretic response of the kidney. His laboratory developed ouabain-sensitive mice by incorporating a mutation in the ouabain receptor domain of the mouse alpha-1 Na/K-ATPase and noted that saline infusion increased the natriuretic response in ouabain-sensitive in comparison to ouabain-resistant mice [54]. More recently, Nascimento showed that bufalin—another derivative of the bufadenolides—required Na/K-ATPase signaling in order to produce natriuretic effects in isolated rat kidneys [55]. Studies from our laboratories also found that high-salt diets cause the endocytosis of Na/K-ATPase in rat proximal tubules, correlating with an increase in Na+ excretion [56]. More recently, we demonstrated that high-salt diets in Dahl salt-resistant mice (R) induced the endocytosis of RPT Na/K-ATPase and NHE3 transporters concurrent with increased Src activity. In contrast, Na/K-ATPase signaling was not activated in Dahl salt-sensitive mice (S) [57].

To re-emphasize, natriuresis due to Na/K-ATPase signaling is a markedly different model from that of the classic pathway. Here, intracellular Na+ is unaffected by the coupling of CTS to the Na/K-ATPase, and instead, signal transduction is responsible for the effects on Na+ transport in RPTs. This alternate pathway also presents distinct tradeoffs from those of the classic pathway (i.e. hypertension). More specifically, natriuresis through CTS-Na/K-ATPase signaling appears to lead to the development of fibrosis in cardiac and renal organs. Of note, previous experiments have already implicated CTS in the hypertrophic growth of cardiac cells [58-65]. Also taking into account the well-established effects of the Src tyrosine kinase in cell growth and differentiation, it is conceivable to suggest a role of CTS in organ remodeling. Remarkably, this phenomenon of fibrosis development has recently been supported by both in vivo and in vitro studies from our laboratory and others.

Using partial (5/6th) nephrectomy models, which have been utilized for many years to simulate renal failure, we noted that the development of cardiac fibrosis in both rats and mice was mediated by an increase in systemic oxidative stress as well as increased levels of circulating MBG [2, 66-68]. Presumably, this suggests that the CTS-induced fibrosis appears to be dependent on Na/K-ATPase signaling leading to the generation of ROS, thus causing oxidative stress to cardiac and renal tissues. This finding in the animal models corresponded to evidence of signaling through the Na/K-ATPase as we detected activation of both Src and MAPK phosphorylation in the fibrotic cardiac tissue [2, 67]. These results were similarly demonstrated in rats subjected to MBG infusion [2, 67]. Remarkably, after adrenalectomy to lower circulating levels of MBG and active immunization against an MBG-albumin conjugate, cardiac fibrosis was significantly reduced in both partial nephrectomy and MBG-infusion experimental groups [2, 66-68].

In a separate set of experiments, Wansapura subjected genetically altered ouabain-sensitive mice (originally developed by Lingrel) to aortic banding in order to simulate a pressure overload model. After four weeks, the ouabain-sensitive group was noted to have developed substantially greater cardiac hypertrophy and fibrosis compared to ouabain-resistant (wild-type) mice. Furthermore, the administration of Digibind to the ouabain-sensitive mice diminished these cardiac changes [69].

Additional in-vivo data support the potential for a more significant reversal of cardiotonic steroid associated hypertension, cardiac hypertrophy and oxidative stress through utilization of a monoclonal antibody (mAb). Haller subjected partially nephrectomized rats demonstrating elevated levels of MBG to mAb with a high affinity for MBG and Digibind. Both treatments resulted in significant improvement in cardiac hypertrophy, hypertension and measures of oxidative stress. While both therapies demonstrated similar responses there were significantly better results with the MGG directed monoclonal antibody [70].

Furthermore, in cultures of rat cardiac and renal fibroblasts as well as human dermal fibroblasts, we found that both ouabain and MBG were able to directly increase collagen production and proline incorporation [67, 71, 72]. By inducing a translocation of PKC to the nucleus, MBG appears to cause the subsequent phosphorylation and degradation of Friend leukemia integration-1 (Fli-1), which Watson and colleagues have demonstrated is a negative regulator of collagen synthesis in dermal fibroblasts [71, 73]. In fact, we found MBG reduced Fli-1 expression and increased procollagen-1 in all three of our fibroblast cell lines (cardiac, renal, dermal) [71]. Furthermore, MBG infusion stimulates the expression and nuclear translocation of Snail, a transcription factor involved in epithelial-mesenchymal transition, which is implicated in renal fibrosis [74].

Similar to the animal studies, these findings in cell culture have corresponded with increased Na/K-ATPase signaling activity and the generation of ROS, which notably was successfully blocked by both ROS scavengers and Src inhibitors [67]. In addition, we examined the effects of spironolactone—known to be a competitive antagonist of CTS binding to the Na/K-ATPase —as well as its major metabolite, canrenone. Corroborating with our hypothesis, we found that spironolactone significantly attenuated cardiac fibrosis in the renal failure models, and both spironolactone and canrenone reduced collagen production in cardiac fibroblasts. It was further demonstrated that MBG-induced Na/K-ATPase signaling was blocked in these experiments [75].

5. Conclusions

Endogenous circulating CTS such as ouabain and MBG are known to be upregulated in the body's stress response towards volume expansion. Binding to its receptor—the Na/K-ATPase —leads to increased sodium excretion in the proximal tubules of the nephron. Whether this is

http://dx.doi.org/10.5772/54722

accomplished through the classic ionic pathway, the alternate signaling pathway, or both is still debated; however, its effect on re-establishing volume homeostasis is undeniable. Like many other physiological processes, the fine-tuning of one pathway may result in unintended consequences elsewhere in the body. In the case of CTS-induced natriuresis through Na/K-ATPase signaling, the tradeoff is apparent in the development of cardiac and renal fibrosis as demonstrated both in vivo and in vitro (Figure 2). Because the fibrosis appears to be dependent on Na/K-ATPase signaling, the generation of ROS, and subsequent oxidative stress to cardiac and renal tissues, this creates the potential for both new and old drugs to target and block the signaling cascade. ROS scavengers, Src inhibitors, spironolactone, and canrenone have already demonstrated exciting possibilities in our experiments. Further research in developing more specific CTS antagonists as well as whether this concept can be extrapolated to humans needs to be explored. Interestingly, in the late 1990's and early 2000's, Pitt and colleagues conducted the Randomized Aldactone Evaluation Study (RALES), followed by the Eplerenone Post–Acute Myocardial Infarction Heart Failure Efficacy and Survival Study (EPHESUS) and determined that spironolactone and eplerenone, respectively, were cardioprotective in patients with advanced stages of congestive heart failure [76, 77]. More recently, the Eplerenone in Mild Patients Hospitalization and Survival Study in Heart Failure (EMPHASIS-HF) and the Anti-Remodeling Effect of Canrenone in Patients with Mild Chronic Heart Failure (AREA IN-CHF) trials found further therapeutic benefit in patients with mild (NYHA Class II) CHF [78, 79]. These clinical studies proposed that the anti-aldosterone effects were primarily responsible for the reduction in morbidity and mortality; however, it is certainly plausible to speculate whether these drugs as Na/K-ATPase signaling inhibitors may have also played a role. Nonetheless, CTS-induced signaling through the Na/K-ATPase is a significant and novel link in balancing the hemodynamics of salt handling and the development of fibrosis.

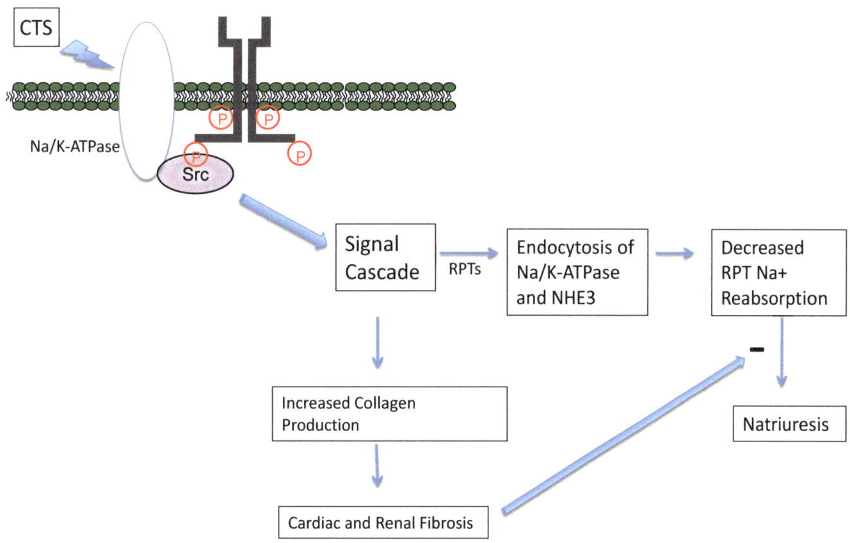

Figure 2. Signaling Pathway: Relationship Between Fibrosis and Natriuresis

Author details

Joe Xie[1], Larry D. Dial[2] and Joseph I. Shapiro[2*]

*Address all correspondence to: shapiroj@marshall.edu

1 The University of Colorado School of Medicine, USA

2 The Joan C. Edwards School of Medicine of Marshall University, USA

References

[1] Sarnak, M. J, et al. Kidney disease as a risk factor for development of cardiovascular disease: a statement from the American Heart Association Councils on Kidney in Cardiovascular Disease, High Blood Pressure Research, Clinical Cardiology, and Epidemiology and Prevention. Hypertension, (2003). , 1050-1065.

[2] Kennedy, D. J, et al. Central role for the cardiotonic steroid marinobufagenin in the pathogenesis of experimental uremic cardiomyopathy. Hypertension, (2006). , 488-495.

[3] Graves, S. W. Endogenous digitalis-like factors. Crit Rev Clin Lab Sci, (1986). , 177-200.

[4] Graves, S. W, & Williams, G. H. Endogenous digitalis-like natriuretic factors. Annu Rev Med, (1987). , 433-444.

[5] Bagrov, A. Y, & Shapiro, J. I. Endogenous digitalis: pathophysiologic roles and therapeutic applications. Nat Clin Pract Nephrol, (2008). , 378-392.

[6] Fedorova, O. V, Shapiro, J. I, & Bagrov, A. Y. Endogenous cardiotonic steroids and salt-sensitive hypertension. Biochim Biophys Acta, (2010). , 1230-1236.

[7] Schrier, R. W, & Berl, T. Nonosmolar factors affecting renal water excretion (first of two parts). N Engl J Med, (1975). , 81-88.

[8] Schrier, R. W, & Berl, T. Nonosmolar factors affecting renal water excretion (second of two parts). N Engl J Med, (1975). , 141-145.

[9] De Wardener, H. E, et al. Evidence for a hormone other than aldosterone which controls urinary sodium excretion. Adv Nephrol Necker Hosp, (1971). , 97-111.

[10] Schrier, R. W, et al. Absence of natriuretic response to acute hypotonic intravascular volume expansion in dogs. Clin Sci, (1968). , 57-72.

[11] Schrier, R. W, et al. Effect of isotonic saline infusion and acute haemorrhage on plasma oxytocin and vasopressin concentrations in dogs. Clin Sci, (1968). , 433-443.

[12] Kramer, H. J, & Gonick, H. C. Effect of extracellular volume expansion on renal Na-K-ATPase and cell metabolism. Nephron, (1974). , 281-296.

[13] Bricker, N. S, et al. On the biology of sodium excretion: The search for a natriuretic hormone. Yale J Biol Med, (1975). , 293-303.

[14] Gruber, K. A, Whitaker, J. M, & Buckalew, V. M. Jr., Endogenous digitalis-like substance in plasma of volume-expanded dogs. Nature, (1980). , 743-745.

[15] Bagrov, A. Y, et al. Characterization of a urinary bufodienolide Na+,K+-ATPase inhibitor in patients after acute myocardial infarction. Hypertension, (1998). , 1097-1103.

[16] Sich, B, et al. Pulse pressure correlates in humans with a proscillaridin A immunoreactive compound. Hypertension, (1996). , 1073-1078.

[17] Hamlyn, J. M, et al. Identification and characterization of a ouabain-like compound from human plasma. Proc Natl Acad Sci U S A, (1991). , 6259-6263.

[18] Komiyama, Y, et al. A novel endogenous digitalis, telocinobufagin, exhibits elevated plasma levels in patients with terminal renal failure. Clin Biochem, (2005). , 36-45.

[19] Lichtstein, D, et al. Identification of digitalis-like compounds in human cataractous lenses. Eur J Biochem, (1993). , 261-268.

[20] Repke, K. New Aspects of Cardiac Glycosides, in First International Pharmacological Meeting(1963). Pergamon Press. New York, NY. , 47-74.

[21] Hamlyn, J. M, et al. A circulating inhibitor of (Na+ + K+)ATPase associated with essential hypertension. Nature, (1982). , 650-652.

[22] Skou, J. C. The influence of some cations on an adenosine triphosphatase from peripheral nerves. Biochim Biophys Acta, (1957). , 394-401.

[23] Kaplan, J. H. Biochemistry of Na,K-ATPase. Annu Rev Biochem, (2002). , 511-535.

[24] Blanco, G, & Mercer, R. W. Isozymes of the Na-K-ATPase: heterogeneity in structure, diversity in function. Am J Physiol, (1998). Pt 2): , F633-F650.

[25] Sweadner, K. J. Isozymes of the Na+/K+-ATPase. Biochim Biophys Acta, (1989). , 185-220.

[26] Lingrel, J. B, Kuntzweiler, T, & Na, K. ATPase. J Biol Chem, (1994). , 19659-19662.

[27] Dostanic-larson, I, et al. The highly conserved cardiac glycoside binding site of Na,K-ATPase plays a role in blood pressure regulation. Proc Natl Acad Sci U S A, (2005). , 15845-15850.

[28] Dostanic-larson, I, et al. Physiological role of the alpha1- and alpha2-isoforms of the Na+-K+-ATPase and biological significance of their cardiac glycoside binding site. Am J Physiol Regul Integr Comp Physiol, (2006). , R524-R528.

[29] Blaustein, M. P. Physiological effects of endogenous ouabain: control of intracellular Ca2+ stores and cell responsiveness. Am J Physiol, (1993). Pt 1): , C1367-C1387.

[30] Blaustein, M. P, & Hamlyn, J. M. Signaling mechanisms that link salt retention to hypertension: endogenous ouabain, the Na(+) pump, the Na(+)/Ca(2+) exchanger and TRPC proteins. Biochim Biophys Acta, (2010). , 1219-1229.

[31] Zhang, J, et al. Sodium pump alpha2 subunits control myogenic tone and blood pressure in mice. J Physiol, (2005). Pt 1): , 243-256.

[32] Liang, M, et al. Identification of a pool of non-pumping Na/K-ATPase. J Biol Chem, (2007). , 10585-10593.

[33] Haas, M, Askari, A, & Xie, Z. Involvement of Src and epidermal growth factor receptor in the signal-transducing function of Na+/K+-ATPase. J Biol Chem, (2000). , 27832-27837.

[34] Haas, M, et al. Src-mediated inter-receptor cross-talk between the Na+/K+-ATPase and the epidermal growth factor receptor relays the signal from ouabain to mitogen-activated protein kinases. J Biol Chem, (2002). , 18694-18702.

[35] Liu, J, et al. Ouabain interaction with cardiac Na+/K+-ATPase initiates signal cascades independent of changes in intracellular Na+ and Ca2+ concentrations. J Biol Chem, (2000). , 27838-27844.

[36] Liu, L, et al. Role of caveolae in signal-transducing function of cardiac Na+/K+-ATPase. Am J Physiol Cell Physiol, (2003). , C1550-C1560.

[37] Tian, J, et al. Binding of Src to Na+/K+-ATPase forms a functional signaling complex. Mol Biol Cell, (2006). , 317-326.

[38] Wang, H, et al. Ouabain assembles signaling cascades through the caveolar Na+/K+-ATPase. J Biol Chem, (2004). , 17250-17259.

[39] Xie, Z, Askari, A, & Na, K. ATPase as a signal transducer. Eur J Biochem, (2002). , 2434-2439.

[40] Yuan, Z, et al. Na/K-ATPase tethers phospholipase C and IP3 receptor into a calcium-regulatory complex. Mol Biol Cell, (2005). , 4034-4045.

[41] Shlipak, M. G, et al. Cardiovascular mortality risk in chronic kidney disease: comparison of traditional and novel risk factors. JAMA, (2005). , 1737-1745.

[42] Chronic Kidney Disease PrognosisC., et al., Association of estimated glomerular filtration rate and albuminuria with all-cause and cardiovascular mortality in general population cohorts: a collaborative meta-analysis. Lancet, (2010). , 2073-2081.

[43] Raj, D. S, et al. Left ventricular morphology in chronic renal failure by echocardiography. Ren Fail, (1997). , 799-806.

[44] Tyralla, K, & Amann, K. Morphology of the heart and arteries in renal failure. Kidney Int Suppl, (2003). , S80-S83.

[45] Mall, G, et al. Diffuse intermyocardiocytic fibrosis in uraemic patients. Nephrol Dial Transplant, (1990). , 39-44.

[46] Mall, G, et al. Myocardial interstitial fibrosis in experimental uremia--implications for cardiac compliance. Kidney Int, (1988). , 804-811.

[47] Aperia, A, Bertorello, A, & Seri, I. Dopamine causes inhibition of Na+-K+-ATPase activity in rat proximal convoluted tubule segments. Am J Physiol, (1987). Pt 2): , F39-F45.

[48] Felder, C. C, et al. Dopamine inhibits Na(+)-H+ exchanger activity in renal BBMV by stimulation of adenylate cyclase. Am J Physiol, (1990). Pt 2): , F297-F303.

[49] Liu, J, et al. Ouabain induces endocytosis of plasmalemmal Na/K-ATPase in LLC-PK1 cells by a clathrin-dependent mechanism. Kidney Int, (2004). , 227-241.

[50] Liu, J, et al. Ouabain-induced endocytosis of the plasmalemmal Na/K-ATPase in LLC-PK1 cells requires caveolin-1. Kidney Int, (2005). , 1844-1854.

[51] Oweis, S, et al. Cardiac glycoside downregulates NHE3 activity and expression in LLC-PK1 cells. Am J Physiol Renal Physiol, (2006). , F997-1008.

[52] Periyasamy, S. M, et al. Salt loading induces redistribution of the plasmalemmal Na/K-ATPase in proximal tubule cells. Kidney Int, (2005). , 1868-1877.

[53] Cai, H, et al. Regulation of apical NHE3 trafficking by ouabain-induced activation of the basolateral Na+-K+-ATPase receptor complex. Am J Physiol Cell Physiol, (2008). , C555-C563.

[54] Loreaux, E. L, et al. Ouabain-Sensitive alpha1 Na,K-ATPase enhances natriuretic response to saline load. J Am Soc Nephrol, (2008). , 1947-1954.

[55] Arnaud-batista, F. J, et al. The natriuretic effect of bufalin in isolated rat kidneys involves activation of the Na+/K+-ATPase-Src kinase pathway. Am J Physiol Renal Physiol, (2012).

[56] Liu, J, et al. Effects of cardiac glycosides on sodium pump expression and function in LLC-PK1 and MDCK cells. Kidney Int, (2002). , 2118-2125.

[57] Liu, J, et al. Impairment of Na/K-ATPase signaling in renal proximal tubule contributes to Dahl salt-sensitive hypertension. J Biol Chem, (2011). , 22806-22813.

[58] Huang, L, Kometiani, P, & Xie, Z. Differential regulation of Na/K-ATPase alpha-subunit isoform gene expressions in cardiac myocytes by ouabain and other hypertrophic stimuli. J Mol Cell Cardiol, (1997). , 3157-3167.

[59] Huang, L, Li, H, & Xie, Z. Ouabain-induced hypertrophy in cultured cardiac myocytes is accompanied by changes in expression of several late response genes. J Mol Cell Cardiol, (1997). , 429-437.

[60] Kometiani, P, et al. Multiple signal transduction pathways link Na+/K+-ATPase to growth-related genes in cardiac myocytes. The roles of Ras and mitogen-activated protein kinases. J Biol Chem, (1998). , 15249-15256.

[61] Peng, M, et al. Partial inhibition of Na+/K+-ATPase by ouabain induces the Ca2+-dependent expressions of early-response genes in cardiac myocytes. J Biol Chem, (1996). , 10372-10378.

[62] Xie, Z, et al. Intracellular reactive oxygen species mediate the linkage of Na+/K+-ATPase to hypertrophy and its marker genes in cardiac myocytes. J Biol Chem, (1999). , 19323-19328.

[63] Ferrandi, M, et al. Organ hypertrophic signaling within caveolae membrane subdomains triggered by ouabain and antagonized by PST 2238. J Biol Chem, (2004). , 33306-33314.

[64] Pierdomenico, S. D, et al. Endogenous ouabain and hemodynamic and left ventricular geometric patterns in essential hypertension. Am J Hypertens, (2001). , 44-50.

[65] Skoumal, R, et al. Involvement of endogenous ouabain-like compound in the cardiac hypertrophic process in vivo. Life Sci, (2007). , 1303-1310.

[66] Hostetter, T. H, et al. Hyperfiltration in remnant nephrons: a potentially adverse response to renal ablation. Am J Physiol, (1981). , F85-F93.

[67] Elkareh, J, et al. Marinobufagenin stimulates fibroblast collagen production and causes fibrosis in experimental uremic cardiomyopathy. Hypertension, (2007). , 215-224.

[68] Kennedy, D. J, et al. Partial nephrectomy as a model for uremic cardiomyopathy in the mouse. Am J Physiol Renal Physiol, (2008). , F450-F454.

[69] Wansapura, A. N, et al. Mice expressing ouabain-sensitive alpha1-Na,K-ATPase have increased susceptibility to pressure overload-induced cardiac hypertrophy. Am J Physiol Heart Circ Physiol, (2011). , H347-H355.

[70] Haller, S. T, et al. Monoclonal antibody against marinobufagenin reverses cardiac fibrosis in rats with chronic renal failure. Am J Hypertens, (2012). , 690-696.

[71] Elkareh, J, et al. Marinobufagenin induces increases in procollagen expression in a process involving protein kinase C and Fli-1: implications for uremic cardiomyopathy. Am J Physiol Renal Physiol, (2009). , F1219-F1226.

[72] El-Okdi, N, et al. Effects of cardiotonic steroids on dermal collagen synthesis and wound healing. J Appl Physiol, (2008). , 30-36.

[73] Czuwara-ladykowska, J, et al. Fli-1 inhibits collagen type I production in dermal fibroblasts via an Sp1-dependent pathway. J Biol Chem, (2001). , 20839-20848.

[74] Fedorova, L. V, et al. The cardiotonic steroid hormone marinobufagenin induces renal fibrosis: implication of epithelial-to-mesenchymal transition. Am J Physiol Renal Physiol, (2009). , F922-F934.

[75] Tian, J, et al. Spironolactone attenuates experimental uremic cardiomyopathy by antagonizing marinobufagenin. Hypertension, (2009). , 1313-1320.

[76] Pitt, B, et al. The effect of spironolactone on morbidity and mortality in patients with severe heart failure. Randomized Aldactone Evaluation Study Investigators. N Engl J Med, (1999). , 709-717.

[77] Pitt, B, et al. Eplerenone, a selective aldosterone blocker, in patients with left ventricular dysfunction after myocardial infarction. N Engl J Med, (2003). , 1309-1321.

[78] Zannad, F, et al. Eplerenone in patients with systolic heart failure and mild symptoms. N Engl J Med, (2011). , 11-21.

[79] Boccanelli, A, et al. Anti-remodelling effect of canrenone in patients with mild chronic heart failure (AREA IN-CHF study): final results. Eur J Heart Fail, (2009). , 68-76.

Chapter 6

Dobutamine-Induced Mechanical Alternans

Akihiro Hirashiki and Toyoaki Murohara

Additional information is available at the end of the chapter

http://dx.doi.org/10.5772/55003

1. Introduction

Mechanical alternans (MA) is a mysterious phenomenon. MA, a condition characterized by beat-to-beat oscillation in the strength of cardiac muscle contraction at a constant heart rate, has been observed in patients with severe heart failure and in animal models of this condition. Although MA is rare under resting conditions in individuals with controlled heart failure, at higher heart rates it is more prevalent and likely to be sustained, as exemplified by pacing-induced MA or dobutamine-induced MA. However, few studies have addressed the clinical implications of dobutamine-induced MA in patients with heart failure. We therefore prospectively examined and compared the prognostic value of dobutamine- and pacing- induced MA in ambulatory patients with idiopathic dilated myocardiopathy (IDCM) in sinus rhythm.[1] Furthermore, this review addresses the clinical circumstances, relevance of MA, current understanding with ideas about its mechanism, and some future perspectives.

2. Mechanical Alternans (MA)

2.1. History of MA

Phenomenon of alternating weak and strong beats observed in a heart which is contracting with constant intervals between beats. It has a long history. Experimental descriptions first appeared over a century ago, and since then there has been a sustained debate among clinicians and physiologists about its origins and clinical significance. A clinical description of an alternating pulse by Traube is often quoted as appearing earlier. [2] However, careful inspection of his figure shows alternating interbeat intervals. In fact, Traube himself commented on the alternation of intervals and used the term "bigeminus" in the title of his report, although the true nature of this arrhythmia can only be guessed at since the electrocardiograms had yet to be invented at the time when Traube reported his case. MA has been studied in the intact human and animal heart, in isolated muscle preparations, and most recently in isolated cardiac muscle cells.

2.2. Induction of MA

The ability to induce MA by rapid driving frequencies appears to be a fundamental property of mammalian ventricular muscle. Experimental studies have shown that by varying the pacing cycle length over a wide range, it is possible to define a critical cycle length (threshold) for the induction of sustained MA.[3] Driving the heart at cycle lengths shorter than the threshold cycle length may increase the amplitude of the beat-to-beat oscillations in contraction strength.

3. Method

3.1. Pacing- and dobutamine- induced MA

It is more prevalent and likely to be sustained, as exemplified by pacing-induced MA. Right atrial pacing was initiated at 80 beats per minute (bpm) and was increased in increments of 10 bpm. We selected steady-state LV pressure data for at least 2 min at the baseline and at each pacing rate for analysis.[4] We calculated the maximum first derivative of LV pressure (LV dP/dt_{max}) as an index of contractility. To evaluate LV isovolumic relaxation, we computed $T_{1/2}$, as previously described.[5] After the hemodynamic values had checked at baseline, dobutamine was infused intravenously at incremental doses of 5, 10, and 15 μg $kg^{-1}min^{-1}$ and hemodynamic measurements were performed at the end of each 5-min infusion period. MA was diagnosed if the pressure difference between the strong and weak beats was ≥4 mmHg continuously in the analyzed LV pressure data, as previously described.[6]

We prospectively followed up all patients for the occurrence of primary events, which were defined as cardiac death (from worsening heart failure or sudden death) or the unscheduled readmission for decompensated heart failure. Noncardiac death was excluded.

4. Results

4.1. Classification of IDCM patients on the basis of dobutamine-induced MA

To identify on the basis of the classification by hemodynamic response to pacing or dobutamine stress testing, patients were classified into three groups: those who exhibited neither pacing- nor dobutamine-induced MA (n = 60, group N), those who manifested only pacing-induced MA (n = 20, group P), and those who developed both pacing- and dobutamine-induced MA (n = 10, group D). All patients who did not develop pacing-induced MA also did not exhibit dobutamine-induced MA. LV pressure waveforms during

http://dx.doi.org/10.5772/55003

atrial pacing at 120 bpm or after dobutamine infusion at 10 μg kg^{-1} min^{-1} are shown for representative patients from each group (Fig. 1).

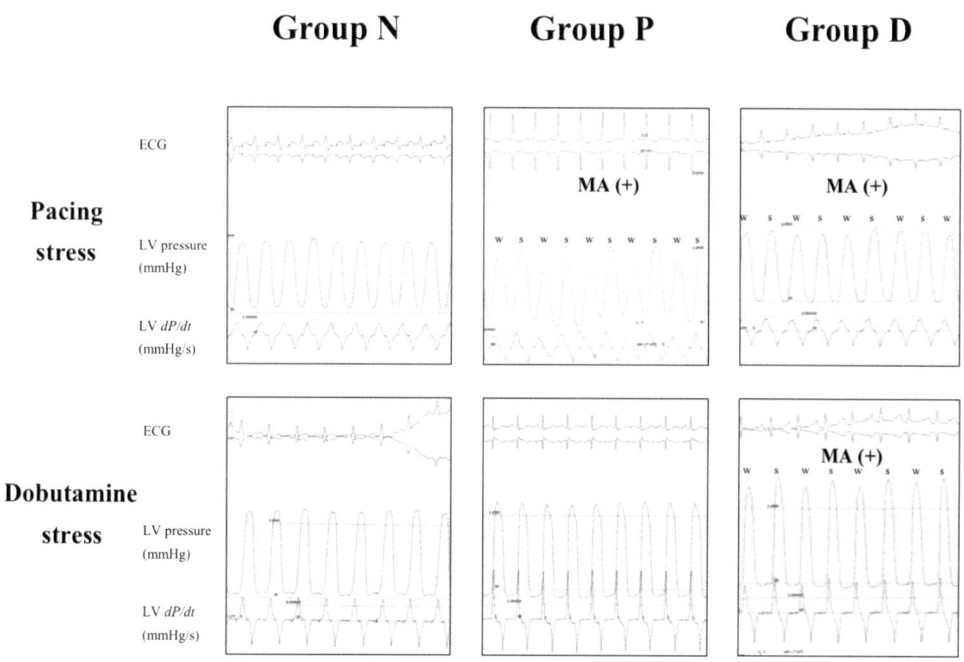

Figure 1. LV pressure waveforms during atrial pacing at 120 bpm and after infusion of dobutamine at a dose of 10 μg kg^{-1} min^{-1} in representative patients of three study groups. The traces represent the lead II electrocardiogram (ECG), LV pressure, and LV *dP/dt*. Both LV dP/dt_{max} and LV dP/dt_{min} showed alternating changes with LV pressure. Strong and weak beats are indicated by s and w, respectively.

4.2. Baseline clinical data

There were no significant differences in age and sex among the three groups of patients (Table 1). All patients were classified as NYHA functional class I or II at the time of cardiac catheterization. The LV ejection fraction (EF) in groups P and D was significantly lower than that in group N. There were also no significant differences in plasma brain natriuretic peptide (BNP) or norepinephrine levels among the three groups.

The abundance of phospholamban mRNA was significantly lower in group D than in group P. The SERCA2a/phospholamban mRNA ratio was significantly higher in group D than in groups N and P (Table 2). The probability of event-free survival in group D was significantly lower than that in groups N or P (P = 0.002) (Fig. 2).

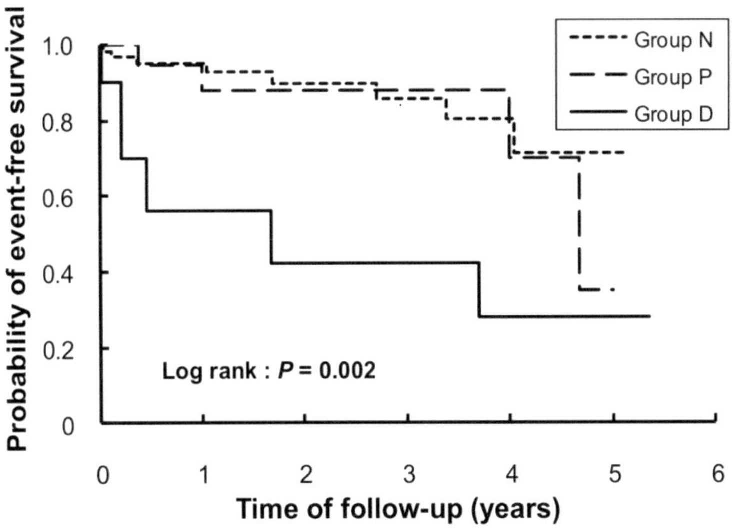

Figure 2. Kaplan-Meier analysis of the cumulative probability of event-free survival of the 90 IDCM study patients. Cardiac events were defined as hospitalization due to worsening heart failure and cardiac death. The probability of event-free survival in group D was significantly lower than that in groups P and N by the log-rank test ($P = 0.002$).

Characteristic	Group N (n = 60)			Group P (n = 20)			Group D (n = 10)		
Age (years)	51	±	12	50	±	13	45	±	11
Sex (M/F)	44	/	16	16	/	4	6	/	4
NYHA functional class I	32		(53%)	9		(45%)	5		(50%)
class II	28		(47%)	11		(55%)	5		(50%)
Medication									
Diuretics	30		(50%)	17*		(85%)	9*		(90%)
ACE inhibitors or ARBs	42		(70%)	19		(95%)	7		(70%)
Beta blockers	22		(37%)	10		(50%)	5		(50%)
PAWP (mmHg)	10.7	±	4.7	14.6	±	6.2*	13.9	±	7.2
Cardiac index (L min^{-1} m^{-2})	3.07	±	0.55	2.83	±	0.58	3.26	±	0.66
LVEF (%)	38.9	±	8.1	32.9	±	9.6*	30.3	±	9.0*
Plasma BNP (pg/mL)	100	±	173	179	±	186	249	±	262
Plasma norepinephrine (pg/mL)	440	±	221	689	±	764	664	±	324

*$P < 0.05$ versus group N. Abbreviations not defined in text: ACE, angiotensin-converting enzyme; ARB, angiotensin-II receptor blocker; PAWP, pulmonary artery wedge pressure.

Table 1. Baseline clinical characteristics of patients in the three study groups.

mRNA ratio	Group N			Group P			Group D		
SERCA2a/GAPDH	0.42	±	0.15	0.41	±	0.13	0.43	±	0.13
Phospholamban/GAPDH	0.82	±	0.45	1.01	±	0.13	0.42	±	0.24*
Ryanodine receptor 2/GAPDH	0.50	±	0.19	0.53	±	0.21	0.75	±	0.17
SERCA2a/phospholamban	0.63	±	0.31	0.59	±	0.40	1.32	±	0.95*†
SERCA2a/Na^+-Ca^{2+} exchanger	0.57	±	0.79	0.50	±	0.56	0.27	±	0.14

*$P < 0.05$ versus group P, †$P < 0.05$ versus group N.

Table 2. Quantitative RT-PCR analysis of the abundance of Ca^{2+}-handling protein mRNAs in endomyocardial biopsy specimens.

4.3. Univariate and multivariate analysis of cardiac events

Univariate analysis revealed that dobutamine-induced MA, pacing-induced MA, NYHA functional class, plasma BNP levels, mitral regurgitation, pulmonary artery wedge pressure, LV end-diastolic volume index, LV end-systolic volume index, LVEF, LV end-diastolic pressure and $T_{1/2}$ were significant predictors of cardiac events (Table 3). Then, stepwise multivariate analysis identified dobutamine-induced MA (odds ratio, 4.05; 95% confidence interval, 1.35 to 12.2) as a significant independent predictor of cardiac events (Table 4). Both $T_{1/2}$ (odds ratio, 1.079; 95% confidence interval, 1.003 to 1.161) and plasma BNP level (odds ratio, 1.002; 95% confidence interval, 1.0004 to 1.0038) were also significant independent predictors of cardiac events, but with smaller odds ratios than that of dobutamine-induced MA.

	Univariate analysis						
Parameter	Event-free group			Cardiac-event group			P
	(n = 72)			(n = 18)			
Dobutamine-induced MA (group D/groups P and N)	4	/	68	6	/	12	0.0019
Pacing-induced MA (groups D and P/group N)	20	/	52	10	/	8	0.04
Age (years)	50	±	12	53	±	14	0.34
Sex (M/F)	53	/	19	13	/	5	0.86
Body mass index (kg/m^2)	24.4	±	4.9	22.5	±	2.6	0.15
NYHA functional class †	1.3	±	0.5	1.6	±	0.4	0.011
QRS duration (ms)	113	±	27	112	±	22	0.88
Beta blockers	55 (76%)			10 (56%)			0.58
Diuretics	52 (72%)			16 (89%)			0.88

Parameter	Univariate analysis						
	Event-free group (n = 72)			Cardiac-event group (n = 18)			*P*
Plasma BNP (pg/mL)	123	±	238	228	±	162	0.0013
eGFR (mL min^{-1} 1.73 m^{-2})	74	±	17	68	±	18	0.089
Plasma norepinephrine (pg/mL)	521	±	452	524	±	292	0.32
E/E'	15.6	±	8.6	24.2	±	8.4	0.227
PAWP (mmHg)	11.5	±	5.3	13.7	±	6.6	0.044
Cardiac index (L min^{-1} m^{-2})	3.02	±	0.57	3.13	±	0.64	0.85
LVEDVI (mL m^{-2})	73	±	52	115	±	79	0.02
LVESVI (mL m^{-2})	43	±	36	84	±	62	0.018
LVEF (%)	38.2	±	8.7	32.8	±	6.8	0.003
Heart rate (bpm)	76	±	17	75	±	14	0.34
LVEDP (mmHg)	12	±	8	15	±	9	0.019
LVSP (mmHg)	119	±	19	116	±	23	0.62
LV dP/dt_{max} (mmHg/s)	1114	±	263	1160	±	263	0.73
$T_{1/2}$ (ms)	39	±	7	44	±	4.7	0.0086

Table 3. Univariate of predictors of cardiac events.

Parameter	Multivariate analysis			
	β	OR	(95% CI)	*P*
Dobutamine-induced MA (group D/groups P and N)	1.4	4.05	(1.35–12.2)	0.013
Plasma BNP (pg/mL)	0.0021	1.002	(1.0004–1.0038)	0.014
$T_{1/2}$ (ms)	0.076	1.079	(1.0033–1.161)	0.041

Table 4. Multivariate analysis of predictors of cardiac events.

5. Impact of dobutamine-induced MA

5.1. Prognosis

The occurrence of dobutamine-induced MA was a clinical predictor of poor prognosis in ambulatory patients with IDCM in sinus rhythm. Although there was no significant difference in LVEF between patients who manifested only pacing-induced MA and those who developed both pacing- and dobutamine-induced MA, the probability of event-free survival in the latter group was significantly lower than that in the former. Multivariate analysis also revealed that the occurrence of dobutamine-induced MA was a significant independent predictor of cardiac events.

5.2. Mechanisms

Three general mechanisms have been proposed to account for the development of MA: alteration of action potential duration, impaired ventricular relaxation, and abnormal intracellular Ca^{2+}-handling.[7] The low relative ratio of phospholamban to SERCA reduces the inhibition of SERCA and increases Ca^{2+}-uptake; this enhances relaxation and contraction in the human atrium. However, humans lacking phospholamban develop lethal IDCM.[8] SERCA2a and ryanodine receptor 2 mRNA levels were similar in all three of our groups, whereas the relative ratio of SERCA to phospholamban was significantly higher in patients with pacing- and dobutamine-induced MA than in those with only pacing-induced MA or with no MA. These results suggest that an imbalance between phospholamban and SERCA mRNA levels in the abundant Ca^{2+}-handling proteins is associated with dobutamine-induced MA. Kobayashi et al. reported that the amounts of mRNAs for the β_1-adrenergic receptor and SERCA2a in the myocardium were smaller in asymptomatic or mildly symptomatic IDCM patients with reduced adrenergic myocardial contractile reserve than in those with preserved adrenergic contractile reserves.[9] The occurrence of dobutamine-induced MA in our patients in the present study might also reflect abnormal β_1-adrenergic receptor signaling in the myocardium. However, steady-state mRNA levels do not necessarily reflect the corresponding protein levels, in particular because both mRNA and protein synthesis or degradation may be altered in the failing heart.[10, 11] Further studies are needed to elucidate these issues.

In patients with heart failure, dobutamine-induced MA is highly prevalent[6] and mechanical and visible T-wave alternans is detectable under tachycardia or catecholamine exposure.[4, 12] Dobutamine-induced MA may be attributed various factors, including an increase in the heart rate as a result of dobutamine infusion, impaired LV contraction, the influence of preload, and abnormal Ca^{2+} under pathophysiological conditions. Dobutamine is a β-stimulator that increases both heart rate and LV contraction. The increase in heart rate, but not that in LV contraction, is likely to be a trigger for the occurrence of dobutamine-induced MA. Therefore, the increased occurrence of dopamine-induced MA in heart failure patients might be related to their poor myocardial contractile reserve.

6. Conclusion

In conclusion, the occurrence of dobutamine-induced MA is a potentially useful clinical predictor of poor prognosis in ambulatory patients with IDCM in sinus rhythm. Recent guidelines for the management of heart failure emphasize the need for earlier identification of and therapy for patients who are at high risk of developing heart failure or who have asymptomatic LV systolic dysfunction.[13] The prevalence of cardiac events or cardiac death was higher in patients with dobutamine- and pacing- induced MA than in those without it. Assessment of dobutamine-induced MA in addition to routine clinical evaluation in patients with IDCM may thus contribute to stratification of individuals into low- or high-risk groups. The identification of pacing- or dobutamine-induced MA requires an invasive examination and time-consuming hemodynamic stress assessment. The current trend in clinical medicine is to find a non-invasive test with prognostic consequences. However, the hemodynamic phenomenon by dobutamine stress testing might be also potentially useful marker for predicting the occurrence of cardiac events.

Author details

Akihiro Hirashiki and Toyoaki Murohara

Department of Advanced Medicine in Cardiopulmonary Disease, University Graduate School of Medicine, Nagoya, Japan

References

[1] Hirashiki, A, Izawa, H, Cheng, X. W, Unno, K, Ohshima, S, & Murohara, T. Dobutamine-induced mechanical alternans is a marker of poor prognosis in idiopathic dilated cardiomyopathy. Clin Exp Pharmacol Physiol (2010)., 37, 1004-1009.

[2] Dries, D. L, Exner, D. V, Gersh, B. J, Domanski, M. J, Waclawiw, M. A, & Stevenson, L. W. Atrial fibrillation is associated with an increased risk for mortality and heart failure progression in patients with asymptomatic and symptomatic left ventricular systolic dysfunction: a retrospective analysis of the SOLVD trials. Studies of Left Ventricular Dysfunction. J Am Coll Cardiol (1998)., 32, 695-703.

[3] Euler, D. E, Guo, H, & Olshansky, B. Sympathetic influences on electrical and mechanical alternans in the canine heart. Cardiovasc Res (1996)., 32, 854-860.

[4] Hirashiki, A, Izawa, H, Somura, F, Obata, K, Kato, T, Nishizawa, T, et al. Prognostic value of pacing-induced mechanical alternans in patients with mild-to-moderate idiopathic dilated cardiomyopathy in sinus rhythm. J Am Coll Cardiol (2006). , 47, 1382-1389.

[5] Mirsky, I. Assessment of diastolic function: suggested methods and future considerations. Circulation (1984)., 69, 836-841.

[6] Kodama, M, Kato, K, Hirono, S, Okura, Y, Hanawa, H, Ito, M, et al. Mechanical alternans in patients with chronic heart failure. J Card Fail (2001)., 7, 138-145.

[7] Lab, M. J, & Lee, J. A. Changes in intracellular calcium during mechanical alternans in isolated ferret ventricular muscle. Circ Res (1990). , 66, 585-595.

[8] Haghighi, K, Kolokathis, F, Pater, L, Lynch, R. A, Asahi, M, Gramolini, A. O, et al. Human phospholamban null results in lethal dilated cardiomyopathy revealing a critical difference between mouse and human. J Clin Invest (2003). , 111, 869-876.

[9] Kobayashi, M I. H. Cheng XW Asano H, Hirashiki A, Unno K, Ohshima S,Yamada T, Murase Y, Kato ST, Obata K, Noda A, Nishizawa T, Isobe S, Nagata K, Matsubara T, Murohara T, Yokota M.. Dobutamine stress testing as a diagnostic tool for evaluation of myocardial contractile reserve in asymptomatic or mildly symptomatic patients with dilated cardiomyopathy. J Am Coll Cardiol Imaging (2008). , 2008, 718-726.

[10] Linck, B, Boknik, P, Eschenhagen, T, Muller, F. U, Neumann, J, Nose, M, et al. Messenger RNA expression and immunological quantification of phospholamban and SR-Ca(2+)-ATPase in failing and nonfailing human hearts. Cardiovasc Res (1996). , 31, 625-632.

[11] Hasenfuss, G. Calcium pump overexpression and myocardial function. Implications for gene therapy of myocardial failure. Circ Res (1998). , 83, 966-968.

[12] Kodama, M, Kato, K, Hirono, S, Okura, Y, Hanawa, H, Yoshida, T, et al. Linkage between mechanical and electrical alternans in patients with chronic heart failure. J Cardiovasc Electrophysiol (2004). , 15, 295-299.

[13] Radford, M. J, Arnold, J. M, Bennett, S. J, Cinquegrani, M. P, Cleland, J. G, Havranek, E. P, et al. ACC/AHA key data elements and definitions for measuring the clinical management and outcomes of patients with chronic heart failure: a report of the American College of Cardiology/American Heart Association Task Force on Clinical Data Standards (Writing Committee to Develop Heart Failure Clinical Data Standards): developed in collaboration with the American College of Chest Physicians and the International Society for Heart and Lung Transplantation: endorsed by the Heart Failure Society of America. Circulation (2005). , 112, 1888-1916.

Section 3

Genetics

Chapter 7

The Role of Genetics in Cardiomyopathy

Luis Vernengo, Alain Lilienbaum,
Onnik Agbulut and Maria-Mirta Rodríguez

Additional information is available at the end of the chapter

http://dx.doi.org/10.5772/55775

1. Introduction

Cardiomyopathies can be defined as disorders of the myocardium which are associated with cardiac dysfunction and are aggravated by arrhythmias, heart failure and sudden death [Ricardson, 2006]. Genetics has played a very important role in the understanding of the different cardiomyopathies since, in 1957, Bridgen cited for the first time the word "cardiomyopathy" and in 1958, Teare, the British pathologist reported nine cases of septum hypertrophy (Teare, 1958).

The American Heart Association (AHA) has classified cardiomyopathies as primary cardiomyopathies (the heart is the only organ affected) and secondary cardiomyopathies (the heart is affected as part of a systemic disease). The European Society of Cardiology (ESC) has classified them according to morphological and functional phenotypes involving their pathophysiology (Maron, 2006; Maron, 2008; Elliott, 2008)

Primary cardiomyopathies are those which and can be genetic, nongenetic or acquired. Secondary cardiomyopathies are those in which the cardiomyopathy is found in a systemic disease. Primary cardiomyopathies can then be classified according to their anatomical and functional impairment in hypertrophic cardiomyopathy, dilated cardiomyopathy (DCM), restrictive cardiomyopathy (RCM), arrhythmogenic right ventricular cardiomyopathy/dysplasia (ARVC/D), ion channel disorders. Secondary cardiomyopathies are those found in muscular dystrophies, mitochondrial disorders among others. The unclassified cardiomyopathies are non-compaction cardiomyopathy and takotsubo cardiomyopathy (Elliott, 2008;)

The genetic diagnosis has a close involvement in the management of primary and secondary cardiomyopathies and its development will have a key role in the understanding of the different molecular mechanisms that lead to a cardiomyopathy.

2. Hypertrophic cardiomyopathy

Hypertrophic cardiomyopathy (HCM) is a familial disease that in fifty percent of the cases is inherited in an autosomal dominant pattern. The disorder shows complete penetrance in most families although it depends on the age and the sex of the patients (Nimura, 1998, Richard, 2003, Richard, 2006).

As the prevalence of HCM is 1: 500, it can be stated that HCM is undoubtedly the most common cardiovascular disorder (Maron, 2002).

HCM has been traditionally described as an unexplained hypertrophy of the left ventricle that develops in the absence of systemic hypertension, valvular heart disease or amyloidosis. The left ventricular hypertrophy (LVH) is usually asymmetric and involves the septum.

The clinical presentation is variable. There can be varying degrees of clinical severity which can range from dyspnea, palpitations, atrial fibrillation, and syncopal episodes to congestive heart failure and sudden death. Many can be asymptomatic throughout their whole life, whereas others may even require heart transplantation. It is the most common cause of death in young athletes while practicing sports.

HCM generally has normal systolic function, impaired diastolic function and outflow obstruction in about 25%. The histopathology shows myocyte disarray, interstitial fibrosis and hypertrophy (Richard, 2006, Ho, 2007).

Mutations in any of the thirteen sarcomeric genes lead to HCM. (See Table 1). The sarcomere has a complex structure where the proteins that form it interact among themselves. The different mechanisms that cause HCM are not yet completely understood. Most mutations in HCM are private of each family and there is clinical heterogeneity within family members (Richard, 2006 Hayashi, 2004; Frank, 2011).

3. Dilated cardiomyopathy

Dilated cardiomyopathy is the most common cause of congestive heart failure in young patients. The prevalence is ~36: 100,000 in the U.S. It is characterized by ventricular chamber enlargement, thin wall thickness, impaired left ventricular systolic function, and there is also, in some cases, secondary diastolic dysfunction. The most common feature is congestive heart failure, though, conduction impairment, syncope and sudden death may also occur. It is an important cause of cardiac transplantation (Sugrue, 1992).

The histological findings are nonspecific and they include myocyte loss and interstitial fibrosis. Familial cases of DCM were initially considered to be quite rare. However, careful screenings have shown that up to 35% of the probands´ relatives have a DCM familial disorder.

In these families, the pattern of inheritance is variable, so the patients present both locus heterogeneity and allelic heterogeneity. Mutations in many genes have been reported to cause

http://dx.doi.org/10.5772/55775

HCM gene	Symbol	Locus name	Chromosome locus	Protein
Beta-myosin heavy chain	*MYH7*	CMH1	14q2	Myosin heavy chain, cardiac muscle beta isoform
Myosin-binding protein C	*MYBPC3*	CMH4	11p11.2	Myosin-binding protein C, cardiac-type
Troponin T	*TNNT2*	CMH2	1q32	TroponinT, cardiac muscle
Troponin I	*TNNI3*	CMH7	19q13.4	TroponinI, cardiac muscle
Alpha-tropomyosin	*TPM1*	CMH3	15q22.1	Tropomyosin1 alpha chain
Regulatory myosin light chain	*MYL2*	CMH10	12q24.3	Myosin regulatory light chain 2, ventricular/ cardiac muscle isoform
Essential myosin light chain	*MYL3*	CMH8	3p21 5	Myosin light polypeptide 3
Actin	*ACTC1*	CMH11	15q14	Actin, alpha cardiac muscle 1
Cardiac troponin C	*TNNC1*	CMH13	3p21.1	Troponin C, slow skeletal and cardiac muscles
Titin	*TTN*	CMH9	2q24.3 2	Titin
Alpha-myosin heavy chain	*MYH6*	CMH14	14q12	Myosin heavy chain, cardiac muscle alpha isoform
Muscle LIM protein	*CSRP3*	CMH12	11p15.	Cysteine and glycine-rich protein 3, muscle LIM protein
Telethonin	*TCAP*	CMH11	17q12 1	Telethonin

Table 1. Sarcomeric genes that cause HCM

different forms of dilated cardiomyopathy. Therefore, autosomal dominant, autosomal recessive, and X-linked inheritance can be observed. (See Table 2) However, the autosomal dominant pattern is the most frequent mode of inheritance. It has been demonstrated that DCM has reduced penetrance. The age of onset shows great variability though it is usually appears in adulthood (Mangin, 1999). When the mutation is in one of the sarcomeric genes the affected patients are usually young adults (Aernout Somsen, 2012).

DCM gene	Symbol	Locus name	Chromosome locus	Protein	Mode of inheritance
Lamin A/C gene	*LMNA*	CMD1A	1q21	lamin A and lamin C	AD
LDB3 gene		CMD1C	10q22-q23	LIM domain-binding protein 3	AD
TNNT2 gene	*TNNT2*	CMD1D	1q32	Troponin T, cardiac muscle	AD
SCN5A		CMD1E	3p	Sodium channel protein type 5 subunit alpha	AD
TTN gene	*TTN*	CMD1G	2q31	Titin	AD
DES gene	*DES*	CMD1I	2q35	Desmin	AD
EYA4 gene	*EYA4*	CMD1J	6q23-q24	Eyes absent homolog 4	AD
SGCD gene	*SGCD*	CMD1L	5q33	Delta-sarcoglycan	AD
CSRP3 gene	*CSRP3*	CMD1M	11p15.1	Cysteine and glycine-rich protein 3	AD
TCAP gene	*TCAP*	CMD1N	17q12;	Telethonin	AD
ABCC9 gene		CMD1O,	on 12p12.1;	ATP-binding cassette, subfamily C, member 9	AD
PLN gene	*PLN*	CMD1P	on 6q22.1;,	Cardiac phospholamban	AD
ACTC1 gene	*ACTC1*	CMD1R	15q14	Actin, alpha cardiac muscle 1	AD
MYH7 gene	*MYH7*	CMD1S	14q12;	Myosin 7	AD
TMPO gene	*TMPO*	CMD1T	12q22	Hymopoietin	AD
PSEN1 gene	*PSEN1*	CMD1U	14q24.3	Presenilin-1	AD
PSEN2 gene	*PSEN2*	CMD1V	1q31-q42;	Presenilin-2	AD
metavinculin VCL		CMD1W	10q22-q23	metavinculin VCL	AD
fukutin	*FKTN*	CMD1X	9q31	Fukutin	AD
TPM1 gene	*Fukutin*	CMD1Y	15q22.1	tropomyosin-1	AD
TNNC1 gene	*TNNC1*	CMD1Z	3p21.3-p14.3	slow troponin-C	AD
ACTN2 gene	*ACTN2*	CMD1AA	1q42-q43;	Alpha-actinin-2	AD
DSG2 gene	*DSG2*	CMD1BB	18q12.1-q12.2;	desmoglein-2	AD
NEXN gene	*NEXN*	CMD1CC	1p31.1	Nelin	AD
RBM20 gene	*RBM20*	CMD1DD	10q25.2;	RNA-Binding motif protein 20	AD
MYH6 gene	*MYH6*	CMD1EE	14q12	Myosin 7	AD

DCM gene	Symbol	Locus name	Chromosome locus	Protein	Mode of inheritance
TNNI3 gene	*TNNI3*	CMD1FF	19q13.4;	Troponin I,	AD
SDHA gene	*SDHA*	CMD1GG	5p15;	Succinate dehydrogenase complex subunit A	AD
BAG3 gene	*BAG3*	CMD1HH	10q25.2-q26.2	BCL2-associated athanogene 3	AD
TNNI3 gene	*TNNI3*	CMD2A,	19q13.42	Troponin I, cardiac muscle	AR
GATAD1 gene.	*GATAD1*	CMD2	7q21.2	GATA zinc finger domain containing protein 1	AR
Dystrophin gene	*DMD*	CMD3B	Xp21.2	dystrophin	X-linked
LAMP2 gene	*LAMP2*	Danon disease	Xq24	lysosome-associated membrane protein-2	X-linked
TAZ gene	*TAZ*		Xq28	dystrophin	X-linked

Table 2. Genes tha cause DCM

Mutations on the following genes *CMD1B* on 9q13; *CMD1H* on 2q14-q22; *CMD1K* on 6q12-q16; and *CMD1Q* on 7q22.3-q31.1 can also cause DCM.

4. Restrictive cardiomyopathy

Familial restrictive cardiomyopathy (RCM) is a rare disease which is inherited in autosomal dominant pattern with incomplete penetrance (Katritsis 1991). The exact prevalence of RCM is unknown (Elliott, 2008). In childhood, RCM accounts for 2–5% of cardiomyopathies and has a grave prognosis (Kaski, 2008.)

RCM is characterized by abnornal diastolic function, which has a restrictive filling pattern, a reduced diastolic volume of one of the ventricles or both ventricles, enlargement of the atria, pulmonary hypertension and heart failure. In the early stages of the disorder the systolic function may be normal, but as the disease progresses, the systolic function generally declines (Kushwaha, 1997).

The familial RCM is linked to the cardiac troponin genes. RCM1 is caused by a mutation in the *TNNI3* gene on chromosome 19q13. This gene encodes the cardiac muscle isoform of troponin 1. RCM2 has been mapped to chromosome 10q23. RCM3 is caused by mutation in the *TNNT2* gene. Mutations in the sarcomere gene, alpha-cardiac actin gene (*ACTC*) have also been reported to cause RCM,

In many cases RCM can be observed overlapping with either HCM or DCM. (Kamisago, 2000; Olson, 2002; Zang, 2005; Kaski, 2008).

5. Arrhythmogenic right ventricular cardiomyopathy / dysplasia

Arrhythmogenic right ventricular cardiomyopathy/dysplasia (ARVC/ARVD) is a commonly inherited disorder with a family history in 30 to 50% of the cases (Klauke, 2010).

The prevalence has been estimated 1:2000 to 1:5000 in the general population (Peters 2006, Cox&Hauer, 2011).

ARVC is characterized by fibro-fatty replacement of the myocardium with a marked involvement of the right ventricle. ARVC can be defined by the presence either sectored or global right ventricular dysfunction. The left ventricular abnormalities which lead to DCM may take place later. Clinical features include tachyarrhythmias, electrocardiographic abnormalities, systolic heart failure, syncope and sudden death. ARVC is a frequent cause of sudden death in young people and athletes (Maron, 2006).

It is transmitted with an autosomal dominant pattern, though autosomal recessive families have also been reported. Incomplete penetrance and great variability in the symptoms have been observed (Hamid, 2002; Awad, 2008; Eliott, 2008; Klauke, 2010, Cox&Hauer, 2011).

Desmosomes are intercellular junctions that link intermediate filaments to the plasma membrane and are essential to tissues that experience mechanical stress such as the myocardium. Mutations in the cardiac desmosome genes are to be held responsible for most of the cases that cause the disorder. (See Table 3)

The mutations p.S13F, p.E114del and p.N116S in the desmin gene have the same ARVC cardiac phenotype. In transfection cells aggresome formation in the cytoplasm was observed (Van Titelen, 2007; Vernengo, 2010; Klauke, 2010). Only recently has it been proven that seven members of the Swedish family with ARVC7 had the p.Pro419Ser mutation in *DES*, instead of a mutation linked to chromosome 10q23.2 (Melberg, 1999; Hedberg, 2012).

Naxos disease and Carvajal disease are ARVC inherited in an autosomal recessive pattern. The former is caused by mutations in the plakoglobin gene on chromosome 17q21,2 and the latter by mutations in the desmoplakin gene on chromosome 6p24 (Protonotarios, 1986; McKoy, 2000; Schonberger, 2001; Cox&Hauer, 2011).

6. Non–compaction cardiomyopathy

Non-compaction cardiomyopathy (NCCM) has been classified as a primary cardiomyopathy with a genetic etiology.The age of onset varies from neonatal to adult hood. There is variability in the clinical features which include heart failure, arrhythmias and thromboembolism, but patients can also be asymptomatic]. The most common congenital heart defects in NCCM are Ebstein's anomaly, septal defects and patent ductus arteriosus,

The patients have a thickened two-layered myocardium with a thin, compact, epicardial layer and a severely thickened endocardial layer with a 'spongy' appearance due to prominent

http://dx.doi.org/10.5772/55775

ARCV gene	Symbol	Locus name	Chromosome locus	Protein
Transforming growth factor beta- 3	*TGFB3*	ARVD1	14q2	Transforming growth factor beta-3
Ryanodine receptor 2	*RYR2*	ARVD2	1q43	RYR2
Unknown	Unknown	ARVD3	14q12-q22	Unknown
Unknown	Unknown	ARVD4	2q32 .1-q32.3	Unknown
transmembrane protein 43	*TMEM43*	ARVD5	3p25 .1	Transmembrane protein 43
Unknown	Unknown	ARVD6	10p14-p12	Unknownn
Desmin	*DES*	ARVD7	2q35	Desmin
Desmoplakin	*DSP*	ARVD8	6p24 .3	Desmoplakin
Plakophilin-2	*PKP2*	ARVD9	12p11 .21	Plakophilin-2
Desmoglein-2	*DSG2*	ARVD10	18q12 .1	Desmoglein-2
Desmocollin-2	*DSC2*	ARVD11	18q12 .1	Desmocollin-2
Junction plakoglobin	*JUP*	ARVD12	17q21 .2	Junction plakoglobin
Desmin	*DES*	ARVC	2q35	Desmin

Table 3. Genes that cause ARVC.

trabeculations and intertrabecular recesses (Hermida-Prieto, 2004; Freedom, 2005; Budde, 2007; Monserrat, 2007; Klaassen, 2008)

The majority of the patients have an autosomal dominant mode of inheritance.

Mutations in several genes coding for sarcomeric proteins have been described in NCCM, such as β-myosin heavy chain (*MYH7*), cardiac myosin-binding protein C (*MYBPC3*), α-cardiac actin (*ACTC1*), cardiac troponin T (*TNNT2*), α-tropomyosin (*TPM1*) and cardiac troponin I (*TNNI3*). MYH7 has been reported to be the most frequent disease gene in NCCM in the absence of HCM (Ichida, 2001; Hermida-Prieto. 2004; Vatta, 2003; Shan, 2008).

7. Takotsubo cardiomyopathy

Takotsubo cardiomyopathy is characterized by an acute but transitient LV systolic dysfunction without atherosclerotic coronary artery disease and it is triggered by psychological stress (Sharkey, 2005; Sealove, 2008).

8. Ion channel disorders

The cell membrane transit of sodium and potassium ions is ruled by the ion channel genes which encode proteins responsible for the right transit of these ions. Mutations in these proteins lead to a group of familial disorders (Aleong, 2007). These ion channel disorders include the Romano-Ward syndrome (long QT syndromes), the short-QT syndrome (SQTS), Brugada syndrome, and the catecholaminergic polymorphic ventricular tachycardia (CPVT). 5% to 10% of the sudden deaths in children can be associated to ion channel disorders (Modell & Lehmann, 2006).

The clinical diagnosis of the ion channelopathies can be often made by identification of alterations found on the ECG (Aleong, 2007; Kass, 2005).

8.1. Romano–Ward syndrome

RWS may be sporadic or transmitted as an autosomal-dominant trait with reduced penetrance. It is the most common form of inherited long QT syndrome. The prevalence of RWS has been estimated to be 1:3000 to 1:7000.

The Romano-Ward syndrome (RWS) is tipically identified in patients that present syncope, seizures, or sudden death due to episodic taquiarrhythmias, QT prolongation and T-wave abnormalities, interval torsade de pointes that lead to ventricular fibrillation and death.

RWS is associated with mutations in the following genes: *KCNQ1* on chromosome 11p15.5-p15.4, *KCNE1* on chromosome 21q22.12, *KCNE2* on chromosome 21q22.11, *KCNH2* on chromosome 7q36.1, *SCN5A* on chromosome *3p22.2, CAV3* on chromosome *3p25.3*, *SCN4B* on chromosome 11q23.3, *AKAP9* on chromosome 7q21.2, *SNTA1* on chromosome 20q11.21 and *KCNJ5* on chromosome *11q24.3* (Schwartz 1993; Schwartz 2001: Schwartz 2011).

8.2. Jervell and Lange–Nielsen syndrome

The Jervell and Lange-Nielsen syndrome (JLNS) is inherited as an autosomal recessive trait. The affected children present symptoms before the age of three and they died before the age of 15 if they are not treated.

The prevalence can vary considerably and it depends on the population studied.

The patients have a more severe QT prolongation (greater than 500 msec) which is associated which tachiarrhythmias including torsade de pointes, ventricular fibrillation, syncope and sudden death.

Mutations in the *KCNQ1* gene on chromosome 11p15.5-p15.4, *KCNE1* gene on chromosome 21q22.12, have been reported in the affected individuals (Schwartz 2000; Schwartz 2006).

8.3. Timothy syndrome

Timothy syndrome is a rare autosomal dominant disorder are due to either a *de novo* mutation or parent germline mosaicism Mutations in the same gene *CACNA1C* cause the two forms of the disorder: the classic, type 1, and type 2. The reported cases of the patients suffering type 1 syndrome have shown complete penetrance (Splawski, 2004).

This complex multisystem disorder has a long QT syndrome associated with syndactily. Various forms of congenital heart defects such as tetralogy of Fallot, hypertrophic cardiomy-

http://dx.doi.org/10.5772/55775

opathy have been observed. The type 2 patients that have been reported did not have syndactily (Splawski, 2005)

Children died at age of 2.5 years due to ventricular tachycardia and ventricular fibrillation, infection or hypoglycemia (Reichenbach, 1992; Marks, 1995a; Marks 1995b; Splawski 2004; Lo-A-Njoe, 2005).

8.4. Brugada syndrome

The Brugada syndrome, which is inherited in an autosomal dominant pattern, is associated with sudden death in young people as the patients have malignant ventricular tachyarrhythmias and sudden cardiac death. The heart is not affected by either a structural heart or systemic disease.

The age of appearance ranges from a two- day- old patient to 85 years (Marks, 1995a; Marks, 1995b; Splawski, 2004; Huang, 2004; Lo-A-Njoe, 2005).

The cardiac differential diagnosis must be made with Duchenne muscular dystrophy, Friedreich ataxia and ARVC.

8.5. Catecholaminergic polymorphic ventricular tachycardia

Catecholaminergic polymorphic ventricular tachycardia (CPVT) is an inherited tachyarrhythmia that is caused by acute adrenergic activation during exercise or acute emotion in young adolescents.

The age of onset varies from 7-9 years to the fourth decade of life.

It presents locus heterogeneity and in only approximatedly 50% of the cases the mutations in the genes causing the disease have been identified.

The prevalence of CPVT in the population is not known, but it could be estimated in approximately 1:10,000.

There is an autosomal dominant form caused by mutations in the RYR2 gene that encodes the ryanodine receptor 2, a calcium-release channel (George, 2003).

The autosomal recessive form is due to mutations in the calsequestrin 2 gene on chromosome 1p13.1 (Wilde, 2008).

8.6. Short–QT syndrome

Short-QT syndrome is a familial disease that is characterized by a high incidence of sudden death. Patients with this disease have QT intervals that are <300 ms, and increased risk of atrial and ventricular arrhythmia.

It is an autosomal dominant inherited disorder that affects patients of 30 years of age, but the fibrillation can even be observed in newborns and young patients.

Missense mutations in the *KCNH2* gene on chromosome 7q36.1, in the *KCNQ1* gene on chromosome 11p15.5-p15.and the *KCNJ2* gene on chromosome 17q24.3 have shown that this is a genetically heterogeneous disease.

9. Cardiomyopathy in muscular dystrophies

Muscular dystrophies are a heterogeneous group of inherited disorders, characterized by progressive weakness and wasting of the skeletal muscles. They are generally associated with cardiomyopathy. In many cases, there is no correlation between the skeletal myopathy and the involvement of the heart. The mutations of the genes that cause muscular dystrophies affect the skeletal and/or cardiac muscles. These include proteins which are associated with the dystrophin–glycoprotein complex, the nuclear lamina or the sarcomere (Hermans, 2012).

Cardiomyopathy occurs in myofibrillar myopathy, myotonic dystrophies, myotonic myopathies, dystrophinopathies, Emery-Dreifuss muscular dystrophy, and limb girdle muscular dystrophies (Hermans, 2012).

They are inherited in autosomal dominant, autosomal recessive and X-linked mode. (See Table 4, Table 5).

The different forms of muscular dystrophies vary in the age of onset with no male or female prevalence and have different clinical features and severity. Mutations in the genes that are involved muscular dystrophies can cause hypertrophic, dilated or restrictive cardiomyopathy, but most cardiomyopathies in patients with a muscular dystrophy are of the dilated type. The progression of the disorders and life expectancy vary widely, even among different members of the same family. Patients die of sudden death due to conduction defects, and heart failure.

In dystrophinopathies, sarcoglycanopathies, and the disorders that are linked to mutations in the fukutin-related protein, the feature that stands out is the cardiomyopathy the patients suffer. In muscular dystrophies, the patients usually have a dilated cardiomyopathy. Hypertrophic cardiomyopathy can be observed in Danon disease, α-B crystallinopathy, and on patients or carriers of DMD and BMD. (De Ambroggi, 1995, Vicart 1998; Nguyen, 1998; Lazarus, 1999; Melacini, 1999; Barresi, 2000; Politano, 2001; Selcen, 2003; Fanin, 2001; Jefferies, 2005; Nakanishi, 2006; Connuck, 2008; Kaspar, 2009; Goldfarb, 2009; Lilienbaum, 2012; Hermans, 2012)

10. Mitochondrial disorders

Mitochondrial disorders are a heterogeneous group of disorders that have common clinical features and are caused by the different mutations found in either the nuclear or mitochondrial DNA (mtDNA) genes which regulate the mitochondrial respiratory chain, the essential final common pathway of aerobic metabolism, tissues and organs. mtDNA is maternally inherited

Disease Name	Gene	Symbol	Locus name	Chromosome locus	Protein	Mode of inheritance
Desminopathy	Desmin	*DES*	MFM1	**2q35**	Desmin	AD/AR
Alpha-B crystallinopathy	CRYAB gene	*CRYAB*	MFM2	11q23.1	alpha-B-crystallin	AR/AD
Myotilinopathy	Myotilin	*MYOT (TTID)*	MFM3	5q31.2	Myotilin (titinmmunoglobulin domain protein)	AD
ZASPopathy	ZASP	*LDB3*	MFM4	**10q23.2**	LIM domain-binding protein 3	AD
Filaminopathy	FilaminC	*FLNC*	MFM5	7q32.1	Filamin C	AD
BAG3-Related Myofibrillar Myopathy	BCL2-associated athanogen 3	*BAG3*	BAG3	***10q26.11***	BAG family molecular chaperone regulator 3	AD
Myotonic dystrophy type 1	myotonin-protein kinase (Mt-PK).	*DMPK*	DMPK	19q13.3	dystrophia myotonica-protein kinase	AD
Myotonic dystrophy type 2	zinc finger protein-9 gene	*CNBP*		*3q21.3*	zinc finger protein-9	AD
Duchenne/Becker muscular dystrophy	dystrophin	*DMD*	DMD	Xp21.2	dystrophin	X-linked
Emery-Dreyfuss Muscular Dystrophy1,X-linked	EMD gene	*EMD*	EMD1	Xq28	emerin	X-linked

Table 4. Genes that cause cardiomyopathy in muscular dystropies

and the disorders can appear at any age. All the mitochondria have multiple copies of their own mtDNA and the mutation rate is much higher than in nuclear DNA (Walter, 2000; Carrasco, 2005; De Jonge, 2011).

Many mitochondrial disorders involve multiple organ systems such as the brain, the heart, the liver, and the skeletal muscles which are, therefore, affected due to the fact they depend on the energy and they are especially susceptible to energy metabolism impairment (Walter, 2000; Carrasco, 2005; De Jonge, 2011).

Mitochondrial dysfunction and clinical symptoms appear when the heteroplasmic levels are above 80%-90% (Walter, 2000; Carrasco, 2005; De Jonge, 2011).

Disease Name	Gene	Symbol	Locus name	Chromosome locus	Protein	Mode of inheritance
LGMD2C	gamma sarcoglycan gene	*SGCG*	SGCG	13q12-q13	gamma sarcoglycan	AR
LGMD2D	alpha sarcoglycan gene	*SGCA*	SGCA	17q21	Alpha sarcoglycan	AR
LGMD2E	Beta sarcoglycan gene	*SGCB*	SGCB	4q12	Beta sarcoglycan	AR
LGMD2F	Delta sarcoglycan gene	*SGCD*	SGCD	5q33-q34	Delta sarcoglycan	AR
LGMD2I	fukutin related protein gene	*FKRP*	FKRP	19q13.32	fukutin related protein	AR

Table 5. Limb-girdle muscular dystrophies

The different mitochondrial cardiomyopathies are a result of the heart being commonly affected. Sometimes, the cardiomyopathy is diagnosed during the first year of life even before the mitochondrial disorder has been diagnosed. Both hypertrophic and dilated cardiomyopathies have been reported (Holmgren, 2003, de Jonge, 2011).

11. Kearns-Sayre syndrome

The Kearns-Sayre syndrome (KSS) is characterized by the triad: onset of the disorder before the age of 20, progressive external ophthalmoplegia and pigmentary retinopathy. A cerebrospinal fluid protein concentration greater than 100 mg/d, and a commonly elevated lactate and pyruvate concentrations in blood and cerebrospinal fluid are found.

The KSS has cardiac involvement with conduction defects such as right bundle branch block, left anterior hemiblock or complete A-V block. These patients can develop a cardiomyopathy usually dilated (Roberts, 1979; Anan, 1995; Carrasco, 2005).

11.1. MELAS

It is a multisystem disorder with onset in childhood with mitochondrial encephalomyopathy, lactic acidosis, and recurrent stroke-like episodes. The variability of symptoms and the severity of the syndrome make it difficult to confirm the diagnosis. MELAS is transmitted by maternal inheritance.

The cardiac involvement is considered to be 18–100% (Hirano, 1994; Vydt, 2007; Wortmann, 2007). The first symptom the affected children have is the cardiomyopathy. The most common feature is a hypertrophic cardiomyopathy, although dilation has also been reported (Okajima, 1998).

Mutations in the nuclear genes that also encode mitochondrial proteins can cause cardiomyopathies. These disorders are sometimes not considered among the group of mitochondrial primary disorders. Two of the most well known disorders are Friedreich´s ataxia and Barth syndrome (de Jonge, 2011).

Friedreich´s ataxia is an autosomal recessive disorder. Frataxin, the protein encoded by *FXN*, is involved in the mitochondrial transport and is needed for the synthesis of the enzymes of the respiratory chain complexes I – III and aconitase. When the protein is mutated in Friederich ´s ataxia, it does not allow the correct respiratory function.

Barth syndrome is a recessive X-linked inherited disease chacterized by cardiomyopathy and neutropenia. The cardiac disease presents a dilated cardiomyopathy, often with a degree of left myocardial thickening and, sometimes, endocardial fibroelastosis. The cardiac disease appears at birth or in the first few months of life

Mutations in the tafazzin gene are to be held responsible for this disorder because of the inhibition of this pathway leads to changes in mitochondrial architecture and function (Spencer, 2006, Schamme, 2006).

12. The impact of genetics in the understanding of cardiomyopathy

Although the diagnosis is based primarily on DNA analysis, a thorough clinical history and examination, blood tests, the ECG, echocardiography, electromyography, and muscle biopsy can also provide information that can be helpful for the diagnosis not only of the patients, but also of the asymptomatic carriers.

With the expansion in number of the different disorders that have myocardial involvement in conjunction with the development of their molecular and biochemical bases, it can be stated that these will play a most important role in the understanding of the pathophysiology of the syndromes.

The exact role and function each mutated protein has and the pathogenic mechanisms that lead to the different disorders still have to be elucidated, in spite of the fact that the mutations that cause them have been found.

It has also been observed that the mutations within the same gene and in the same family can give rise to distinct phenotypes in HCM, DCM and RCM. The pathogenesis of the three major types of cardiomyopathy can be linked to the the genetic mutations in the different sarcomeric proteins. These gene mutations are responsible to trigger the different pathways that lead to the remodeling of the heart. The mechanisms why this occurs are still unclear and the animal models are markedly distinct.

Since HCM is an autosomal dominant disorder most of the patients suffering from it are heterozygous. Mutations in MYH7 and/or MYBPC3 genes account for 80% of the mutations (Richard, 2006).

In some cases, patients have two different mutations, usually in *MYH7* and/or *MYBPC3* genes. These mutations result in the patients being compound heterozygous. The double heterozygotes that have also been observed have mutations in the *MyBP-C/ β –MHC, MyBP-C/ TNNT2, MyBP-C/TNNT3, MyBP-C/TPM, β-MHC/TNNT2* genes. Sometimes, the patients can be homozygous for a mutation in the genes *MyBP-C, β -MHC*, and *TNNT2* (Richard, 1999; Richard 2003; Van Driest, 2004; Ingles, 2005; Richard 2006).

The genotype-phenotype correlations have been linked to specific mutations (Richard, 2006).

The different mutations in the *MYH7*gene show great variability in symptomatology. Patients with the R403Q, R719W and R719Q mutations have complete penetrance, severe hypertrophy and short life expectancy, whereas those with the V606M mutation have a mild progression (Ho, 2000; Richard, 2006; Overeem, 2007; Uro-Coste, 2009).

All the patients that have mutations in the *TNNT2* gene seem to have a more severe course. In most cases, the affected patients carrying the mutations R92W, R92Q, I79N are young, and even though they have a mild LVH, they died of sudden death. The F110I mutation does not seem to have a so severe development as the rest of the mutations in this gene (Watkins, 1995; Arian, 1998; Tardiff, 2005, Richard, 2006).

It is believed that patients having double mutations have a greater severity of the disorder due to a double dose effect (Ingles, 2005).

Incomplete or reduced penetrance has been observed in many cases (20 to 30%) as there are parents that are carriers of the mutations, but they have not developed the disease. It is unknown whether carriers will develop the disorder at a certain age of their lives or will remain asymptomatic. Symptoms show a great variability among the patients that have the same mutation and suffer the disorder. These may be due to gene interaction, environmental factors and modifier genes (Michels, 1992; Mestroni, 1999; Criley, 2003; Richard, 2006).

In many cases RCM can be observed overlapping with either HCM or DCM. An autosomal dominant cardiomyopathy has been described where the single sarcomere *TNNT2* gene mutation can cause idiopathic RCM in some patients, or HCM or DCM in others.

All affected members of a RCM-associated family have the I79N mutation in the *TNNT2* gene, thus showing the variability of the disorders (Peddy, 2006; Menon, 2008).

It is very difficult to assess the genotype-phenotype correlation in NCCM. It seems that when there are mutations in the alpha-dystrobrevin gene (*DTNA)* on chromosome 18q12.1 and taffazin gene (*TAZ)* on chromosome Xq28 (Bleyt, 1997). It has been observed that when the mutations are in a sarcomeric gene, they give rise to a truncated protein and the onset of the disorder is during childhood. When there is an adult onset, there can be multiple mutations in a non sarcomeric gene thus the phenotype is more severe

As soon as the patients are diagnosed with the myopathies mentioned above they should be cardiologically checked-up, and should be treated immediately as the cardiac therapy improves the cardiac involvement and life expectancy

In Timothy syndrome the molecular diagnosis of *CACNA1C* should be performed in several tissues, including sperm.

It has been observed that mutations in the lamin A/C gene cause CMD1A, LGMD1B or EDMD2 in the same family (Becane, 2000; Brodsky, 2000)

The mitochondrial deletion syndromes are generally not inherited. The *de novo* deletions that take place in the mother's oocytes during germline development or in the embryo during embryogenesis are to be held responsible for these syndromes. 90% of the patients with KSS have deletions of mtDNA. The deletions are present in all tissues in individuals with KSS. There is no correlation between the size or the location of the mtDNA deletion and the phenotype and penetrance because there are related to the mutation load.

It has suggested that the mutations in the nuclear gene *RRM2B* gene cause cause KSS following a Mendelian mode of inheritance. The patient had multiple mtDNA deletions and a normal left ventricular function with an increased thickness of the interventricular septum and left posterior ventricular wall (Pitceathly, 2012).

Approximately 80% of cases of MELAS are due to mutations in the mtDNA gene *MT-TL1* which encodes tRNA leucine. The mutations in *MT-ND5* gene which encodes the NADH-ubiquinone oxidoreductase subunit 5 have also been found in individuals with MELAS or with overlap syndromes (Di Mauro,2005).

13. What should the genetic counseling be in cardiomyopathy?

To provide genetic counseling to an individual that has a cardiomyopathy is not an easy task.

When a patient or a relative that has been diagnosed with cardiomyopathy comes for genetic counseling, the geneticist has to be forthright and explain that there are all sorts of disorders that cause it, locus heterogeneity and clinical variability.

It is very important that when a numerical value is provided the patient and/or his family understand what has been explained to them. It is necessary to be very clear that chance does not have a memory. It would be embarrassing to face a family that comes with a second affected child because they have misinterpreted the information provided to them.

It should also be pointed out that the molecular diagnosis of a disorder it is not only time consuming and a very expensive process, but also that, sometimes, there is not a specific mutation that stands out in the different disorders that cause a cardiomyopathy. Many patients do not have an identified causing gene defect.

Opinions differ about procedures when consultants are under 18 and asymptomatic, and at risk of having the disorder when adults, and there is not a causal treatment. Therefore, running the molecular test of the disorder would be inappropriate. If a mutation is found, the children will not longer lead a normal life and it will also have a negative effect on family life.

In HCM, the first step the geneticist should take is to order the molecular analyses of *MYH7* and *MYBPC3*, the two genes that carry most of the mutations.

Should the mutations not be in these two genes, the genetic analyses of *TNNT2, TNNT3, MYL2, MYL3, TPM1* and *ACTC* might clarify other cases.

Sometimes, if no mutations are found in any of the genes tested, the disorder cannot be ruled out because it is likely that a new gene not yet discovered can be the cause.

In DCM the mode of inheritance has to be defined in other to provide a correct counseling as the there is locus and allelic heterogeneity.

In the autosomal dominant cardiomyopathies most individuals diagnosed have an affected parent. However, the index case may have the disorder as the result of a *de novo* mutation.

In HCM, it is not known the number of cases that are caused by these *de novo* gene mutations. While in Brugada syndrome and in RWS *de novo* mutations are low, and in CPVT is almost 40%.

Timothy syndrome is due to either a *de novo* mutation or parental germline mosaicism. They do not live long enough to reproduce.

Only the siblings are at risk of inheriting the disorder.

When there is a *de novo* mutation, alternate paternity and maternity as well as whether the patient is adopted have to be ruled out.

The offspring of a patient suffering autosomal dominant familial cardiomyopathy has a 50% chance of inheriting the mutation. Families in which penetrance appears to be incomplete or reduced have been observed; therefore a parent with a mutation that causes the disorder is not affected whereas the son or daughter is. The severity and age of onset cannot be predicted.

The siblings of the index case depend on the genetic condition of their parents. If a parent is affected or has the mutation that causes the disorder, the risk to inherit the mutated allele is 50%.

In the cases reported where more than one mutation in one the genes encoding a sarcomere protein has been identified in a patient with HCM, it is very difficult to assess the mode of inheritance and makes it arduous for the geneticist to give an accurate risk assessment to another family member.

It is essential to provide patients and relatives that are at risk, the potential risk their offspring might have in these disorders and the reproductive options they have.

In the autosomal recessive traits the parents are obligate carriers. The offspring of a patient suffering an autosomal recessive familial cardiomyopathy will be obligate carriers. The siblings have a 25% chance of inheriting the mutation.

The deletions in mtDNA are usually due to *de novo* mutations, so there is only one family member affected. The offspring of a male patient are not at risk whereas all females' offspring are at risk of inheriting the mutation. There is not risk that any other family member will inherit the disease.

When there are multiple mtDNA deletions the analysis of *RRM2B* should be performed because it conditions the genetic counseling.

A prenatal diagnosis for those patients there are at risk for any cardiomyopathy is possible, if the mutation carried by the parents or the proband has been previously identified.

Preimplantation genetic diagnosis (PGD) may be available for families in which the mutation that causes the disorder has already been identified.

14. Conclusion

In spite of the fact that there has been considerable improvement in the molecular diagnosis of the different mutations that lead to cardiomyopathies, we still have to learn more about the pathophysiology of these sometimes deadly disorders.

Author details

Luis Vernengo[1], Alain Lilienbaum[2], Onnik Agbulut[2] and Maria-Mirta Rodríguez[1]

1 Clinical Unit, Department of Genetics, Faculty of Medicine, University of the Republic, Montevideo, Uruguay

2 University Paris Diderot-Paris , Unit of Functional and Adaptive Biology (BFA) affiliated with CNRS (EAC), Laboratory of Stress and Pathologies of the Cytoskeleton, Paris, France

References

[1] Aernout Somsen, Kees Hovingh G, Tulevski I. Familial dilated cardiomyopathy. In Baars H, van der Smagt, J, Doevendans P, editors. Clinical Cardiogenetics: Springer 2011; p. 63-78.

[2] Aleong, R.G., Milan, D.J. & Ellinor, P.T. (2007). The diagnosis and treatment of cardiac ion channelopathies: congenital long QT syndrome and Brugada syndrome. Cur Treat Opt in Cardio Med 2007; 9; 5:364-371.

[3] Al-Jassar C, Knowles T, Jeeves M et al. The nonlinear structure of the desmoplakin plakin domain and the effects of cardiomyopathy-linked mutations. J Mol Biol. 2011 411:1049-1061.

[4] Annan R, Nakagawa M, Miyata M et al. Cardiac involvement in mitocondrial disease. A study of 17 patients with documental mitochondrial DNA defects. Circulation 1995; 91:955-961.

[5] Awad M, Calkins H, Judge D. Mechanisms of disease: molecular genetics of arrhythmogenic right ventricular dysplasia/cardiomyopathy.Nat Clin Pract Cardiovasc (2008);5:258-67

[6] Baig M, Goldman J, Caforio A et al. Familial dilated cardiomyopathy: cardiac abnormalities are common in asymptomatic relatives and may represent early disease. J Am Coll Cardiol 1998; 3:195–201.

[7] Bahl A, Saikia U & Khullar Madhu. Idiopathic restrictive cardiomyopathy- perspectives from genetics studies. Is it time to Redefine these disorders. Cardiogenetics 2012: 2e4.

[8] Barresi R, Di Blasi C, Negri T, et al. Disruption of heart sarcoglycan complex and severe cardiomyopathy caused by beta sarcoglycan mutations. J Med Genet 2000; 37:102–107.

[9] Becane H, Bonne G, Varnous S et al. High incidence of sudden death with conduction system and myocardial disease due to lamins A and C gene mutation. Pacing Clin Electrophysiol 2000; 23:1661–6.

[10] Begoña B, Brugada J et al. The Brugada syndrome. In Baars H, van der Smagt, J, Doevendans P, editors. Clinical Cardiogenetics: Springer 2011; p.165-188.

[11] Budde B, Binner P, Waldmuller S et al. Noncompaction of the ventricular myocardium is associated with a de novo mutation in the beta-myosin heavy chain gene. PLoS One.2007; 2:e1362.

[12] Brodsky G, Muntoni F, Miocic S et al. Lamin A/C gene mutation associated with dilated cardiomyopathy with variable skeletal muscle involvement. Circulation 2000; 101:473–6.

[13] Carrasco L, Vernengo L, Mesa R et al. Síndrome de Kearns-Sayre. Presentación de un caso clínico y revisión de la bibliografía. Arch. Inst. Neurol. 2005; 8(2):31-35. [Article in Spanish. Abstract in English].

[14] Christiaans I & Carrier L. Hypertrophic cardiomyopathy In Baars H, van der Smagt, J, Doevendans P, editors. Clinical Cardiogenetics: Springer 2011; p.47-61.

[15] Connuck D, Sleeper L, Colan S et al. Characteristics and outcomes of cardiomyopathy in children with Duchenne or Becker muscular dystrophy: a comparative study from the Pediatric Cardiomyopathy Registry. Am Heart J 2008; 155:998–1005.

[16] Cox M & Hauer R. Arrhythmogenic right ventricular dysplasia/ cardiomyopathy from desmosome to disease. In Baars H, van der Smagt, J, Doevendans P, editors. Clinical Cardiogenetics: Springer 2011; p 80-96.

[17] Crilley J, Boehm E, Blair E et al. Hypertrophic cardiomyopathy due to sarcomeric gene mutations is characterized by impaired energy metabolism irrespective of the degree of hypertrophy. J Am Coll Cardiol 2003;41:1776–1787.

[18] De Ambroggi L, Raisaro A, Marchiano V, Radice S, Meola G. Cardiac involvement in patients with myotonic dystrophy: characteristic features of magnetic resonance imaging. Eur Heart J 1995;16:1007–10.

[19] Danek A, Rubio J, Rampoldi L et al. McLeod neuroacanthocytosis: genotype and phenotype. Ann Neurol 2001; 50:755–764.

[20] De Jonge N & Kirkels J. Restrictive cardiomyopathy. In Baars H, van der Smagt, J, Doevendans P, editors. Clinical Cardiogenetics: Springer 2011; p.123-128.

[21] Di Mauro S, Bonilla E, Zeviani M et al. Mitochondrial myopathies. Ann Neurol 1985; 17:521-538.

[22] Dooijes D, Hoedemaekers Y, Michels M et al. Left ventricular noncompaction cardiomyopathy: disease genes, mutation spectrum and diagnostic implications. Submitted. 2009.

[23] Elliott, P. Cardiomyopathy. Diagnosis and management of dilated cardiomyopathy. Heart 2000 84; 1; 106-112.

[24] Elliott P, Andersson, B, Arbustini E et al. Classification of the cardiomyopathies: a position statement from the European Society Of Cardiology Working Group on Myocardial and Pericardial Diseases. Euro Heart Journal 2008; 29:270-276.

[25] Fanin M, Melacini P, Boito C et al. LGMD2E patients risk developing dilated cardiomyopathy. Neuromuscul Disord 2003;13:303–309.

[26] Frank D & Frey N. Cardiac Z-disc Signaling Network. JBC 2011 286; 12: 9897–9904

[27] Freedom, R, Yoo, S, Perrin D et al. The morphological spectrum of ventricular noncompaction. Cardiology in the Young 2005; 15:345-364.

[28] Ga Overeem S, Schelhaas H, Blijham P et al. Symptomatic distal myopathy with cardiomyopathy due to a MYH7 mutation. Neuromuscul Disord 2007;17:490–3.

[29] George C, Higgs G, Lai F. Ryanodine receptor mutations associated with stress-induced ventricular tachycardia mediate increased calcium release in stimulated cardiomyocytes. Circ Res. (2003); 93:531–534.

[30] Goodwin JF.Cardiomyopathies and specific heart muscle diseases. Definitions, terminology, classifications and new and old approaches. Postgrad Med J. 1992;68 Suppl 1:S3-6.

[31] Goldfarb L, Dalakas M. Tragedy in a heartbeat: malfunctioning desmin causes skeletal and cardiac muscle disease. J Clin Invest 2009; 119:1806–1813.

[32] Hamid M, Norman M, Quraishi A, et al. Prospective evaluation of relatives for familial arrhythmogenic right ventricular cardiomyopathy/dysplasia reveals a need to broaden diagnostic criteria. J Am Coll Cardiol. 2002;40:1445-1450.

[33] Hayashi T, Arimura T, Itoh-Satoh M, et al. Tcap gene mutations in hypertrophic cardiomyopathy and dilated cardiomyopathy. J Am Coll Cardiol. 2004;44:2192-2201.

[34] Hedberg C, Melberg A, Kuhl A et al. Autosomal dominant myofibrillar myopathy with arrhythmogenic right ventricular cardiomyopathy 7 is caused by a DES mutation. Eur J Hum Genet 2012; 20:984-985.

[35] Hermida-Prieto MML, Castro-Beiras A, Laredo R et al. Familial dilated cardiomyopathy and isolated left ventricular noncompaction associated with Lamin A/C gene mutations. Am J Cardiol. 2004; 94:50 –54.

[36] Ho C, Lever H, DeSanctis R, Farver C et al. Homozygous mutation in cardiac troponin T: implications for hypertrophic cardiomyopathy. Circulation 2000;102:1950-1955.

[37] Hoedemaekers Y, Caliskan K, Michels M. The importance of genetic counseling, DNA diagnostics and cardiologic family screening in left ventricular noncompaction cardiomyopathy. Circ Cardiovasc Genet. 2010; 3:232-239.

[38] Hoedemaekers Y, Caliskan K, Majoor-Krakauer D. Non-compaction cardiomyopathy. In Baars H, van der Smagt, J, Doevendans P, editors. Clinical Cardiogenetics: Springer 2011; P.98-122.

[39] Holgrem D, Wahlander H, Eriksson, B et al. Cardiomyopathy in children with mitochondrial disease: clinical course and cardiologigal findings. Eur Heart J 2003; 24:280-288..

[40] Ichida F, Tsubata S, Bowles KR et al. Novel gene mutations in patients with left ventricular noncompaction or Barth syndrome. Circulation. 2001;103:1256 –1263.

[41] Ingles J, Doolan A, Chiu C et al. Compound and double mutations in patients with hypertrophic cardiomyopathy: implications for genetic testing and counselling. J Med Genet. 2005;42:e59.

[42] Jefferies, J & Towbin, J. (2010). Dilated cardiomyopathy. Lancet 2010; 375:752-762.

[43] Jefferies J, Eidem B, Belmont J et al. Genetic predictors and remodeling of dilated cardiomyopathy in muscular dystrophy. Circulation 2005; 112:2799–804.

[44] Kamisago M, Sharma S, DePalma S et al. Mutations in sarcomere protein genes as a cause of dilated cardiomyopathy. New Eng. J. Med. 2000; 343: 1688-1696

[45] Kass, R.S. The channelopathies: novel insights into molecular and genetic mechanisms of human disease J Clin Invest 2005; 115: 1986-1989,

[46] Katritsis D, Wilmshurst P, Wendon J et al. Primary restrictive cardiomyopathy: clinical and pathologic characteristics. J Am Coll Cardiol 1991;18:1230-1235

[47] Klaassen S, Probst S, Oechslin E et al. Thierfelder L. Mutations in sarcomere protein genes in left ventricular noncompaction. Circulation 2008; 117:2893–2901

[48] Kaski J, Syrris P, Burch M, Tomé-Esteban M et al. Idiopathic restrictive cardiomyopathy in children is caused by mutations in cardiac sarcomere protein genes. Heart 2008; 94:1478–1484.

[49] Kaspar R, Allen H, Ray W et al. Alvarez CE, Kissel JT, Pestronk A, et al. Analysis of dystrophin deletion mutations predicts age of cardiomyopathy onset in Becker muscular dystrophy. Circ Cardiovasc Genet 2009; 2:544–51.

[50] Kirkels J & de Jonge N.Mitochondrial cardiomyopathy. In Baars H, van der Smagt, J, Doevendans P, editors. Clinical Cardiogenetics: Springer 2011; p123-128.

[51] Kirkels J & de Jonge N. Restrictive cardiomyopathy. In In Baars H, van der Smagt, J, Doevendans P, editors. Clinical Cardiogenetics: Springer 2011; p130-139.

[52] Klauke B, Kossmann S, Gaertner A et al. De novo desmin-mutation N116S is associated with arrhythmogenic right ventricular cardiomyopathy. Hum Mol Genet 2010; 19; 4595–4607.

[53] Kumar Singh B, Kolappa Pilla K et al. Classification and definitions of cardiomyopathies. In Joseph Veselka, editor.: Cardiomyopathies –from basic research to clinical management InTech 2012; p.3-20.

[54] Kushwaha S, Narula J, Narula N et al.Pattern of changes over time in myocardial blood flow and microvascular dilator capacity in patients with normally functioning cardiac allografts. Am J Cardiol. (1998); 82:1377-81.

[55] Lazarus A, Varin J, Ounnoughene Z et al. Relationships among electrophysiological findings and clinical status, heart function, and extent of DNA mutation in myotonic dystrophy. Circulation 1999; 99:1041–6.

[56] Lilienbaum A & Vernengo L. Cardiomyopathies associated with myofibrillar myopathies .In Joseph Veselka, editor.: Cardiomyopathies –from basic research to clinical management InTech 2012; p.353-382.

[57] Lo-A-Njoe SM, Wilde AA et al. Syndactyly and long QT syndrome (CaV1.2 missense mutation G640R) is associated with hypertrophic cardiomyopathy. Heart Rhythm. 2005; 2:1365–1368.

[58] Mangin L, Charron P, Tesson F et al. Familial dilated cardiomyopathy: clinical features in French families.. Eur J Heart Fail 1999; 1 4: 353-361.

[59] Marian A, Roberts R. The molecular genetic basis for hypertrophic cardiomyopathy. J Mol Cell Cardiol 2001; 33:655.

[60] Marks M, Trippel D, Keating M. Long QT syndrome associated with syndactyly identified in females. Am J Cardiol. 1995a;76:744–5.

[61] Marks ML, Whisler SL, Clericuzio C, Keating M. A new form of long QT syndrome associated with syndactyly. J Am Coll Cardiol. 1995b; 25:59–64.

[62] Maron, BJ. Cardiology patient pages. Hypertrophic cardiomyopathy. Circulation (2002); 106:2419-2421,

[63] Maron BJ, Towbin JA, Thiene G et al.. Contemporary definitions and classification of the cardiomyopathies. An American Heart Association scientific statement from the Council on Clinical Cardiology, Heart Failure and Transplantation Committee; Quality of Care and Outcomes Research and Functional Genomics and Translational Biology Interdisciplinary Working Groups; and Council on Epidemiology and Prevention. Circulation (2006). 1;113:1807–1816.

[64] Maron, B.J. (2008). The 2006 American Heart Association classification of cardiomyopathies is the gold standard. Circulation Heart Failure (2008). 1; 72-75.

[65] McKoy G, Protonotarios N, Crosby A et al. Identification of a deletion in plakoglobin in arrhythmogenic right ventricular cardiomyopathy with palmoplantar keratoderma and woolly hair (Naxos disease). Lancet. (2000); 355:2119-2124.

[66] Melacini P, Fanin M, Duggan D et al. Heart involvement in muscular dystrophies due to sarcoglycan gene mutations. Muscle Nerve 1999; 22:473–479.

[67] Melberg A, Oldfors, A, Blomstrom-Lundqvist C et al. Autosomal dominant myofibrillar myopathy with arrhythmogenic right ventricular cardiomyopathy linked to chromosome 10q .Ann. Neurol. 46: 684-692, 1999.

[68] Menon S., Michels V, Pellikka et al. Cardiac troponin T mutation in familial cardiomyopathy with variable remodeling and restrictive physiology. Clin. Genet. 2008; 74: 445-454.

[69] Mestroni L, Rocco C, Gregori D, et al. Familial dilated cardiomyopathy: evidence for genetic and phenotypic heterogeneity. Heart Muscle Disease Study Group. J Am Coll Cardiol 1999; 34:181–90.

[70] Michels V, Moll P, Miller F et al. The frequency of familial dilated cardiomyopathy in a series of patients with idiopathic dilated cardiomyopathy. N Engl J Med 1992; 326:77– 82.

[71] Modell, S.M. & Lehmann, M.H. (2006).The long QT syndrome family of cardiac ion channelopathies: a HuGE review. . Genet in Med 2006; 8;143-155

[72] Moolman J, Corfield V, Posen B et al. Sudden death due to troponin T mutations. J Am Coll Cardiol 1997;29:549.

[73] Monserrat L, Hermida-Prieto M, Fernandez X et al. Mutation in the alpha-cardiac actin gene associated with apical hypertrophic cardiomyopathy, left ventricular noncompaction, and septal defects. Eur Heart J. 2007; 28:1953–1961.

[74] Nakanishi T, Sakauchi M, Kaneda Y et al. Cardiac involvement in Fukuyama-type congenital muscular dystrophy. Pediatrics 2006;117:e1187–119.

[75] Nguyen H, Wolfe 3rd J, Holmes Jr D, Edwards W. Pathology of the cardiac conduction system in myotonic dystrophy: a study of 12 cases. J Am Coll Cardiol 1988; 11:662–71.

[76] Nimura H, Bachinski L, Sangwatanaroj S et al. Mutations in the gene for cardiac myosin-binding protein C and late-onset familial hypertrophic cardiomyopathy. N Engl J Med 1998;338:1248–57.

[77] Nimura H, Patton K, McKenna W et al. Sarcomere protein gene mutations in hypertrophic cardiomyopathy of the elderly. Circulation. 2002;105:446–51

[78] Norgett E, HatsellS, Carvajal-Huerta L et al. Recessive mutation in desmoplakin disrupts desmoplakin-intermediate filament interactions and causes dilated cardiomyopathy, woolly hair and keratoderma. Hum. Mol. Genet 2000; 9:2761-2766.

[79] Okajima Y, Tanabe Y, Takayanagi M, Aotsuka H. A follow up study of myocardial involvement in patients with mitochondrial encephalomyopathy, lactic acidosis and strokelike episodes (MELAS). Heart. (1998); 80:292-295.

[80] Olson T; Illenberger S, Kishimoto N et al. Metavinculin mutations alter actin interaction in dilated cardiomyopathy. Circulation. 2002; 105: 431-437.

[81] Peddy S, Vricella L, Crosson J et al. Infantile restrictive cardiomyopathy resulting from a mutation in the cardiac troponin T gene. Pediatrics 2006; 117:1830-1833.

[82] Peters S. Advances in the diagnostic management of arrhythmogenic right ventricular dysplasia-cardiomyopathy. Int J Cardiol. 2006;113:4–11.

[83] Politano L, Nigro V, Passamano L et al. Evaluation of cardiac and respiratory involvement in sarcoglycanopathies. Neuromuscul Disord 2001;11:178–185.

[84] Protonotarios N, Tsatsopoulou A, Patsourakos P et al. Cardiac abnormalities in familial palmoplantar keratosis. Brit. Heart J. 56: 321-326, 1986.

[85] Richard P, Isnard R, Carrier L, et al. Double heterozygosity for mutations in the betamyosin heavy chain and in the cardiac myosin binding protein C genes in a family with hypertrophic cardiomyopathy. J Med Genet. 1999;36:542-545.

[86] Richard P, Charron P, Carrier L, et al. Hypertrophic cardiomyopathy: distribution of disease genes, spectrum of mutations, and implications for a molecular diagnosis strategy. Circulation. 2003;107:2227-2232.

[87] Richard P, Villard E, Charron P, Isnard R. The genetic bases of cardiomyopathies. J Am Coll Cardiol. 2006;48:A79–8

[88] Richardson P, McKenna W, Bristow M, et al. Report of the 1995 World Health Organization/International Society and Federation of Cardiology Task Force on the Definition and Classification of Cardiomyopathies. Circulation 1996;93:841–842.

[89] Roberts N, Perloff J, Kark R. A follow up study of myocardial involvement in patients with mitochondrial encephalomyopathy, lactic acidosis, and stroke-like episodes (MELAS). Heart (1998);80:292-2955.

[90] Sealove B, Tiyyagura S, & Fuster, V. Takotsubo cardiomyopathy. J of Gen Intern Med, 2008; 23; 1904-1908.

[91] Schlame M, Ren M. Barth syndrome, a human disorder of cardiolipin metabolism. FEBS Lett. (2006) ;580:5450-5455.

[92] Schonberger J, Seidman CE. Many roads lead to a broken heart: the genetics of dilated cardiomyopathy. Am. J. Hum. Genet. 69: 249-260, 2001.

[93] Schoser B, Ricker, K, Schneider-Gold C et al. Sudden cardiac death in myotonic dystrophy type 2. Neurology 2004; 63: 2402-2404.

[94] Schwartz P, Moss A, Vincent G, Crampton R. Diagnostic criteria for the long QT syndrome. An update. Circulation. (1993); 88:782–784.

[95] Schwartz P, Priori S, Spazzolini C et al. Genotype-phenotype correlation in the long-QT syndrome: gene-specific triggers for life-threatening arrhythmias. Circulation. (2001);103:89–95.

[96] Schwartz P, Crotti L. QTc behavior during exercise and genetic testing for the long-QT syndrome. Circulation. (2011); 124:2181–2184.

[97] Selcen D, Engel AG. Myofibrillar myopathy caused by novel dominant negative alpha B-crystallin mutations. Ann Neurol 2003; 54:804–810.

[98] Shan L, Makita N, Xing Y et al. SCN5A variants in Japanese patients with left ventricular noncompaction and arrhythmia. Mol Genet Metab. 2008;93:468–474.

[99] Sharkey S., Lesser J, Zenovich et al.. Acute and reversible cardiomyopathy provoked by stress in women from the United States. Circulation 2005; 111:472-479

[100] Spencer C, Bryant R, Day J et al. Cardiac and clinical phenotype in Barth syndrome. Pediatrics 2006;118:e337–346.

[101] Splawski I, Timothy K, Sharpe L et al. Ca(V)1.2 calcium channel dysfunction causes a multisystem disorder including arrhythmia and autism. Cell (2004); 119:19-31.

[102] Splawski I, Timothy KW, Decher N et al. Severe arrhythmia disorder caused by cardiac L-type calcium channel mutations. Proc Natl Acad Sci USA. (2005); 102:8089–8096.

[103] Sugrue DD, Rodeheffer RJ, Codd MB, et al. The clinical course of idiopathic dilated cardiomyopathy: a population-based study. Ann Intern Med (1992);117:117–123.

[104] Tardiff JC. Sarcomeric proteins and familial hypertrophic cardiomyopathy: linking mutations in structural proteins to complex cardiovascular phenotypes. Heart Fail Rev 2005;10:237

[105] Teare D.Asymmetrical hypertrophy of the heart Br heart J 1958;20:1-8 Postgrad Med J 1992;68 Suppl 1:S3-6.

[106] Thierfelder, L., Watkins, H., MacRae, C et al .Alpha-tropomyosin and cardiac troponin T mutations cause familial hypertrophic cardiomyopathy: a disease of the sarcomere, Cell 1994; 77: 701-712,

[107] Uro-Coste E, Arne-Bes M, Pellissier J et al. Striking phenotypic variability in two familial cases of myosin storage myopathy with a MYH7 Leu1793pro mutation. Neuromuscul Disord 2009; 19:163–1636.

[108] Van der Werf C & Wilde A. Catecholaminergic polymorphic ventricular tachycardia. In Baars H, van der Smagt, J, Doevendans P, editors. Clinical Cardiogenetics: Springer 2011; p.197-206.

[109] Van der Zwaag, P, Jongbloed J, van den Berg M et al. A genetic variants database for arrhythmogenic right ventricular dysplasia/cardiomyopathy. Hum Mutat 2009; 30:1278–1283.

[110] Van Driest SL, Vasile VC, Ommen SR, Will ML, Jamil Tajik A, Gersh BJ,Ackerman MJ. Myosin binding protein C mutations and compoundheterozygosity in hypertrophic cardiomyopathy. J Am Coll Cardiol2004;44:1903–1016 ;

[111] Van Tintelen J, Van Gelder I, Asimaki A et al. Severe cardiac phenotype with right ventricular predominance in a large cohort of patients with a single missense mutation in the DES gene. Heart Rhythm 2009; 6: 1574–1583.

[112] Vatta M, Mohapatra B, Jimenez S et al. Mutations in Cypher/ZASP in patients with dilated cardiomyopathy and left ventricular noncompaction. J Am Coll Cardiol 2003;42:2014 –2027.

[113] Vernengo L, Choubargi O, Panuncio A et al. Desmin myopathy with severe cardiomyopathy in a Uruguayan family due to a codon deletion in a new location within the desmin 1A rod domain. Neuromuscul Disord 2010; 20:178-187.

[114] Vicart P, Caron A, Guicheney P et al. A missense mutation in the alphaB-crystallin chaperone gene causes a desmin-related myopathy. Nat Genet 1998; 20:92–95.

[115] Walter L, Nogueira V, Leverve X et al. Three classes of ubiquinone analogs regulate the mitochondrial permeability transition pore through a common site. J Biol Chem (2000); 275:29521-29527.

[116] Watkins H, McKenna WJ, Thierfelder L, et al. Mutations in the genes for cardiac troponin T and alpha-tropomyosin in hypertrophic cardiomyopathy. N Engl J Med 1995;332:1058.

[117] Wilde A, Bhuiyan Z, Crotti L et al Left cardiac sympathetic denervation for catecholaminergic polymorphic ventricular tachycardia. N Engl J Med. (2008); 358:2024–2029.

[118] Wolpert C, Veltmann C et al. Short QT syndrome. In Baars H, van der Smagt, J, Doevendans P, editors. Clinical Cardiogenetics: Springer 2011; p.189-196.

[119] Zhang, J., Kumar, A., Stalker, H et al.Clinical and molecular studies of a large family with desmin-associated restrictive cardiomyopathy.Clin. Genet. 2001; 59:248-256.

[120] Zhang J, Kumar A, Kaplan L et al. Genetic linkage of a novel autosomal dominant restrictive cardiomyopathy locus. J Med Genet 2005;42:663-665.

Chapter 8

Specific Forms of Cardiomyopathy: Genetics, Clinical Presentation and Treatment

M. Obadah Al Chekakie

Additional information is available at the end of the chapter

http://dx.doi.org/10.5772/55628

1. Introduction

Ischemic heart disease is the most common cause of cardiomyopathy and has been the subject of intense research and study. However, other rare forms of cardiomyopathy exist and represent a diagnostic as well as a therapeutic challenge for the clinician. This chapter aims to review the rare forms of cardiomyopathy, from genetic abnormalities, clinical presentation to treatment and sudden death prevention.

2. Cardiac sarcoidosis

2.1. Introduction

Sarcoidosis is a multisystem disease characterized by noncaseating granulomas involving multiple organ systems. Cardiac involvement is relatively rare and ranges from 5 to 40%. Clinically, patients could have palpitations, atrioventricular block, syncope, shortness of breath, left ventricular dysfunction and sudden cardiac death. Early recognition and treatment is important since cardiac involvement portends a poor prognosis and is the second cause of death in patients with sarcoidosis [1].

2.2. Epidemiology

Sarcoidosis is common in Japan, Ireland, Scandanavia and the United States. Females are more commonly affected than males. In the United States, African Americans are more commonly affected and in general have more severe forms of the disease. The age adjusted annual incidence is highest for African American females in the age group of 30 to 39 years and is at 107 per 100,000 [2]. Clinical cardiac involvement is reported to be 5%, while subclinical cardiac involvement detected by imaging studies is in the range of 30-40%, which matches autopsy series.

2.3. Environmental and genetic factors

The etiology of sarcoidosis remains unknown. The presence of noncaseating granulomas in the lungs, skin and eyes and clustering of cases in certain occupations (navy personnel, firefighters at the world trade center) point to an immunological response to environmental agents or infectious exposure [3, 4]. Mycobacterial DNA and RNA have been found in sarcoid tissue using polymerase chain reaction, especially the DNA of the mycobacterium tuberculosis catalase-peroxidase (mKatG) gene [5].

There is familial clustering of the disease, and patients are more likely to have an affected member but there is little concordance in organs involved. Class I HLA-B8 and Class II HLA-DRB1 and HLA-DQB1 alleles have been consistently associated with sarcoidosis [6, 7]. Genome-wide scans for loci associated with sarcoidosis showed the strongest signals in chromosomes 5p and 5q in African Americans [8]. The strongest signals in Germans were found in chromosome 6p, which helped identify the butyrophillin-like 2 (BTLN2) gene. This gene is a negative co-stimulatory molecule within the major histocompatibility complex region [9]. Chromosome 18q22 has a strong link to the presence of cardiac or renal sarcoidosis [10]. Likely there is an interaction between environmental exposure and certain susceptibility genes leading to the development of sarcoidosis. Further research is needed to clarify such interactions.

2.4. Pathology

The hallmark of sarcoidosis is the presence of noncaseating granulomas. These are compact collections of macrophages and epithelioid cells with minimal inflammation and multinucleated giant cells. Even though clinical involvement of the heart is reported to be 5%, autopsy series show cardiac involvement in 25 to 40% of patients [11, 12]. Several recent imaging studies show that delayed enhancement magnetic resonance imaging (DE MRI) in patients with histology proven extra-cardiac sarcoidosis could detect cardiac involvement even in patients with normal electrocardiograms, with cardiac involvement in these studies ranging from 26-32%, which matches autopsy series [13, 14]. The ventricles are commonly affected, especially the left ventricular (LV) free wall, basal LV, inter-ventricular septum and conduction system. The heart could be involved among other systems, but isolated cardiac disease does occur. Endomyocardial biopsy has a low yield (~20%) given the patchy involvement of the heart muscle. However, it is still needed at times in diagnosis especially when other diseases are suspected.

2.5. Clinical features of cardiac sarcoidosis

The heart could be the only organ affected or could be involved in combination with other systems. The degree of lung involvement does not predict cardiac involvement and cardiac involvement can be subclinical without any apparent symptoms. Patients might have non-specific symptoms like shortness of breath and fatigue. Palpitations are common and could be due to atrial tachycardia, atrial fibrillation, premature ventricular contractions, sustained and non-sustained ventricular tachycardia. Rarely patients could present with pericarditis and cardiac tamponade. The most common criteria used for diagnosing cardiac sarcoidosis is the 2006 revised guidelines of the Japanese Ministry of Health and Wellness [15]. Table 1 gives a summary of these guidelines.

Advanced atrioventricular block in young patients should prompt search for cardiac sarcoidosis especially in females [16]. Patients with extra-cardiac sarcoidosis and abnormalities in the electrocardiogram (ECG) should have at least an echocardiogram performed to look for left ventricular function, especially when symptoms suggestive of heart failure are present. However, the JMHW guidelines are not very sensitive and cardiac involvement could be present even in patients with normal electrocardiograms [17]. There is no consensus about the best way to screen patients with sarcoidosis for cardiac involvement. In a recent Delphi study on diagnosing cardiac sarcoidosis, a survey of a group of sarcoidosis experts from different subspecialties including pulmonologists, cardiologist and electrophysiologists showed a wide range of practices with most experts utilizing history, physical examination and ECG for screening. About 75% of experts would not do any further testing in the absence of symptoms or signs of cardiac involvement along with normal ECG. But when Cardiac sarcoidosis is suspected, most experts would perform ECG, TTE and cardiac MRI and 67% would order Holter monitor and cardiac fluorodeoxy-glucose (FDG) PET scan [18]. This reflects the wide range of clinical practice and the fact that sarcoidosis in general can mimic other diseases and could stay subclinical. However, it is clear from recent cardiac MRI studies that cardiac involvement can be present in patients with no cardiac symptoms and a normal ECG in 30% of patients with biopsy proven extracardiac sarcoidosis [17]. Smedema et al study suggests that the combination of ECG and MRI is the most cost effective for screening [14]. It is important to diagnose cardiac sarcoidosis, as patients with cardiac involvement die for heart failure or sudden cardiac death.

2.6. Laboratory investigations

Laboratory testing in sarcoidosis is non-specific. Patient can have anemia and some might have hypercalcemia due to activation of vitamin D by macrophages present in granulomas [19]. Elevated angiotensin converting enzyme levels were proposed initially as a diagnostic test and to follow treatment response. However, there is a wide range of normal in healthy subjects and it is a poor therapeutic guide [20].

2.7. Electrocardiography (ECG)

The ECG has been used as a screening tool for cardiac involvement in patients with sarcoidosis. Abnormalities noted include right bundle branch block (RBBB), which can be seen in 20-25% of patients. Premature ventricular contractions (PVCs), non-sustained ventricular tachycardia (NSVT) and sustained ventricular tachycardia (VT) could also occur. Inflammation and scar formation lead to slow conduction and reentry, which is the mechanism of VT in these patients

Histologic diagnosis group	Cardiac sarcoidosis is confirmed when endomyocardial biopsy specimens demonstrate noncaseating epithelioid granulomas.
Clinical diagnosis group*	Cardiac sarcoidosis is diagnosed in the absence of an endomyocardial biopsy specimen or in the absence of typical granulomas on cardiac biopsy when extracardiac sarcoidosis has been proven and a combination of majore or minor diagnostic criteria has been satisfied: 1. More than 2 of the 4 major diagnostic criteria are met OR 2. One of the 4 major criteria and 2 or more of the minor criteria are met. Major Criteria: 1. Advanced AV block 2. Basal thinning of the ventricular septum 3. Positive cardiac gallium uptake 4. Left ventricular ejection fraction < 50%. Minor Criteria: 1. Abnormal electrocardiogram findings including ventricular tachycardia, multifocal frequent premature ventricular contractions, complete right bundle branch block, pathologic Q waves or abnormal axis deviation 2. Abnormal echocardiogram demonstrating regional wall motion abnormalities, ventricular aneurysm or unexplained increase in wall thickness. 3. Perfusion defects detected by myocardial scintigraphy 4. Delayed godalinium enhancement of the myocardium on cardiac MRI scanning 5. Interstitial fibrosis or monocyte infiltration greater than moderate grade by endomyocardial biopsy.

Table 1. Modified Guidelines for the Diagnosis of Cardiac Sarcoidosis from the Japanese Ministry of Health and Wellness

[21]. Left bundle branch block and Q waves have been described [22]. Advanced atrioventricular block (AVB) and complete heart block could occur in up to 20-30% of patients due to the involvement of the basal LV septum as well as involvement of the AV nodal artery and they portend a poor prognosis [16]. In patients with symptomatic cardiac sarcoidosis, Shuller et al showed that fragmentation of the QRS occurs in up to 75% of patients and when combined with bundle branch block, has 90% sensitivity in detecting cardiac involvement, however, the study was limited to symptomatic patients [22]. Mehta et al showed that ECG sensitivity could be as low as 8%. Using 24 hours holter monitoring could help detect abnormalities including AV block, PVCs and NSVT and has more sensitivity compared to the 12 lead electrocardiogram (50% vs 8% respectively) [17].

2.8. Endomyocardial biopsy

The presence of noncaseating granulomas in endomyocardial biopsy is diagnostic of sarcoidosis. However, endomyocardial biopsy is not sensitive, since the disease is usually patchy and most commonly involves the left ventricle. Of the 28 patients with clinical

http://dx.doi.org/10.5772/55628

systematic sarcoidosis with documented cardiomyopathy who underwent endomyocardial biopsy at John Hopkins, only 7 had noncasesating granulomas. If sarcoidosis is suspected, it is often recommended to obtain biopsy from other organs like the paratracheal lymphnodes, skin and even the liver. PET scanning could help detect disease activity and potential sites for biopsy [23].

The main differential diagnosis to sarcoidosis histologically is giant cell myocarditis. In a series comparing 42 patients with cardiac sarcoidosis to 73 patients with giant cell myocarditis, nearly a third of the patients finally diagnosed with cardiac sarcoidosis had no extracardiac involvement. Underscoring the fact that isolated cardiac involvement does occur [24]. Table 2 lists the features that help differentiate cardiac sarcoidosis from giant cell myocarditis. Rarely, cardiac sarcoidosis could only be diagnosed at the time of heart transplantation, further scoring the difficulties of establishing the diagnosis [25].

	Sarcoidosis	**Giant Cell Myocarditis**
African American race	31%	4%
Syncope	31%	5%
AV block	50%	15%
Clinical Presentation	AV block or heart failure symptoms of > 9 weeks duration	Usually acute heart failure presentation
Histology	Granulomas and fibrosis	Eosinophils, myocyte damage and foci of lymphocytic myocarditis

Table 2. Clinical and Histological features comparing Sarcoidosis to Giant Cell Myocarditis.

2.9. Imaging studies in cardiac sarcoidosis

2.9.1. Chest x-ray

Bilateral hilar lymphadenopathy is the most common finding on chest x-ray (CXR). However, bilateral hilar fullness could be also a sign of pulmonary dilatation secondary to cardiac involvement or pulmonary hypertension. Cardiomegaly is sometimes noted. When bilateral hilar lymphadenopathy is found and sarcoidosis is suspected, then high resolution computed tomography scan is indicated to detect pulmonary parenchymal involvement [19].

2.9.2. Echocardiography

Transthoracic echocardiography (TTE) could be useful in detecting cardiac involvement in patients diagnosed with extracardiac sarcoidosis. Segmental wall motion abnormalities with thinning of the ventricular wall and LV dysfunction are common but non-specific findings. The presence of basal septal thinning in the LV should lead the clinician to consider sarcoidosis highly in the differential diagnoses especially in young patients with conduction abnormalities [26]. Aneurysms could be seen especially in the inferior wall. Regional hypertrophy could also be found due to inflammation and edema. Right ventricular dysfunction is also seen and in later stages of pulmonary sarcoidosis, pulmonary hypertension and tricuspid regurgitation are seen. Mitral regurgitation and rarely pericardial effusion with tamponade physiology could be the first presentation in patients with sarcoidosis [27]. The sensitivity of TTE in detecting cardiac involvement in patients with extracardiac sarcoidosis is poor, and ranges from 14-25% [17, 28].

2.9.3. Magnetic Resonance Imaging (MRI)

Cardiac MRI has emerged as a sensitive modality to detect clinical and subclinical cardiac sarcoidosis. It has great spatial resolution and can help detect disease activity, presence or absence of fibrosis, wall motion abnormalities, pericardial involvement as well as right ventricular involvement. Increased signal intensity on T2 weighted images signifies edema and inflammation. Focal myocardial thickening can also be due to edema. Delayed enhancement using godalinium is likely due to fibrosis. The basal and lateral LV walls are most commonly affected, especially the basal septum [29]. Delayed enhancement MRI is more sensitive than ^{201}Thallium imaging and ^{67}Ga imaging in detecting subclinical cardiac sarcoidosis. In a study of 10 patients by Tadamura et al, only 50% of patients with sarcoidosis exhibited abnormalities on ^{201}Thallium imaging and only 20% had ^{67}Ga uptake while a 100% of these patients had abnormalities detected by cardiac MRI [30]. Smedema et al studied 58 patients with biopsy proven extracardiac sarcoidosis using the JMHW 1993 criteria as gold standard. Other modalities studied included ECG, TTE, ^{201}Thallium scintigrams and DE MRI. Cardiac MRI had a sensitivity of 78-100% and specificity of 64-89% in detecting cardiac involvement. Cardiac MRI was noted to detect cardiac involvement even in patients with normal ECG, Echocardiography and ^{201}Thallium Scintigrams [14].

Mehta et al studied 62 patients with extracardiac sarcoidosis using a systematic approach including ECG, Holter monitoring, TTE, ^{18}F-FDG PET scanning and cardiac MRI. The prevalence of cardiac sarcoidosis was 39%. The modified JMHW criteria had a sensitivity of 33% and specificity of 97%. Holter monitoring was superior of ECG in detecting conduction system abnormalities as well as other ventricular arrhythmias. In the 22 patients who had both cardiac MRI and ^{18}F-FDG PET scans done, 32% had delayed enhancement and 5% had edema on T2 images while abnormalities on ^{18}F-FDG PET scan was observed in 86% of the patients. Cardiac MRI and PET scans can be reasonably done in patients with suspected cardiac sarcoidosis and can detect subclinical involvement and are more sensitive than the JWHW criteria [17]. Patel et al studied 81 patients with biopsy proven extracardiac sarcoidosis and used the JMHW modified criteria as well as DE MRI to look for cardiac involvement. The JMHW identified 10 patients (12%) with cardiac involvement while DE MRI identified cardiac involvement in 21 patients (26%), only 8 patients overlapped. The median extent of damage detected by DE MRI was 6.1% of the left ventricle. The basal and mid ventricular septum showed delayed enhancement in 76% of patients. Furthermore, of the 4 patients with positive endomyocardial biopsy, all the 4 patients (100%) had abnormalities detected by DE MRI, while only 2 patients (50%) met the diagnostic criteria of the JMHW. Patients with DE MRI had 11-fold increase risk of death compared to patients without DE MRI findings [13]. Furthermore, delayed enhancement correlated with disease duration, regional wall motion abnormalities, ventricular function, severity of mitral regurgitation and presence of ventricular tachycardia [31].

2.9.4. Radionuclide scintigraphy

^{201}Thallium has been used to detect cardiac involvement in patients with sarcoidosis. Segmental areas of decreased perfusion at rest that improve with stress imaging (areas with reverse distribution) are seen in patients with cardiac sarcoidosis but are not necessarily specific, since they are also seen in other forms of cardiomyopathy. ^{201}Thallium is more sensitive than ^{67}Ga scanning in detecting cardiac sarcoidosis, but ^{67}Ga is more specific for sarcoidosis since it accumulates in inflamed areas and could be used to predict response to therapy and follow disease activity [32]. ^{67}Ga scanning has the advantage of detecting cardiac as well as extracardiac sarcoidosis and could guide to areas that are more amenable to biopsy [33]. Both modalities suffer from poor spatial resolution and both are less sensitive than DE MRI in detecting cardiac sarcoidosis [13, 30]. ^{99m}Tc-sestamibi has been used in combination with ^{67}Ga scanning and could help in showing that areas with increased ^{67}Ga uptake are due to cardiac as opposed to extracardiac involvement [34].

18- fluoro-2-deoxy-D-glucose PET scanning (^{18}F-FDG PET) has been shown to be of great value in detecting cardiac involvement in patients with sarcoidosis. ^{18}F-FDG PET is taken up by the macrophages, lymphocytes and epitheloid cells which are present in the granulomas and is helpful in detecting active inflammation and following response to corticosteroids treatment. In a series of 17 patients with biopsy proven extracardiac sarcoidosis, ^{18}F-FDG PET was found to be the more sensitive in detecting cardiac involvement compared to both ^{201}Thallium and ^{67}Ga scintigraphy. While ^{67}Ga scintigraphy was the least sensitive modality in detecting cardiac involvement, possibly because of it has a lower spatial resolution compared to ^{18F}-FDG PET. Most of the abnormalities noted on ^{18}F-FDG PET were found in the basal, mid anteroseptal and lateral walls and disappeared after treatment with corticosteroids [35]. In another study, PET and DE MRI were performed in patients with biopsy proven extracardiac sarcoidosis. In these series, 22 patients had both ^{18}F-FDG PET and DE MRI performed. Of these, abnormalities in ^{18}F-FDG PET were observed in 86% of the patients while MRI abnormalities were observed in 36% of the patients. It is possible that the apparent high sensitivity of ^{18}F-FDG PET is due to its ability to detect active inflammation while DE MRI could only detect edema and scar and is unable to detect active inflammation [17].

2.10. Therapy

Therapy for cardiac sarcoidosis aims at treating and preventing heart failure, treatment of conduction system disease and prevention of sudden cardiac death. It is important to recognize cardiac involvement in patients with sarcoidosis, since sudden cardiac death could be the first presentation and is the second leading cause of death in patients with sarcoidosis [1].

2.10.1. Medical therapy

Similar to other forms of cardiomyopathy, treatment with angiotensin converting enzyme inhibitors and angiotensin receptor blockers is important since they have anti-fibrotic properties and have been shown to improve survival. β -blockers were also shown to improve survival in patients with heart failure. Since the initial cardiac lesions are due to granuloma formation which could progress with time to fibrosis, early recognition and initiation of corticosteroid treatment is important and could lead to improvement in LV function as well as achieve control of the arrhythmias [36]. In a Japanese retrospective study of 48 patients with cardiac sarcoidosis, only patients with pretreatment LVEF > 30% had improvement in their LV function with corticosteroid therapy, while those with pretreatment LVEF of < 30% showed little improvement [37]. The exact dose of corticosteroids and the duration of therapy are not well defined due to the absence of randomized controlled trials. In general, initial dose of 30 to 60 milligrams/day of prednisone is started for 8-12 weeks; with gradual taper to a daily dose of 5-10 mgs/day of prednisone over 6-12 months is recommended. Relapses could occur in up to 25% of patients [19, 38]. Use of Methotrexate, cyclosporine or hydroxychoroquine has been described and could be considered especially in patients with side effects to corticosteroids or who are not responding to therapy [38].

2.10.2. Device based therapy and the role of electrophysiology study

Patients presenting with heart block due to cardiac sarcoidosis could see improvement with corticosteroids therapy [36]. However, permanent pacemaker implantation is recommended even if there is a transient improvement in heart block with corticosteroids therapy [39]. Patients with depressed LVEF < 35%who do not improve with steroid therapy and patients who present with VT or survive cardiac arrest should undergo defibrillator (ICD) implantation [39]. Some experts advocate ICD implantation in patients with AVB due to cardiac sarcoidosis with extensive cardiac involvement on imaging studies even if the LVEF is still preserved [40]. The 2008 guidelines for device based therapy recommend consideration for defibrillator implantation to be based on LV function, presence of spontaneous or induced ventricular tachycardia, heart failure status and syncope. Patients with depressed LVEF < 35%, NYHA Class II-IV heart failure and wide QRS of > 120 milliseconds are candidates for biventricular defibrillator implantation (BiV ICD) [39].

For patients with LVEF of 35-55%, programmed electrical stimulation (PES) could help in the risk stratification of these patients. In a study by Mehta et al, PES helped identify patients at risk of ventricular arrhythmias and only 1 of the 68 patients with negative PES died over 5 yrs [41]. In another series by Aizer et al, PES was predictive of arrhythmic events and ICD therapy; however 2 of the 20 patients with negative PES died or had spontaneous sustained VT during follow up [42]. Currently, PES is used for risk stratification, but the negative predictive value of programmed electrical stimulation needs further study and the clinician needs to utilize knowledge of the published literature as well as clinical judgment when considering ICD therapy for primary prevention of SCD in sarcoidosis patients with LVEF of 35-55%.

There are no randomized trials for the prevention of sudden cardiac death in patients with cardiac sarcoidosis, and most of the efficacy is obtained from the experience of tertiary care

http://dx.doi.org/10.5772/55628

centers. In a retrospective study of patients with sarcoidosis who received ICD therapy, inappropriate shocks were low (13.3%) and appropriate shocks occurred in 37.8%, with an annual incidence of 15% per year. Most of the event occurred in the first 3 years post implantation [43]. In another study of 112 patients with cardiac sarcoidosis that had ICD implantation, 32% had appropriate ICD therapy and 14% had VT storm. Inappropriate therapies occurred in 11% of patients [44]. Depressed LVEF, Depressed RVEF and complete heart block were important predictors of appropriate ICD therapies [44].

For patients who have frequent shocks due to ventricular tachycardia, catheter ablation could be used for treatment of these VTs. The mechanism of VT in patients with sarcoidosis is mostly due to reentry or triggered activity. Reentry is the most common mechanism and could be due to slow conduction from active inflammation or from scar formation. Most of these circuits are near the basal right ventricle near the tricuspid valve area and most patients have a dramatic decrease in the VT burden or complete elimination of the VTs following ablation [45].

Some patients with cardiac sarcoidosis progress to advanced heart failure and might need heart transplantation. Patients with sarcoidosis have a good 1 and 5-year survival rates post transplantation [46]. Some of the patients were only diagnosed with cardiac sarcoidosis at the time of transplantation, underscoring the difficulties clinicians face in establishing the diagnosis of cardiac sarcoidosis [25].

3. Arrhythmogenic Right Ventricular Dysplasia/ Cardiomyopathy (ARVD/C)

3.1. Epidemiology

Arrhythmogenic right ventricular Dysplasia/ Cardiomyopathy (ARVD/C) is an inherited myopathy characterized by fibrofatty infiltration of the right ventricular (RV) wall, with left ventricular involvement over time in some patients [47, 48]. Males are more commonly affected than females. The true prevalence of the disease is unknown, but familial involvement is seen in up to 50%, which means screening family members is essential. The overall incidence is thought to be 1:1000 to 1:5000, with certain regions in Greece and Italy having increased prevalence compared to the rest of the world [49].

3.2. Environmental and genetic factors

There is no clear environmental cause of ARVD/C, and the etiology is not fully understood. Family members of patients with ARVD/ C are affected in 30-50% of the time, and the disease has autosomal dominant inheritance with variable penetrance. Several genetic loci have been identified, and mostly are mutations in cardiac desmosomes. Desmosomes are membrane structures composed of plasma cell membrane proteins that are responsible for force transmission between the cells. Abnormal function of these structures leads to cell detachment, death and inflammatory reaction leading to fibrosis and fatty infiltration. The most common mutation involves the PKP2 gene, encoding the plakophilin 2. Other desomsomal mutations were identified in DSP gene, encoding desmoplakin, DSG2 gene, encoding desmgelin 2 and DSC2 gene, encoding desmocolin 2. Desmosomal mutations occur in 52% of North Americans with ARVD/C and are associated with ventricular tachycardia and younger age of presentation [50]. There is genetic variability that occurs in healthy subjects, and has been noted to be as high as 16%. However, certain mutations make the diagnosis of ARVD/C more likely, including radical mutations as well as certain missense mutations that are rare in Caucasians [51]. The autosomal recessive form is associated with woolly hair and palmoplantar keratosis, the so-called Naxos disease, since it was discovered in the Greek island of Naxos. This gene encodes plakoglobin and desmoplakin. This autosomal recessive form has been mapped to chromosome 17q21. In addition, the cardiac ryanodine receptor gene RyR2 may be involved in the disease and causes juvenile sudden death with minimal RV wall motion abnormalities [52]. Mutations in the transforming growth factor B3 (TGF-B3) were also found in a large family in ARVD/C [53].

3.3. Pathology

The hallmark of ARVD/C is fibrofatty infiltration of the RV wall. This occurs in the epicardial layers first and moves endocardially. The RV inflow, RV apex and RV outflow are typically affected, forming what is called the triangle of dysplasia. With time, the interventricular septum is affected too. LV involvement has been described and could be seen in up to 76% of patients [54]. It usually parallels right ventricular involvement and is associated with worse prognosis [55]. Table 3 shows the major and minor pathological criteria used by the Task Force for diagnosis [56]. Endomyocardial biopsy doesn't have high sensitivity, since it is usually performed in the interventricular septum rather than the RV free wall. However, endomyocardial biopsy might help exlude other disease that could mimic ARVD/C, especially sarcoidosis. [57]

3.4. Clinical presentation

The clinical course is variable and most patients present before age 40. Patients with ARVD/C can be asymptomatic for years. The most common clinical presentation is with palpitations (due to frequent ventricular ectopy and ventricular tachycardia), chest pain, syncope and sudden cardiac death. In fact sudden cardiac death could be the first manifestation of the disease [54]. With time patients might develop RV dilatation leading to symptoms and signs of right-sided heart failure including fatigue, abdominal fullness and lower extremity edema. LV involvement leads to systolic heart failure and is associated with worse prognosis [58].

3.5. Electrocardiographic changes in ARVD/C

Patients with ARVD usually have sinus rhythm. The Task force criteria specify some depolarization abnormalities as major criteria for diagnosis, namely the presence of Epsilon wave (which could be seen in up to 30%, very specific but is not sensitive). If the ECG is highly amplified, Epsilon potentials could be detected in as many as 77% of patients with ARVD [59]. Repolarization abnormalities considered to be major criteria are inverted T waves in V1 to V3 or beyond in the absence of right bundle branch block (RBBB) [56, 60]. T wave inversion in V1

http://dx.doi.org/10.5772/55628

to V4 in the presence of RBBB is considered minor criteria for diagnosis. QRS fragmentation, defined as deflections at the beginning of the QRS, on top of the R wave or at the nadir of the S wave, could be found in as many as 85% of patients with ARVD/C and it correlates with LV involvement [59]. Signal average electrocardiography is simple and non-invasive method that could be used for screening. Abnormalities on signal average ECG considered to be minor criteria are listed in Table 3.

Patients with ARVD/C can have ventricular tachycardia and frequent premature ventricular contractions (PVCs). Ventricular tachycardia in general has left bundle branch morphology and is caused by macro-reentry. There is evidence that adrenergic stimulation acts as a trigger for these arrhythmias [61]. Exercise testing can induce these arrhythmias in 50-60% of ARVD/C patients. These arrhythmias could lead to syncope and SCD. In fact, ARVC/D accounts for 3 to 10% of death occurring in patients younger than 65 years [62] and is one of the causes of sudden cardiac death in athletes [63]. Patients with ARVD/D should not participate in moderate to high intensity exercise [64].

Ventricular tachycardia with left bundle branch (LBB) morphology and inferior axis is considered minor criteria, while VT with LBB morphology and superior axis is considered major criteria. Hoffmayer et al proposed criteria to differentiate idiopathic right ventricular outflow tract VT from ventricular tachycardia caused by ARVD/C. Since both conditions could present with ventricular tachycardia with left bundle branch morphology with inferior axis. In multivariate analysis, prolonged QRS duration in Lead I > 120 msec and transition in V5 or later predicted ARVD/C as the cause of VT [65]. Table 3 lists major and minor electrocardiographic and arrhythmia criteria for diagnosis of ARVD/C [56].

	Major Criteria	**Minor Criteria**
Global and/or regional dysfunction and structural alterations	By 2D echo: 1) Regional RV akinesia, dyskinesia, or aneurysm 2) and 1 of the following (end diastole): • PLAX RVOT ≥32 mm (corrected for body size [PLAX/BSA] ≥19 mm/m^2) • PSAX RVOT ≥36 mm (corrected for body size [PSAX/BSA] ≥21 mm/m^2) • fractional area change ≤33% By MRI: 1) Regional RV akinesia or dyskinesia or dyssynchronous RV contraction 2) and 1 of the following: • Ratio of RV end-diastolic volume to BSA ≥110 mL/m^2 (male) or ≥100 mL/m^2 (female) • RV ejection fraction ≤40% By RV angiography:	By 2D echo: 1) Regional RV akinesia or dyskinesia 2) and 1 of the following (end diastole): • PLAX RVOT ≥29 to <32 mm (corrected for body size [PLAX/BSA] ≥16 to <19 mm/m^2) • PSAX RVOT ≥32 to <36 mm (corrected for body size [PSAX/BSA] ≥18 to <21 mm/m^2) • fractional area change >33% to ≤40% By MRI: 1) Regional RV akinesia or dyskinesia or dyssynchronous RV contraction 2) and 1 of the following: • Ratio of RV end-diastolic volume to BSA ≥100 to <110 mL/m^2 (male) or ≥90 to <100 mL/m^2 (female) • RV ejection fraction >40% to ≤45%

	Major Criteria	Minor Criteria
	Regional RV akinesia, dyskinesia, or aneurysm	
Tissue characterization of walls	1) Residual myocytes <60% by morphometric analysis (or <50% if estimated), with fibrous replacement of the RV free wall myocardium in ≥1 sample, with or without fatty replacement of tissue on endomyocardial biopsy	1) Residual myocytes 60% to 75% by morphometric analysis (or 50% to 65% if estimated), with fibrous replacement of the RV free wall myocardium in ≥1 sample, with or without fatty replacement of tissue on endomyocardial biopsy
Repolarization abnormalities	1) Inverted T waves in right precordial leads (V_1, V_2, and V_3) or beyond in individuals >14 years of age (in the absence of complete right bundle-branch block QRS ≥120 ms)	1) Inverted T waves in leads V_1 and V_2 in individuals >14 years of age (in the absence of complete right bundle-branch block) or in V_4, V_5, or V6 2) Inverted T waves in leads V1, V2, V3, and V4 in individuals >14 years of age in the presence of complete right bundle-branch block
Depolarization/ conduction abnormalities	1) Epsilon wave (reproducible low-amplitude signals between end of QRS complex to onset of the T wave) in the right precordial leads (V_1 to V_3)	1) Late potentials by SAECG in ≥1 of 3 parameters in the absence of a QRS duration of ≥110 ms on the standard ECG 2) Filtered QRS duration (fQRS) ≥114 ms 3) Duration of terminal QRS <40 µV (low-amplitude signal duration) ≥38 ms 4) Root-mean-square voltage of terminal 40 ms ≤20 µV 5) Terminal activation duration of QRS ≥55 ms measured from the nadir of the S wave to the end of the QRS, including R′, in V_1, V_2, or V_3, in the absence of complete right bundle-branch block
Arrhythmias	1) Nonsustained or sustained ventricular tachycardia of left bundle-branch morphology with superior axis (negative or indeterminate QRS in leads II, III, and aVF and positive in lead aVL)	1) Nonsustained or sustained ventricular tachycardia of RV outflow configuration, left bundle-branch block morphology with inferior axis (positive QRS in leads II, III, and aVF and negative in lead aVL) or of unknown axis 2) >500 ventricular extrasystoles per 24 hours (Holter)
Family history	1) ARVC/D confirmed in a first-degree relative who meets current Task Force criteria 2) ARVC/D confirmed pathologically at autopsy or surgery in a first-degree relative 3) Identification of a pathogenic mutation[†] categorized as associated or probably	1) History of ARVC/D in a first-degree relative in whom it is not possible or practical to determine whether the family member meets current Task Force criteria 2) Premature sudden death (<35 years of age) due to suspected ARVC/D in a first-degree relative

http://dx.doi.org/10.5772/55628

Major Criteria	Minor Criteria
associated with ARVC/D in the patient under evaluation	3) ARVC/D confirmed pathologically or by current Task Force Criteria in second-degree relative

PLAX indicates parasternal long-axis view; RVOT, RV outflow tract; BSA, body surface area; PSAX, parasternal short-axis view

Table 3. Revised Task Force Criteria for the diagnosis of ARVD/C.

3.6. Imaging in ARVD/C

3.6.1. Right ventricular contrast angiography

Right ventricular angiography could detect wall motion abnormalities, RV dilatation and even aneurysm formation in patients with ARVD/C. However, due to its invasive nature, difficulty in visually assessing RV wall motion abnormalities especially in the presence of premature contractions makes it less attractive as a diagnostic modality.

3.6.2. Echocardiography

In patients with ARVD/C, the RV could be dilated with RV wall motion abnormalities and decreased RV function. Aneurysms could form in the RV free wall but also could be found in the inferior wall and apex. If adequate visualization of the walls is not possible because of poor windows, contrast injection could help overcome difficulties in delineating the RV wall. Right ventricular outflow (RVOT) enlargement is the most common abnormality found on TTE in patients with ARVD, and RVOT long axis dimension > 30 mm has the best sensitivity (89%) and specificity (86%) for diagnosing ARVD/C. Trabecular derangement, sacculations and hyper-reflective moderator band are less commonly found. Attention to regional RV wall motion abnormalities is important and could be seen in up to 80% of patients. Impaired RV function is seen in up to 67% of patients [66]. Occasionally, trans-esophageal echocardiography and intracardiac echocardiography could be used for diagnosis in patients with difficult images; however, they are more invasive. TTE is widely available, simple and non-invasive which makes it suitable as a primary diagnostic modality and should be performed in patients with PVCs and VT with left bundle branch block and inferior axis. Major and minor echocardiographic criteria for diagnosing ARVD/C are listed in Table 3 [56].

3.6.3. Radioisotope imaging

Cardiac sympathetic innervation is decreased in patients with ARVD/C, and radioisotopes with specific affinity to the ß receptors in the heart could help in early diagnosis. However, it has poor spatial resolution and the sensitivity and specificity of this modality is not well established [67]. Myocardial perfusion imaging could show decreased areas of radioisotope uptake in the RV, which could help in patients presenting with RVOT type VT. However, it is not widely used and doesn't have high sensitivity or specificity. Because of all this, radioisotope imaging is not considered as first line diagnostic imaging in patients with ARVD/C.

3.6.4. *Magnetic resonance imaging*

Cardiac MRI has high resolution and helps in assessment of anatomy, function and hemodynamics of the right and left ventricle in patients with ARVD/C. Dilatation of the RVOT area, RV wall motion abnormalities, RV aneurysms, depress RV function and presence of fat infiltration of the RV wall all have been described in patients with ARVD/C [68-70]. However, MRI cannot be used in patients who have defibrillators and it depends on the experience of the center and reader [69]. Tagged MRI helps detect regional wall motion abnormalities in the RV and LV walls. Jain et al found that regional wall motion in the LV parallels the degree of RV function and is present in patients with grossly normal LV function [55]. LV abnormalities include intramyocardial fat as well as wall motion abnormalities, and could be seen in up to 27% of patients (Figure 1). Delayed enhancement MRI (DE MRI) has great sensitivity and could show increased signal in the RV (most commonly the basal sub-tricuspid region extending anteriorly to the RV outflow) in up to 67% of patients with ARVD/C. It is important to differentiate epicardial fat from fat infiltration of the RV wall. In patients with ARVD/C, areas of fat infiltration are most commonly dyskinetic. Relying on fat infiltration alone without wall motion or quantitative assessment of the RV and without adequate testing and attention to the task force criteria could lead to over diagnosis of ARVD/C [69]. Fat infiltration is very sensitive (84%) but has low specificity (79%) while regional RV wall motion abnormalities and RV enlargement are very specific but less sensitive [71]. Table 3 lists the major and minor MRI criteria used for diagnosing ARVD/C.

3.7. Electrophysiology study and three dimensional electro-anatomical mapping

Electrophysiologic testing with programmed electrical stimulation (PES) is used for risk stratification of sudden cardiac death in patients with ARVD/C but it has poor positive predictive value (35 to 49%) and limited negative predictive value (49 to 74%) in predicting arrhythmias and appropriate ICD shocks [72-74]. Electroanatomical mapping could help in detecting areas of scar in patients with ARVD/C. Corrado et al demonstrated that scar could accurately be localized in patients with ARVD/C and usually correlates with areas with wall motion abnormalities and fibrofatty infiltration at endomyocardial biopsy. Areas with low voltage of < 0.5 mV are considered scar areas, while healthy tissue usually has a voltage of > 1.5 mV [75]. Areas with voltage between 0.5 and 1.5 mV are considered transitional zone. It is important to insure appropriate contact using either fluoroscopy or intracardiac echocardiography and to obtain multiple points in the same area to confirm that it is a low voltage area. Furthermore, fractionated signals can be found in areas with low voltage and is evidence of slow conduction and could be part of the ventricular tachycardia circuit. Voltage mapping can help delineate the substrate for macro-reentrant VT in patients with ARVD [75]. Low voltage areas indicating scar are noted in the anterolateral RV free wall, apex, and inflow and outflow tracts of the RV and correlate with MRI findings [76]. Even in patients with ARVD and minimal scar, prolonged endocardial activation could be noted. In a study of 25 patients with left bundle branch VT, Tandri et al showed that patients with ARVD/C had prolonged endocardial activation > 65 msec while none of the patients with idiopathic RVOT VT had prolonged endocardial activa-

http://dx.doi.org/10.5772/55628

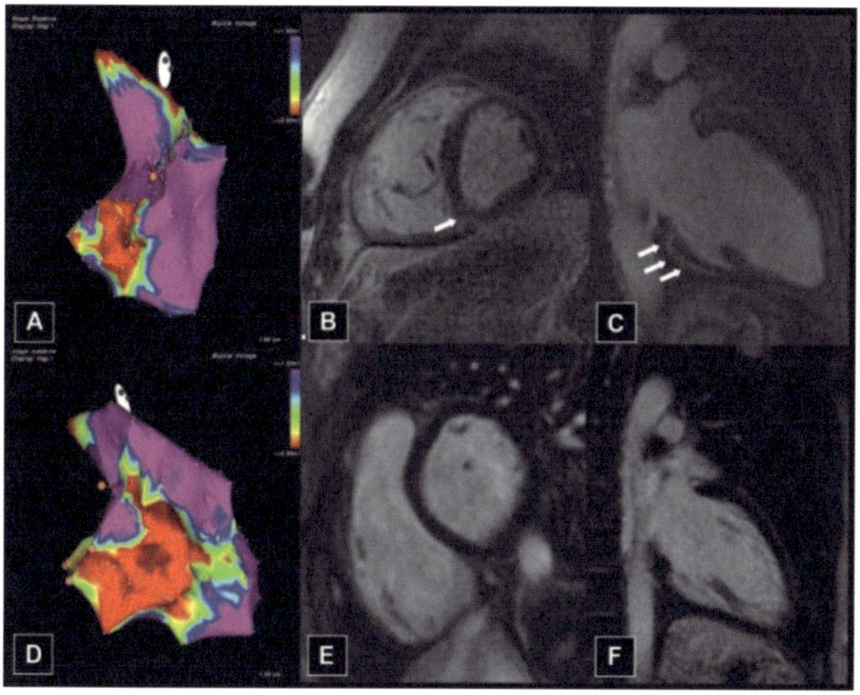

Figure 1. Representative cases of discordance between endocardial voltage mapping (EVM) and contrast-enhanced magnetic resonance (DE-MRI). **A**, Lateral view of the right ventricular (RV) EVM showing electroanatomical scar (EAS) in the RV inferobasal region and outflow tract. **B** and **C**, Basal short- and long-axis views of DE-MRI sequences showing no signs of delayed contrast enhancement (DE) in the RV free wall. Subepicardial DE is visible in the inferior and inferoseptal regions of the left ventricle (LV; white arrows). **D**, Lateral view of EVM showing a large EAS affecting the inferobasal, anterolateral, and, partly, RV outflow tract region. **E** and **F**, Basal short- and long-axis views of DE MRI showing neither RV nor LV DE. (From Martina Perazzolo Marra, MD, PhD et al "Imaging Study of Ventricular Scar in Arrhythmogenic Right Ventricular Cardiomyopathy / Clinical Perspective : Comparison of 3D Standard Electroanatomical Voltage Mapping and Contrast-Enhanced Cardiac Magnetic Resonance" Circulation: Arrhythmia and Electrophysiology. 2012; 5: 91-100, With Permission)

tion [77]. Electroanatomical mapping is actually more sensitive than DE MRI in detecting areas with scar, (Figure 1). especially if the scar area is < 20% of the total RV area [78].

3.8. Diagnosis of ARVD/C

Diagnosis of ARVD/C is based on the Modified Task Force Criteria published in 2010 [56]. These criteria are specific and rely on the demonstration of structural, functional and electrophysiological changes to diagnose the disease. To diagnose ARVD/C, 2 major criteria, one major and two minor criteria or 4 minor criteria need to be fulfilled. The modified criteria are more sensitive in detecting the disease in first-degree relatives of affected members without compromising specificity and incorporate certain pathogenic mutations as major criteria for diagnosis. Furthermore, it offers more quantitative parameters in imaging studies for diagnosis compared to the original 1994 criteria. Table 3 lists the modified criteria.

3.9. Therapy

Therapy of ARVD/C aims at suppressing ventricular arrhythmias, prevention of sudden cardiac death and treatment of right and/or left ventricular heart failure. Family members should be screened for the disease since most of the cases have autosomal dominant inheritance.

Patients with ARVD/C should not participate in competitive sports and should avoid moderate to high intensity exercise. And since the occurrence of ventricular tachycardia is related to adrenergic stimulation, most of the patients with ARVD/C with sustained and NSVT are typically treated with β-blockers and given antiarrhythmic drugs. Sotalol was thought to suppress ventricular arrhythmias in patients with ARVD/C and is widely used in this population [79]. However, a recent publication from the North American ARVD/C registry showed that sotalol did not suppress ventricular arrhythmias or prevent ICD therapies while amiodarone had a better efficacy but only 10 patients received amiodarone in this registry [80]. In patients with heart failure, β-blockers, angiotensin converting enzyme inhibitors and angiotensin receptor blockers are indicated. Catheter ablation for ventricular arrhythmias is used to treat sustained ventricular tachycardia that lead to syncope and ICD shocks in patients with ARVD/C. Both activation mapping as well as substrate mapping could be used to delineate the VT circuit [81]. The success rate of catheter ablation ranges from 32 to 88%, and most patients require two or three ablation procedures [82, 83]. For prevention of sudden cardiac death, implantable cardioverter defibrillators (ICDs) are clearly indicated in patients with ARVD/C who survive cardiac arrest or have sustained VT. It is considered a class IIa indication in ARVD/C patients with one or more risk factors of sudden cardiac death (unexplained syncope, presence of nonsustained VT on ambulatory monitoring, extensive RV involvement, LV involvement and positive EPS study) [39]. However, there is no clear consensus on the risk factors for SCD in patients with ARVD/C, and the physician needs to utilize knowledge, experience and clinical judgment when considering ICD implantation for patients with this disease.

Since this is a young population, they are also likely to experience inappropriate shocks due to sinus tachycardia or other supraventricular arrhythmias especially atrial fibrillation. Inappropriate shocks occur frequently and could happen in 16 to 24% of patients [72-74]. Appropriate ICD shocks occur in 25 to 50% of patients with no prior VT or VF [74, 84]. Most therapies are clustered early, especially in the first 2 years [43]. Syncope, inducibility at EP study, left ventricular involvement, presence of non-sustained ventricular tachycardia or > 1000 PVCs at holter monitoring are important predictors of appropriate ICD therapy [73, 84]. Furthermore, due to the progressive nature of the disease, lead complications could occur late and lead repositioning or implantation of a new lead are not uncommon and could occur in 14% to 21% of patients [72, 73]. In general ICD therapy is life saving and is well tolerated and has become accepted standard of care in patients with ARVD/C who experience cardiac arrest, sustained VT, unexplained syncope or marked RV dilatation or LV involvement [39].

Prognosis is dependent on the rate of progression of the disease, presence of heart failure and the degree of LV involvement [85]. The diagnosis of ARVD/C should prompt genetic testing to identify the mutation involved and guide the screening of family members. Heart Transplantation is indicated in patients with advanced right and/or left sided heart failure.

4. Isolated left ventricular non-compaction

4.1. Introduction

Noncompaction of the left ventricular myocardium is a rare disorder that occurs in isolation or with other congenital cardiac defects. It is caused by the arrest of compaction of the myocardial fibers, leading to prominent trabeculations giving the myocardium a spongy appearance. Patients can be asymptomatic and could present with syncope, chest pain, palpitations, shortness of breath and sudden cardiac death. Management of patients with isolated left ventricular non-compaction (ILVNC) involves treating heart failure, protection from sudden cardiac death, anticoagulation to prevent thromboembolic events, and screening of family members.

4.2. Epidemiology

The true prevalence of isolated LV noncompaction is unknown, as most cases are referred to tertiary care centers. In clinical series, the prevalence ranges from 0.05 to 0.25%. The median age at diagnosis ranges from 90 days to 45 years and males are more commonly affected than females [86-89].

4.3. Pathology

Noncompaction of the left ventricular myocardium is caused by the arrest of intrauterine compaction of the myocardial fibers, leading to prominent trabeculations giving the myocardium a spongy appearance [90]. It is often associated with other congenital cardiac anomalies, especially obstruction of the right or left ventricular outflow tracts. However, the deep intertrabecular recesses that persist in these cases are in communication with the ventricular cavity and the coronary circulation [87]. In contrast, the intertrabecular recesses in isolated LV noncompaction are in communication with the LV cavity only and not with the coronary circulation. Histologically, there is myocardial thickening as well as interstitial and subendocardial fibrosis [91]. Microcirculatory dysfunction is present in both compacted and noncompacted segments which might explain the subendocarial scar noted on biopsies as well as the wall motion abnormalities noted in imaging [92].

4.4. Genetics

Familial involvement was high in initial reports describing isolated LV noncompaction [93] In later series involving adults, the familial recurrence ranged from 12 to 44%. Some mutations involving the G4.5 gene have X linked Inheritance [94, 95]. However, autosomal dominant inheritance has also been reported with mutations in chromosome 11p15 [95, 96].

Sarcomere protein gene defects are also found in patients with ILVNC. Mutations in cipher/ ZASP, a gene encoding for the Z-band, can cause dilated cardiomyopathy as well as ILVNC [97]. In a study of 63 unrelated patients with ILVNC, mutations in genes encoding sarcomere proteins were identified in 11 patients. These genes include β myosin heavy chain (MYH7), α-cardiac actin and cardiac troponin T. Similar sarcomere gene mutations, especially in MYH7 are also found in patients with hypertrophic and dilated cardiomyopathies [98]. These sarcomere mutations could account for up to 29% of mutations in ILVNC, but they do not predict clinical outcome [99].

4.5. Clinical presentation

Patients with isolated LV noncompaction can be asymptomatic for years and eventually could present with heart failure, arrhythmias, embolic events and sudden cardiac death. The clinical course is variable, with patients who are asymptomatic having a more stable clinical course, while patients presenting with heart failure having a progressive clinical course with heart failure and ventricular arrhythmias [100]. Most patients have some degree of LV dysfunction, which has been reported in up to 60% of patients in the four largest reports of LV noncompaction [86, 87, 93, 101]. However, presentation as congestive heart failure with dyspnea on exertion has ranged from 30–68%. Patients could have systolic as well as diastolic dysfunction. Microcirculatory dysfunction could lead to ischemia and scar causing wall motion abnormalities and systolic heart failure. While impaired filling and abnormal relaxation from prominent trabeculations could lead to diastolic heart failure [92]. Several arrhythmias have been reported with ILVNC, including atrial fibrillation (5–29% in major reports), atrial tachycardia, premature ventricular complexes and ventricular tachycardia (18–47% in major reports). Sudden cardiac death accounted for 50% of deaths in ILVNC. Presence of subendocardial scar can act as a substrate of reentry in these patients. Embolic complications in ILVNC could be due to thrombus formation in the recesses of the trabeculations, due to stagnant flow from severely depressed LV function or from atrial fibrillation. These emboli can go to the cerebrovascular circulation, peripheral circulation, or pulmonary circulation. The incidence of embolization has ranged from 21–38%. Anticoagulation to prevent thromboembolic complications is very important in ILVNC [91].

4.6. Electrocardiogram

Abnormalities noted in the electrocardiogram in patients with ILVNC include left bundle branch block, right bundle branch block, left ventricular hypertrophy with repolarization abnormalities, and AV block. Wolff-Parkinson-White syndrome has been described in children with ILVNC. Atrial fibrillation, frequent premature ventricular contractions with sustained and non-sustained ventricular tachycardia could be present and could be the first presentation of the disease. There is a high prevalence of early repolarization in patients with ILVNC, especially in those patients who present with malignant arrhythmias [86, 87, 102].

http://dx.doi.org/10.5772/55628

4.7. Imaging in isolated left ventricular non-compaction

4.7.1. Echocardiography

Transthoracic echocardiography is the modality most commonly used to diagnose ILVNC [103]. The most common criteria used for diagnoses have been proposed by Jenni et al, with a ratio of noncompacted to compacted LV myocardium of 2 to 1 considered diagnostic [104]. This is typically measured at end systole in the parasternal short axis view. Deep intertrabecular recesses that are supplied from the LV cavity and absence of other congenital anomalies are part of Jenni's criteria. However, some experts suggest the ratio of noncompacted to compacted myocardium should be measured but in the parasternal short axis view at end diastole [103]. Chin et al proposed a measurement of compacted myocardium (C) to the total thickness of both compacted and noncompacted layers (C + NC) at end diastole, with the ratio of C/ (NC+C) of < 0.5 considered diagnostic. However, there is poor agreement between readers when it comes to the ratio of noncompated to compacted myocardium, with only 74% of agreement noted and there is poor agreement between these two criteria for diagnosis [105]. Jenni's criteria are more specific while Chin's criteria are more sensitive. In general the noncompacted segments most commonly involve the apex more than the base, and are seen mostly in the inferior wall and also in the lateral wall [104]. Multiple segments are usually involved (Figure 2). The right ventricle is involved in 40% of the cases [89, 105]. Wall motion abnormalities, impaired diastolic filling as measured from mitral inflow velocities are also seen. Depressed LV ejection fraction is noted in a lot of patients with LV noncompaction, and patients with severe LV dysfunction have a poor prognosis. It is important to differentiate ILVNC from hypertrophic cardiomyopathy (especially the apical variant), dilated cardiomyopathy, arrhythmogenic right ventricular dysplasia and endocardial fibroelastosis. But in isolated LVNC, perfused recesses and hypokinetic segments are very specific, and the wall thickening noted is confined to certain walls of the LV. Visualization of the trabecular recesses could be enhanced using contrast. Transesophageal echocardiography could also be used in diagnoses in patients with difficult windows.

4.7.2. Magnetic Resonance Imaging (MRI)

Magnetic resonance imaging (MRI) has been also used for diagnosis. Delayed gadolinium enhancement has been seen in both compacted and noncompacted myocardium. In compacted myocardium, delayed enhancement correlated well with fibrosis, while in the noncompacted segments, delayed enhancement correlated with fibrosis as well as mucoid degeneration of the endocardium [106]. MRI offers better spatial resolution and can help assess LV and RV functions, wall motion abnormalities, as well as the ratio of compacted and noncompacted segments, which has been shown to be an important predictor of major adverse cardiac events, including heart failure, ventricular arrhythmias and thromboembolism. A ratio of noncompacted to compacted myocardium of > 2.3 at end diastole had the best sensitivity (86%) and specificity (99%) in diagnosing ILVNC [107]. However, 140 patients (43%) of 323 patients in the MESA cohort had at least one area with trabeculated to compact ratio of > 2.3 and the authors advised caution in using these criteria alone for diagnosis of ILVNC [108]. The

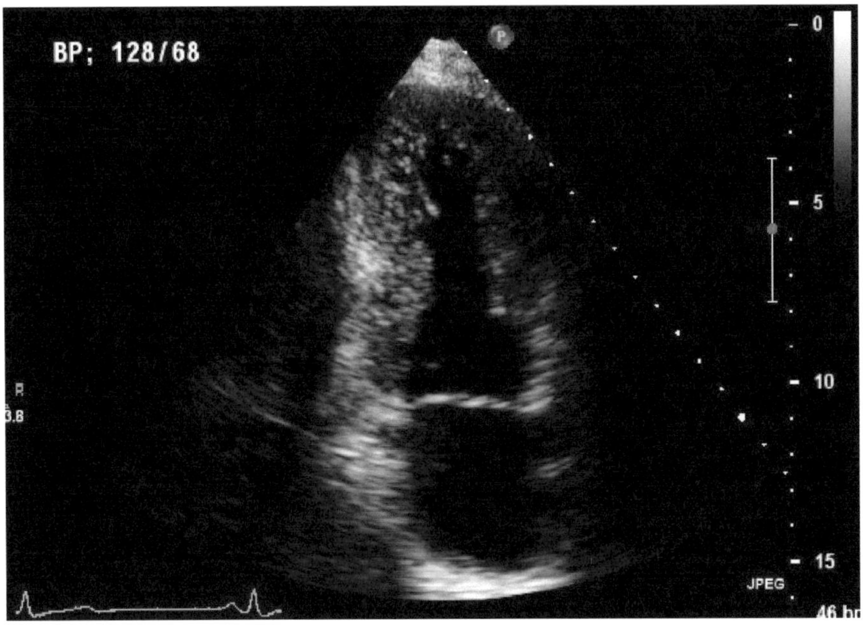

Figure 2. Apical 2 chamber view showing prominent trabeculations in the apex and inferior walls consistent with Isolated Left Ventricular Non-Compation.

calculation of trabeculated LV mass using MRI could help also in the diagnosis of ILVNC, with trabeculated LV mass of >20% of the total LV mass having the highest sensitivity and specificity (93.7%) in diagnosing ILVNC [109].

4.7.3. Other imaging modalities

Computed tomography scan could be used to diagnose ILVNC and has high spatial resolution. Prominent trabeculations as well as deep intertrabecular recesses are typically seen [103]. Contrast ventriculography could also be used but is invasive. PET scan could show decreased myocardial flow reserve in noncompacted areas as well as microcirculatory dysfunction in both compacted and noncompacted myocardium but this has limited utility in establishing the diagnosis [92, 110]. To date, Echocardiography and MRI remain the most common modalities used for diagnosing ILVNC.

4.8. Therapy

Management of patients with ILVNC involves treating heart failure, protection from sudden cardiac death, anticoagulation to prevent thromboembolic events, and screening of family members. β-blockers, angiotensin converting enzyme inhibitors and angtiotensin receptor blockers are used and have been reported to improve symptoms and the LVEF [111]. Anticoagulation with coumadin is recommended in all patients, even if they don't have atrial fibrillation. Electrophysiology testing to predict the risk of sudden cardiac death has not yielded great results. Currently, the decision to implant a defibrillator (ICD) or biventricular defibrillator (BiV ICD) is clear in patients who have survived a cardiac arrest or in patients with LVEF <35% who qualify for an ICD or BIV ICD according to the current guidelines [39]. In a series of 30 patients with ILVNC who received ICDs or BiV ICDs according to the current guidelines, Kobza et al showed that appropriate ICD therapy (either shocks or antitachycardia pacing) occurred in 37% of cases with a mean follow up of 21 ± 16 months. Inappropriate shocks occurred in 13% of cases. In patients who received ICD therapy for primary prevention, 33% had appropriate ICD therapy with mean follow up of 27 ± 33 months. There were no predictors of appropriate ICD therapy [112].

The prognosis of ILVNC varies. Initial reports were based on the experience in tertiary care centers led to the belief that the prognosis is poor, with progressive heart failure leading to death or transplantation in 47% of adults with ILVNC followed for 44 ± 39 months [91]. However, recent reports challenge this and asymptomatic patients in general have a good prognosis [113]. Certain clinical characteristics are more common in non-survivors compared to survivors, including higher LV end-diastolic diameter, New York Heart Association class III–IV heart failure, left bundle branch block, and persistent atrial fibrillation. Patients with such clinical characteristics need frequent follow up, with strong consideration for more aggressive treatment [86]. Family screening is important, with transthoracic echocardiography being the most common screening modality. Family members may have other forms of cardiomyopathy, like dilated or hypertrophic cardiomyopathy [113]. Recent advances in genetic testing will allow identification of the genetic mutation in the proband and help narrow the search for the genetic mutations.

5. Conclusion

Cardiac Sarcoidosis, arrhythmogenic right ventricular dysplasia and isolated left ventricular noncompaction are rare forms of cardiomyopathy that affect young patients and put them at risk of sudden cardiac death. Early recognition and treatment is important. In the absence of clear guidelines to prevent sudden cardiac death in this young population, the clinician should use current knowledge, clinical judgment and expertise when treating these patients. Advances in diagnostic imaging as well as genetic testing will help early diagnosis and identification of affected family members.

Author details

M. Obadah Al Chekakie

University of Colorado, Cheyenne Regional Medical Center, Cheyenne, Wyoming, USA

References

[1] Gideon NM, Mannino DM. Sarcoidosis mortality in the United States 1979-1991: an analysis of multiple-cause mortality data. Am J Med. 1996;100(4):423-427.

[2] Rybicki BA, Major M, Popovich J, Jr., Maliarik MJ, Iannuzzi MC. Racial differences in sarcoidosis incidence: a 5-year study in a health maintenance organization. Am J Epidemiol. 1997;145(3):234-241.

[3] Morgenthau AS, Iannuzzi MC. Recent advances in sarcoidosis. Chest.139(1):174-182.

[4] Izbicki G, Chavko R, Banauch GI, Weiden MD, Berger KI, Aldrich TK, et al. World Trade Center "sarcoid-like" granulomatous pulmonary disease in New York City Fire Department rescue workers. Chest. 2007;131(5):1414-1423.

[5] Song Z, Marzilli L, Greenlee BM, Chen ES, Silver RF, Askin FB, et al. Mycobacterial catalase-peroxidase is a tissue antigen and target of the adaptive immune response in systemic sarcoidosis. J Exp Med. 2005;201(5):755-767.

[6] Rossman MD, Thompson B, Frederick M, Maliarik M, Iannuzzi MC, Rybicki BA, et al. HLA-DRB1*1101: a significant risk factor for sarcoidosis in blacks and whites. Am J Hum Genet. 2003;73(4):720-735.

[7] Iannuzzi MC, Maliarik MJ, Poisson LM, Rybicki BA. Sarcoidosis susceptibility and resistance HLA-DQB1 alleles in African Americans. Am J Respir Crit Care Med. 2003;167(9):1225-1231.

[8] Iannuzzi MC, Iyengar SK, Gray-McGuire C, Elston RC, Baughman RP, Donohue JF, et al. Genome-wide search for sarcoidosis susceptibility genes in African Americans. Genes Immun. 2005;6(6):509-518.

[9] Schurmann M, Reichel P, Muller-Myhsok B, Schlaak M, Muller-Quernheim J, Schwinger E. Results from a genome-wide search for predisposing genes in sarcoidosis. Am J Respir Crit Care Med. 2001;164(5):840-846.

[10] Rybicki BA, Sinha R, Iyengar S, Gray-McGuire C, Elston RC, Iannuzzi MC. Genetic linkage analysis of sarcoidosis phenotypes: the sarcoidosis genetic analysis (SAGA) study. Genes Immun. 2007;8(5):379-386.

[11] Silverman KJ, Hutchins GM, Bulkley BH. Cardiac sarcoid: a clinicopathologic study of 84 unselected patients with systemic sarcoidosis. Circulation. 1978;58(6):1204-1211.

[12] Roberts WC, McAllister HA, Jr., Ferrans VJ. Sarcoidosis of the heart. A clinicopathologic study of 35 necropsy patients (group 1) and review of 78 previously described necropsy patients (group 11). Am J Med. 1977;63(1):86-108.

[13] Patel MR, Cawley PJ, Heitner JF, Klem I, Parker MA, Jaroudi WA, et al. Detection of myocardial damage in patients with sarcoidosis. Circulation. 2009;120(20):1969-1977.

[14] Smedema JP, Snoep G, van Kroonenburgh MP, van Geuns RJ, Dassen WR, Gorgels AP, et al. Evaluation of the accuracy of gadolinium-enhanced cardiovascular magnetic resonance in the diagnosis of cardiac sarcoidosis. J Am Coll Cardiol. 2005;45(10): 1683-1690.

[15] Dubrey SW, Falk RH. Diagnosis and management of cardiac sarcoidosis. Prog Cardiovasc Dis.52(4):336-346.

[16] Kandolin R, Lehtonen J, Kupari M. Cardiac sarcoidosis and giant cell myocarditis as causes of atrioventricular block in young and middle-aged adults. Circ Arrhythm Electrophysiol.4(3):303-309.

[17] Mehta D, Lubitz SA, Frankel Z, Wisnivesky JP, Einstein AJ, Goldman M, et al. Cardiac involvement in patients with sarcoidosis: diagnostic and prognostic value of outpatient testing. Chest. 2008;133(6):1426-1435.

[18] Hamzeh NY, Wamboldt FS, Weinberger HD. Management of cardiac sarcoidosis in the United States: a Delphi study. Chest.141(1):154-162.

[19] Iannuzzi MC, Rybicki BA, Teirstein AS. Sarcoidosis. N Engl J Med. 2007;357(21): 2153-2165.

[20] Studdy PR, Bird R. Serum angiotensin converting enzyme in sarcoidosis--its value in present clinical practice. Ann Clin Biochem. 1989;26 (Pt 1):13-18.

[21] Soejima K, Yada H. The work-up and management of patients with apparent or subclinical cardiac sarcoidosis: with emphasis on the associated heart rhythm abnormalities. J Cardiovasc Electrophysiol. 2009;20(5):578-583.

[22] Schuller JL, Olson MD, Zipse MM, Schneider PM, Aleong RG, Wienberger HD, et al. Electrocardiographic characteristics in patients with pulmonary sarcoidosis indicating cardiac involvement. J Cardiovasc Electrophysiol.22(11):1243-1248.

[23] Ardehali H, Howard DL, Hariri A, Qasim A, Hare JM, Baughman KL, et al. A positive endomyocardial biopsy result for sarcoid is associated with poor prognosis in patients with initially unexplained cardiomyopathy. Am Heart J. 2005;150(3):459-463.

[24] Okura Y, Dec GW, Hare JM, Kodama M, Berry GJ, Tazelaar HD, et al. A clinical and histopathologic comparison of cardiac sarcoidosis and idiopathic giant cell myocarditis. J Am Coll Cardiol. 2003;41(2):322-329.

[25] Milman N, Andersen CB, Mortensen SA, Sander K. Cardiac sarcoidosis and heart transplantation: a report of four consecutive patients. Sarcoidosis Vasc Diffuse Lung Dis. 2008;25(1):51-59.

[26] Uemura A, Morimoto S, Kato Y, Hiramitsu S, Ohtsuki M, Kato S, et al. Relationship between basal thinning of the interventricular septum and atrioventricular block in patients with cardiac sarcoidosis. Sarcoidosis Vasc Diffuse Lung Dis. 2005;22(1): 63-65.

[27] Cross B, Nicolarsen J, Bullock J, Sugeng L, Bardo D, Lang R. Cardiac sarcoidosis presenting as mitral regurgitation. J Am Soc Echocardiogr. 2007;20(7):906 e909-913.

[28] Burstow DJ, Tajik AJ, Bailey KR, DeRemee RA, Taliercio CP. Two-dimensional echocardiographic findings in systemic sarcoidosis. Am J Cardiol. 1989;63(7):478-482.

[29] Vignaux O. Cardiac sarcoidosis: spectrum of MRI features. AJR Am J Roentgenol. 2005;184(1):249-254.

[30] Tadamura E, Yamamuro M, Kubo S, Kanao S, Saga T, Harada M, et al. Effectiveness of delayed enhanced MRI for identification of cardiac sarcoidosis: comparison with radionuclide imaging. AJR Am J Roentgenol. 2005;185(1):110-115.

[31] Smedema JP, Snoep G, van Kroonenburgh MP, van Geuns RJ, Cheriex EC, Gorgels AP, et al. The additional value of gadolinium-enhanced MRI to standard assessment for cardiac involvement in patients with pulmonary sarcoidosis. Chest. 2005;128(3): 1629-1637.

[32] Okayama K, Kurata C, Tawarahara K, Wakabayashi Y, Chida K, Sato A. Diagnostic and prognostic value of myocardial scintigraphy with thallium-201 and gallium-67 in cardiac sarcoidosis. Chest. 1995;107(2):330-334.

[33] Alavi A, Palevsky HI. Gallium-67-citrate scanning in the assessment of disease activity in sarcoidosis. J Nucl Med. 1992;33(5):751-755.

[34] Nakazawa A, Ikeda K, Ito Y, Iwase M, Sato K, Ueda R, et al. Usefulness of dual 67Ga and 99mTc-sestamibi single-photon-emission CT scanning in the diagnosis of cardiac sarcoidosis. Chest. 2004;126(4):1372-1376.

[35] Yamagishi H, Shirai N, Takagi M, Yoshiyama M, Akioka K, Takeuchi K, et al. Identification of cardiac sarcoidosis with (13)N-NH(3)/(18)F-FDG PET. J Nucl Med. 2003;44(7):1030-1036.

[36] Kato Y, Morimoto S, Uemura A, Hiramitsu S, Ito T, Hishida H. Efficacy of corticosteroids in sarcoidosis presenting with atrioventricular block. Sarcoidosis Vasc Diffuse Lung Dis. 2003;20(2):133-137.

[37] Winters SL, Cohen M, Greenberg S, Stein B, Curwin J, Pe E, et al. Sustained ventricular tachycardia associated with sarcoidosis: assessment of the underlying cardiac anatomy and the prospective utility of programmed ventricular stimulation, drug therapy and an implantable antitachycardia device. J Am Coll Cardiol. 1991;18(4): 937-943.

[38] Hamzeh NY, Wamboldt FS, Weinberger HD. Management of cardiac sarcoidosis in the United States: a Delphi study. Chest. 2012;141(1):154-162.

[39] Epstein AE, DiMarco JP, Ellenbogen KA, Estes NA, 3rd, Freedman RA, Gettes LS, et al. ACC/AHA/HRS 2008 Guidelines for Device-Based Therapy of Cardiac Rhythm Abnormalities: a report of the American College of Cardiology/American Heart Association Task Force on Practice Guidelines (Writing Committee to Revise the

ACC/AHA/NASPE 2002 Guideline Update for Implantation of Cardiac Pacemakers and Antiarrhythmia Devices): developed in collaboration with the American Association for Thoracic Surgery and Society of Thoracic Surgeons. Circulation. 2008;117(21):e350-408.

[40] Kim JS, Judson MA, Donnino R, Gold M, Cooper LT, Jr., Prystowsky EN, et al. Cardiac sarcoidosis. Am Heart J. 2009;157(1):9-21.

[41] Mehta D, Mori N, Goldbarg SH, Lubitz S, Wisnivesky JP, Teirstein A. Primary prevention of sudden cardiac death in silent cardiac sarcoidosis: role of programmed ventricular stimulation. Circ Arrhythm Electrophysiol. 2011;4(1):43-48.

[42] Aizer A, Stern EH, Gomes JA, Teirstein AS, Eckart RE, Mehta D. Usefulness of programmed ventricular stimulation in predicting future arrhythmic events in patients with cardiac sarcoidosis. Am J Cardiol. 2005;96(2):276-282.

[43] Betensky BP, Tschabrunn CM, Zado ES, Goldberg LR, Marchlinski FE, Garcia FC, et al. Long-term follow-up of patients with cardiac sarcoidosis and implantable cardioverter-defibrillators. Heart Rhythm. 2012;9(6):884-891.

[44] Schuller JL, Zipse M, Crawford T, Bogun F, Beshai J, Patel AR, et al. Implantable cardioverter defibrillator therapy in patients with cardiac sarcoidosis. J Cardiovasc Electrophysiol. 2012;23(9):925-929.

[45] Jefic D, Joel B, Good E, Morady F, Rosman H, Knight B, et al. Role of radiofrequency catheter ablation of ventricular tachycardia in cardiac sarcoidosis: report from a multicenter registry. Heart Rhythm. 2009;6(2):189-195.

[46] Zaidi AR, Zaidi A, Vaitkus PT. Outcome of heart transplantation in patients with sarcoid cardiomyopathy. J Heart Lung Transplant. 2007;26(7):714-717.

[47] Sen-Chowdhry S, Lowe MD, Sporton SC, McKenna WJ. Arrhythmogenic right ventricular cardiomyopathy: clinical presentation, diagnosis, and management. Am J Med. 2004;117(9):685-695.

[48] Gemayel C, Pelliccia A, Thompson PD. Arrhythmogenic right ventricular cardiomyopathy. J Am Coll Cardiol. 2001;38(7):1773-1781.

[49] Thiene G, Basso C. Arrhythmogenic right ventricular cardiomyopathy: An update. Cardiovasc Pathol. 2001;10(3):109-117.

[50] den Haan AD, Tan BY, Zikusoka MN, Llado LI, Jain R, Daly A, et al. Comprehensive desmosome mutation analysis in north americans with arrhythmogenic right ventricular dysplasia/cardiomyopathy. Circ Cardiovasc Genet. 2009;2(5):428-435.

[51] Kapplinger JD, Landstrom AP, Salisbury BA, Callis TE, Pollevick GD, Tester DJ, et al. Distinguishing arrhythmogenic right ventricular cardiomyopathy/dysplasia-associated mutations from background genetic noise. J Am Coll Cardiol.57(23):2317-2327.

[52] Tiso N, Stephan DA, Nava A, Bagattin A, Devaney JM, Stanchi F, et al. Identification of mutations in the cardiac ryanodine receptor gene in families affected with arrhyth-

mogenic right ventricular cardiomyopathy type 2 (ARVD2). Hum Mol Genet. 2001;10(3):189-194.

[53] Nattel S, Schott JJ. Arrhythmogenic right ventricular dysplasia type 1 and mutations in transforming growth factor beta3 gene regulatory regions: a breakthrough? Cardiovasc Res. 2005;65(2):302-304.

[54] Corrado D, Basso C, Thiene G, McKenna WJ, Davies MJ, Fontaliran F, et al. Spectrum of clinicopathologic manifestations of arrhythmogenic right ventricular cardiomyopathy/dysplasia: a multicenter study. J Am Coll Cardiol. 1997;30(6):1512-1520.

[55] Jain A, Shehata ML, Stuber M, Berkowitz SJ, Calkins H, Lima JA, et al. Prevalence of left ventricular regional dysfunction in arrhythmogenic right ventricular dysplasia: a tagged MRI study. Circ Cardiovasc Imaging.3(3):290-297.

[56] Marcus FI, McKenna WJ, Sherrill D, Basso C, Bauce B, Bluemke DA, et al. Diagnosis of arrhythmogenic right ventricular cardiomyopathy/dysplasia: proposed modification of the task force criteria. Circulation.121(13):1533-1541.

[57] Vasaiwala SC, Finn C, Delpriore J, Leya F, Gagermeier J, Akar JG, et al. Prospective study of cardiac sarcoid mimicking arrhythmogenic right ventricular dysplasia. J Cardiovasc Electrophysiol. 2009;20(5):473-476.

[58] Kies P, Bootsma M, Bax J, Schalij MJ, van der Wall EE. Arrhythmogenic right ventricular dysplasia/cardiomyopathy: screening, diagnosis, and treatment. Heart Rhythm. 2006;3(2):225-234.

[59] Peters S, Trummel M, Koehler B. QRS fragmentation in standard ECG as a diagnostic marker of arrhythmogenic right ventricular dysplasia-cardiomyopathy. Heart Rhythm. 2008;5(10):1417-1421.

[60] Jain R, Dalal D, Daly A, Tichnell C, James C, Evenson A, et al. Electrocardiographic features of arrhythmogenic right ventricular dysplasia. Circulation. 2009;120(6): 477-487.

[61] Leclercq JF, Potenza S, Maison-Blanche P, Chastang C, Coumel P. Determinants of spontaneous occurrence of sustained monomorphic ventricular tachycardia in right ventricular dysplasia. J Am Coll Cardiol. 1996;28(3):720-724.

[62] Tabib A, Loire R, Chalabreysse L, Meyronnet D, Miras A, Malicier D, et al. Circumstances of death and gross and microscopic observations in a series of 200 cases of sudden death associated with arrhythmogenic right ventricular cardiomyopathy and/or dysplasia. Circulation. 2003;108(24):3000-3005.

[63] Maron BJ. Sudden death in young athletes. N Engl J Med. 2003;349(11):1064-1075.

[64] Maron BJ, Chaitman BR, Ackerman MJ, Bayes de Luna A, Corrado D, Crosson JE, et al. Recommendations for physical activity and recreational sports participation for

young patients with genetic cardiovascular diseases. Circulation. 2004;109(22): 2807-2816.

[65] Hoffmayer KS, Machado ON, Marcus GM, Yang Y, Johnson CJ, Ermakov S, et al. Electrocardiographic comparison of ventricular arrhythmias in patients with arrhythmogenic right ventricular cardiomyopathy and right ventricular outflow tract tachycardia. J Am Coll Cardiol.58(8):831-838.

[66] Yoerger DM, Marcus F, Sherrill D, Calkins H, Towbin JA, Zareba W, et al. Echocardiographic findings in patients meeting task force criteria for arrhythmogenic right ventricular dysplasia: new insights from the multidisciplinary study of right ventricular dysplasia. J Am Coll Cardiol. 2005;45(6):860-865.

[67] Wichter T, Schafers M, Rhodes CG, Borggrefe M, Lerch H, Lammertsma AA, et al. Abnormalities of cardiac sympathetic innervation in arrhythmogenic right ventricular cardiomyopathy : quantitative assessment of presynaptic norepinephrine reuptake and postsynaptic beta-adrenergic receptor density with positron emission tomography. Circulation. 2000;101(13):1552-1558.

[68] Tandri H, Saranathan M, Rodriguez ER, Martinez C, Bomma C, Nasir K, et al. Noninvasive detection of myocardial fibrosis in arrhythmogenic right ventricular cardiomyopathy using delayed-enhancement magnetic resonance imaging. J Am Coll Cardiol. 2005;45(1):98-103.

[69] Bomma C, Rutberg J, Tandri H, Nasir K, Roguin A, Tichnell C, et al. Misdiagnosis of arrhythmogenic right ventricular dysplasia/cardiomyopathy. J Cardiovasc Electrophysiol. 2004;15(3):300-306.

[70] Fattori R, Tricoci P, Russo V, Lovato L, Bacchi-Reggiani L, Gavelli G, et al. Quantification of fatty tissue mass by magnetic resonance imaging in arrhythmogenic right ventricular dysplasia. J Cardiovasc Electrophysiol. 2005;16(3):256-261.

[71] Tandri H, Castillo E, Ferrari VA, Nasir K, Dalal D, Bomma C, et al. Magnetic resonance imaging of arrhythmogenic right ventricular dysplasia: sensitivity, specificity, and observer variability of fat detection versus functional analysis of the right ventricle. J Am Coll Cardiol. 2006;48(11):2277-2284.

[72] Piccini JP, Dalal D, Roguin A, Bomma C, Cheng A, Prakasa K, et al. Predictors of appropriate implantable defibrillator therapies in patients with arrhythmogenic right ventricular dysplasia. Heart Rhythm. 2005;2(11):1188-1194.

[73] Corrado D, Leoni L, Link MS, Della Bella P, Gaita F, Curnis A, et al. Implantable cardioverter-defibrillator therapy for prevention of sudden death in patients with arrhythmogenic right ventricular cardiomyopathy/dysplasia. Circulation. 2003;108(25): 3084-3091.

[74] Corrado D, Calkins H, Link MS, Leoni L, Favale S, Bevilacqua M, et al. Prophylactic implantable defibrillator in patients with arrhythmogenic right ventricular cardiomy-

opathy/dysplasia and no prior ventricular fibrillation or sustained ventricular tachycardia. Circulation.122(12):1144-1152.

[75] Corrado D, Basso C, Leoni L, Tokajuk B, Bauce B, Frigo G, et al. Three-dimensional electroanatomic voltage mapping increases accuracy of diagnosing arrhythmogenic right ventricular cardiomyopathy/dysplasia. Circulation. 2005;111(23):3042-3050.

[76] Boulos M, Lashevsky I, Reisner S, Gepstein L. Electroanatomic mapping of arrhythmogenic right ventricular dysplasia. J Am Coll Cardiol. 2001;38(7):2020-2027.

[77] Tandri H, Asimaki A, Abraham T, Dalal D, Tops L, Jain R, et al. Prolonged RV endocardial activation duration: a novel marker of arrhythmogenic right ventricular dysplasia/cardiomyopathy. Heart Rhythm. 2009;6(6):769-775.

[78] Santangeli P, Hamilton-Craig C, Dello Russo A, Pieroni M, Casella M, Pelargonio G, et al. Imaging of scar in patients with ventricular arrhythmias of right ventricular origin: cardiac magnetic resonance versus electroanatomic mapping. J Cardiovasc Electrophysiol.22(12):1359-1366.

[79] Wichter T, Borggrefe M, Haverkamp W, Chen X, Breithardt G. Efficacy of antiarrhythmic drugs in patients with arrhythmogenic right ventricular disease. Results in patients with inducible and noninducible ventricular tachycardia. Circulation. 1992;86(1):29-37.

[80] Marcus GM, Glidden DV, Polonsky B, Zareba W, Smith LM, Cannom DS, et al. Efficacy of antiarrhythmic drugs in arrhythmogenic right ventricular cardiomyopathy: a report from the North American ARVC Registry. J Am Coll Cardiol. 2009;54(7): 609-615.

[81] Arbelo E, Josephson ME. Ablation of ventricular arrhythmias in arrhythmogenic right ventricular dysplasia. J Cardiovasc Electrophysiol.21(4):473-486.

[82] Dalal D, Jain R, Tandri H, Dong J, Eid SM, Prakasa K, et al. Long-term efficacy of catheter ablation of ventricular tachycardia in patients with arrhythmogenic right ventricular dysplasia/cardiomyopathy. J Am Coll Cardiol. 2007;50(5):432-440.

[83] Borger van der Burg AE, de Groot NM, van Erven L, Bootsma M, van der Wall EE, Schalij MJ. Long-term follow-up after radiofrequency catheter ablation of ventricular tachycardia: a successful approach? J Cardiovasc Electrophysiol. 2002;13(5):417-423.

[84] Bhonsale A, James CA, Tichnell C, Murray B, Gagarin D, Philips B, et al. Incidence and predictors of implantable cardioverter-defibrillator therapy in patients with arrhythmogenic right ventricular dysplasia/cardiomyopathy undergoing implantable cardioverter-defibrillator implantation for primary prevention. J Am Coll Cardiol. 58(14):1485-1496.

[85] Lemola K, Brunckhorst C, Helfenstein U, Oechslin E, Jenni R, Duru F. Predictors of adverse outcome in patients with arrhythmogenic right ventricular dysplasia/cardiomyopathy: long term experience of a tertiary care centre. Heart. 2005;91(9):1167-1172.

[86] Oechslin EN, Attenhofer Jost CH, Rojas JR, Kaufmann PA, Jenni R. Long-term follow-up of 34 adults with isolated left ventricular noncompaction: a distinct cardiomyopathy with poor prognosis. J Am Coll Cardiol. 2000;36(2):493-500.

[87] Ichida F, Hamamichi Y, Miyawaki T, Ono Y, Kamiya T, Akagi T, et al. Clinical features of isolated noncompaction of the ventricular myocardium: long-term clinical course, hemodynamic properties, and genetic background. J Am Coll Cardiol. 1999;34(1):233-240.

[88] Pignatelli RH, McMahon CJ, Dreyer WJ, Denfield SW, Price J, Belmont JW, et al. Clinical characterization of left ventricular noncompaction in children: a relatively common form of cardiomyopathy. Circulation. 2003;108(21):2672-2678.

[89] Peters F, Khandheria BK, dos Santos C, Matioda H, Maharaj N, Libhaber E, et al. Isolated left ventricular noncompaction in sub-Saharan Africa: a clinical and echocardiographic perspective. Circ Cardiovasc Imaging.5(2):187-193.

[90] Dusek J, Ostadal B, Duskova M. Postnatal persistence of spongy myocardium with embryonic blood supply. Arch Pathol. 1975;99(6):312-317.

[91] Weiford BC, Subbarao VD, Mulhern KM. Noncompaction of the ventricular myocardium. Circulation. 2004;109(24):2965-2971.

[92] Jenni R, Wyss CA, Oechslin EN, Kaufmann PA. Isolated ventricular noncompaction is associated with coronary microcirculatory dysfunction. J Am Coll Cardiol. 2002;39(3):450-454.

[93] Chin TK, Perloff JK, Williams RG, Jue K, Mohrmann R. Isolated noncompaction of left ventricular myocardium. A study of eight cases. Circulation. 1990;82(2):507-513.

[94] Bleyl SB, Mumford BR, Brown-Harrison MC, Pagotto LT, Carey JC, Pysher TJ, et al. Xq28-linked noncompaction of the left ventricular myocardium: prenatal diagnosis and pathologic analysis of affected individuals. Am J Med Genet. 1997;72(3):257-265.

[95] Ichida F, Tsubata S, Bowles KR, Haneda N, Uese K, Miyawaki T, et al. Novel gene mutations in patients with left ventricular noncompaction or Barth syndrome. Circulation. 2001;103(9):1256-1263.

[96] Sasse-Klaassen S, Probst S, Gerull B, Oechslin E, Nurnberg P, Heuser A, et al. Novel gene locus for autosomal dominant left ventricular noncompaction maps to chromosome 11p15. Circulation. 2004;109(22):2720-2723.

[97] Vatta M, Mohapatra B, Jimenez S, Sanchez X, Faulkner G, Perles Z, et al. Mutations in Cypher/ZASP in patients with dilated cardiomyopathy and left ventricular noncompaction. J Am Coll Cardiol. 2003;42(11):2014-2027.

[98] Klaassen S, Probst S, Oechslin E, Gerull B, Krings G, Schuler P, et al. Mutations in sarcomere protein genes in left ventricular noncompaction. Circulation. 2008;117(22): 2893-2901.

[99] Probst S, Oechslin E, Schuler P, Greutmann M, Boye P, Knirsch W, et al. Sarcomere gene mutations in isolated left ventricular noncompaction cardiomyopathy do not predict clinical phenotype. Circ Cardiovasc Genet.4(4):367-374.

[100] Fazio G, Sutera L, Corrado G, Novo S. The chronic heart failure is not so frequent in non-compaction. Eur Heart J. 2007;28(10):1269; author reply 1269-1270.

[101] Ritter M, Oechslin E, Sutsch G, Attenhofer C, Schneider J, Jenni R. Isolated noncompaction of the myocardium in adults. Mayo Clin Proc. 1997;72(1):26-31.

[102] Caliskan K, Ujvari B, Bauernfeind T, Theuns DA, Van Domburg RT, Akca F, et al. The prevalence of early repolarization in patients with noncompaction cardiomyopathy presenting with malignant ventricular arrhythmias. J Cardiovasc Electrophysiol. 23(9):938-944.

[103] Paterick TE, Umland MM, Jan MF, Ammar KA, Kramer C, Khandheria BK, et al. Left ventricular noncompaction: a 25-year odyssey. J Am Soc Echocardiogr.25(4):363-375.

[104] Jenni R, Oechslin E, Schneider J, Attenhofer Jost C, Kaufmann PA. Echocardiographic and pathoanatomical characteristics of isolated left ventricular non-compaction: a step towards classification as a distinct cardiomyopathy. Heart. 2001;86(6):666-671.

[105] Kohli SK, Pantazis AA, Shah JS, Adeyemi B, Jackson G, McKenna WJ, et al. Diagnosis of left-ventricular non-compaction in patients with left-ventricular systolic dysfunction: time for a reappraisal of diagnostic criteria? Eur Heart J. 2008;29(1):89-95.

[106] Chaowu Y, Li L, Shihua Z. Histopathological features of delayed enhancement cardiovascular magnetic resonance in isolated left ventricular noncompaction. J Am Coll Cardiol.58(3):311-312.

[107] Petersen SE, Selvanayagam JB, Wiesmann F, Robson MD, Francis JM, Anderson RH, et al. Left ventricular non-compaction: insights from cardiovascular magnetic resonance imaging. J Am Coll Cardiol. 2005;46(1):101-105.

[108] Kawel N, Nacif M, Arai AE, Gomes AS, Hundley WG, Johnson WC, et al. Trabeculated (noncompacted) and compact myocardium in adults: the multi-ethnic study of atherosclerosis. Circ Cardiovasc Imaging.5(3):357-366.

[109] Jacquier A, Thuny F, Jop B, Giorgi R, Cohen F, Gaubert JY, et al. Measurement of trabeculated left ventricular mass using cardiac magnetic resonance imaging in the diagnosis of left ventricular non-compaction. Eur Heart J.31(9):1098-1104.

[110] Junga G, Kneifel S, Von Smekal A, Steinert H, Bauersfeld U. Myocardial ischaemia in children with isolated ventricular non-compaction. Eur Heart J. 1999;20(12):910-916.

[111] Toyono M, Kondo C, Nakajima Y, Nakazawa M, Momma K, Kusakabe K. Effects of carvedilol on left ventricular function, mass, and scintigraphic findings in isolated left ventricular non-compaction. Heart. 2001;86(1):E4.

http://dx.doi.org/10.5772/55628

[112] Kobza R, Steffel J, Erne P, Schoenenberger AW, Hurlimann D, Luscher TF, et al. Implantable cardioverter-defibrillator and cardiac resynchronization therapy in patients with left ventricular noncompaction. Heart Rhythm.7(11):1545-1549.

[113] Murphy RT, Thaman R, Blanes JG, Ward D, Sevdalis E, Papra E, et al. Natural history and familial characteristics of isolated left ventricular non-compaction. Eur Heart J. 2005;26(2):187-192.

Section 4

Sudden Death

Chapter 9

Sudden Cardiac Death

Prabhat Kumar and J Paul Mounsey

Additional information is available at the end of the chapter

http://dx.doi.org/10.5772/55636

1. Introduction

Sudden cardiac death (SCD) is a major cause of death in the USA and accounts for almost half of all cardiovascular deaths. The estimated annual incidence of SCD in the USA stands at 300,000 to 350,000. A significant fraction of the patients who die from SCD have underlying cardiovascular pathology, most commonly some form of cardiomyopathy but, often the disease remains unrecognized presenting with SCD as the first event. Ischemic heart disease is overwhelmingly the commonest cause of SCD but other forms of cardiomyopathy become more important cause of SCD in younger population. Although the patients with cardiomyopathy account for a small fraction of population burden of SCD, a subset of these patients are at high risk and this rationalizes aggressive preventive strategy in them (figure 1). Lower prevalence of ischemic heart disease in younger population makes other forms of cardiomyopathy more important in that population. Moreover, the relative contribution of SCD in the population has changed as the epidemiology, natural course and outcomes of lifestyle related cardiovascular diseases, particularly ischemic heart disease, have changed. In this chapter we will review sudden cardiac death in patients with cardiomyopathies focusing on epidemiology and risk stratification of SCD, and approaches for primary and secondary prevention strategies in them.

2. Sudden cardiac death and various forms of cardiomyopathy

Most cardiomyopathies with primary myocardial pathology predispose to sudden cardiac death. These include dilated cardiomyopathy (DCM), hypertrophic cardiomyopathy (HCM), left ventricular noncompaction and arrhythmogenic right ventricular cardiomyopathy (ARVC). Apart from the primary pathologies involving the myocardium, various other conditions can affect the myocardium secondarily due to myocardial stress, ischemia and

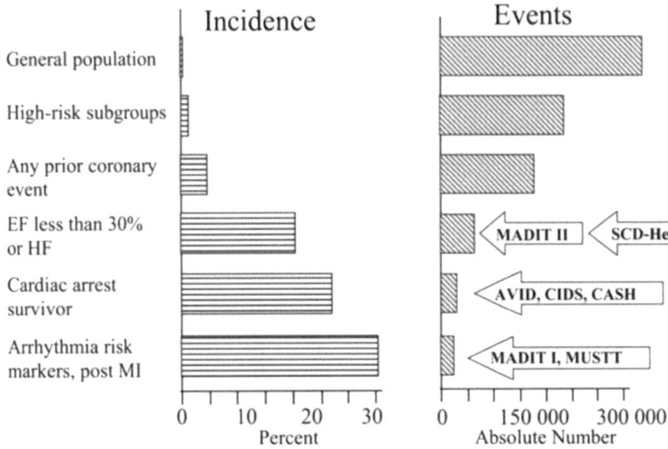

Figure 1. Absolute numbers of events and event rates of SCD in the general population and in specific subpopulations over 1 y. General population refers to unselected population age greater than or equal to 35 y, and high-risk subgroups to those with multiple risk factors for a first coronary event. Clinical trials that include specific subpopulations of patients are shown in the right side of the figure. AVID _ Antiarrhythmics Versus Implantable Defibrillators; CASH _ Cardiac Arrest Study Hamburg; CIDS _ Canadian Implantable Defibrillator Study; EF _ ejection fraction; HF _ heart failure; MADIT _ Multicenter Automatic Defibrillator Implantation Trial; MI _ myocardial infarction; MUSTT _ Multicenter UnSustained Tachycardia Trial; SCD-HeFT _ Sudden Cardiac Death in Heart Failure Trial. (Adapted with permission from reference 165)

infiltration. These conditions though not strictly classifiable as cardiomyopathies, but are important and common causes of SCD in the setting of myocardial dysfunction. They include ischemic heart disease, hypertension, valvular heart disease, and myocardial involvement with conditions like sarcoidosis, amyloidosis.

3. Etiopathogenesis and pathophysiology of sudden cardiac death

The commonest mechanism of SCD is a ventricular arrhythmia, most often ventricular tachycardia leading to vemntricular fibrillation. This accounts for 75-80% of all SCDs; the remainder are the result of bradyarrhythmias. [1] Bradyarrhythmias including high grade AV block and sinus node dysfunction may potentially be a mechanism of sudden death in cardiomyopathies. However, assessing the exact electrophysiological mechanism of sudden death may be complex since ventricular fibrillation may arise as an aftermath of a bradyarrhythmia. Futhermore patients having suffered a VF arrest may be found to be in asystole (the end stage of all arrhythmic sudden death) when first coming to medical attention, so both mechanisms may be involved either as an initiator or as perpetuator in the event of sudden death. In the Implanted Cardioverter Defibrillator (ICD) era with aborted sudden deaths due to ICD shocks, bradyarrhythmic mechanisms of sudden death may be masked effectively by back up bradycardia pacing by the ICDs.

Ventricular arrhythmias associated with cardiomyopathies result from primary electrical defects inherent to the cardiomyopathy and activation of the neuro-humoral system in the

http://dx.doi.org/10.5772/55636

body as a compensatory hemodynamic mechanism. The efficacy of neuro-humoral blockers like beta-blocker and renin-angiotensin-aldosterone axis blockers in effectively reducing the risk of sudden cardiac death in cardiomyopathy, and relation of the risk of sudden cardiac death to degree of hemodynamic jeopardy with cardiomyopathy suggest the latter mechanism. In the following sections we will discuss the current knowledge of mechanisms of sudden death in various forms of cardiomyopathies.

3.1. Ischemic cardiomyopathy

Ischemic cardiomyopathy is by far the most common cardiomyopathy leading to SCD Commonest cause of SCD in these patients is ventricular tachyarrhythmia. Beyond the early post-MI period, when recurrent MI and associated complications (mechanical and arrhythmic) are more likely, almost three-fourth of patient deaths among those with prior MI (more than three months old) and LV dysfunction are sudden and presumably arrhythmic, most likely due to ventricular arrhythmias. [2] Susceptibility to ventricular arrhythmia in these patients has multiple mechanisms. Scar resulting from myocardial infarction provides substrate for reentrant ventricular tachycardia. Re-entry circuits involve areas of residual viable relatively slowly conducting myocardial tissue inside the scars. These tracks of slowly conducting myocardial tissue inside a scar, called isthmus, connecting two healthy or relatively healthy areas form a full circuit for re-entrant arrhythmia. Patients with larger myocardial scar are more likely to have reentrant circuit. [3] Moreover, larger scars also lead to more ventricular remodeling and LV dysfunction, leading to activation of compensatory neuro-humoral factors in the setting of left ventricular dysfunction and heart failure. These factors lead to changes in repolarization and conduction properties of myocardial cells and abnormalities in intracellular calcium homeostasis which are potentially arrhythmogenic by promoting triggered activity and facilitating reentry. [4] Moreover, patients with ischemic cardiomyopathy have areas of ischemic myocardium which predispose to the arrhythmia by changes in the myocyte automaticity, excitability and refractoriness leading to dispersion of repolarization. The border zones of the myocardial scars are important substrates for arrhythmia as they are composed of fibrotic tissue as well as viable myocardium which are often ischemic. Heterogeneity of infarct tissue as assessed by magnetic resonance imaging has been shown to predispose to arrhythmia. Additionally, myocardial infarction leads to disturbances in the autonomic innervation of the myocardium in the area surrounding the post-infarct scar which makes the surrounding myocardium more susceptible to arrhythmia due to prolongation of refractory periods in the denervated myocardium. [5] Apart from these, a patient with ischemic heart disease is predisposed to SCD due to acute coronary syndrome.

3.2. Hypertrophic cardiomyopathy

Studies of HCM patients with ICDs have suggested that ventricular arrhythmias are the major causes of SCD in this group of patients, [6], [7] although availability of back up pacing for bradyarrhythmia precludes the ability of an ICD study to exclude the possibility of a bradyarrhythmic etiology. [6] Bradyarrhythmias are, however, reported rarely in HCM so this seems an unlikely possibility. Multiple pathologic, molecular and physiologic mechanisms could contribute to the causation of ventricular arrhythmias in patients with HCM. HCM is characterized pathologically by hypertrophied myocardium along with increased fibrosis and myocardial disarray (figure 2). [8-10] Apart from these histopathological features that predispose to ventricular arrhythmias, there are also abnormalities of calcium handling at molecular level. Cardiomyocytes in patients with systolic and diastolic heart failure have impaired ability of calcium cycling due to altered expression and phosphorylation of sarcoplasmic calcium ATPase 2(SERCA 2) and ryanodine receptor 2, key proteins involved in intracellular calcium handling. [11], [12] Perturbed calcium fluxes have also been seen in HCM. [13], [14] Inefficient energy utilization in some of the HCM associated mutations of troponin lead to insufficient energy for the cardiomyocytes to maintain cellular calcium hemostasis, leading to increased risk of arrhythmia especially during exercise. [15], [16] Microvascular dysfuction with myocardial ischemia along with increased energy needs is another important factor contributing to the arrhythmogenicity in HCM. [17], [18] Left ventricular outflow tract obstruction (LVOTO) and altered systolic blood pressure response to exercise may mechanistically predispose to SCD by electromechanical dissociation and demand ischemia. Hence arrhythmogenic substrates in HCM potentially include altered cellular handling of calcium, with myocardial ischemia, patchy myocardial fibrosis and hypertrophy maintaining the arrhythmias. Moreover, presence of systolic or diastolic heart failure itself may contribute to the risk by neuro-humoral activation. Apart from these intrinsic predispositions to arrhythmogenesis in the natural course of disease, there has been recent concern of iatrogenic arrhythmias in patients undergoing alcohol septal ablation, which leaves a large ventricular septal scar predisposing to scar-related re-entrant ventricular arrhythmias. [19]-[21]

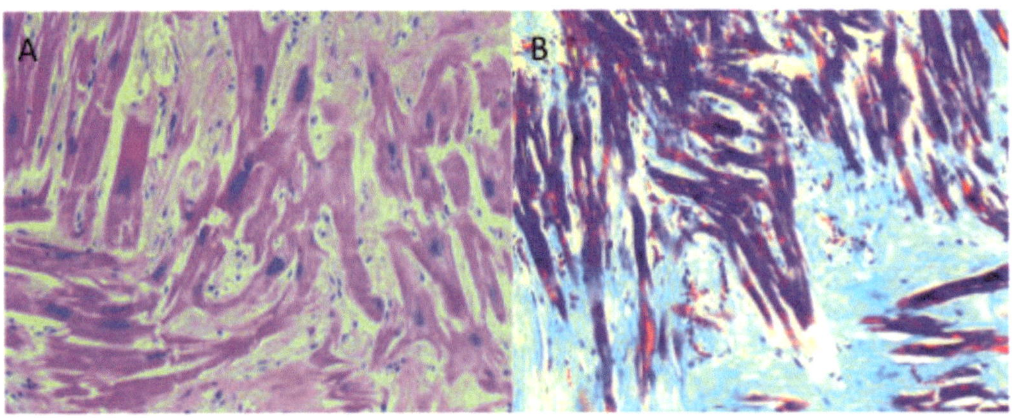

Figure 2. Photomicrographs showing hematoxyline and eosin-stained section with florid myocyte disarray and fibrosis in familial HCM. Disarray is characterized by hypertrophic myocytes with enlarged and pleomorphic nuclei aligned at odd angles to one another (panel A). Photomicrograph showing Masson's trichrome stain with marked increase in interstitial fibrosis, a hallmark of HCM (panel B). **Adapted with permission from chapter 'Cardiomyopathy' by Sian Hughes from the book 'Cardiac PatholOlgy: A Guide to Current Practice' eds' S. Kim Suvarna ISBN: 978-1-4471-2406-1 (Print) 978-1-4471-2407-8 (Online) (Springer).**

http://dx.doi.org/10.5772/55636

3.3. Arrhythmogenic cardiomyopathy

The hallmark of arrhythmogenic cardiomyopathy (previously called arrhythmogenic right ventricular cardiomyopathy) is a defect in cell-cell adhesion caused by genetic defects most commonly affecting the desmosomal proteins. Such defects lead to myocyte loss with fibrofatty replacement of the myocardial tissue (figure 3), most commonly involving the right ventricle, with left ventricular and biventricular involvement less commonly. This provides a substrate for ventricular tachycardia from re-entry around the fibrous scar. [22] Reports of ventricular arrhythmia in subjects harboring the genes of arrhythmogenic cardiomyopathy even in the absence of detectable histopathological and MRI changes in the myocardium suggest an additional electrical substrate distinct from simple reentry involving perhaps intracellular signaling process or heterogeneity in conduction. Gap junction remodeling with paucity of gap junctions in the myocardial cells of affected patients may also provide a substrate for arrhythmia. [23]

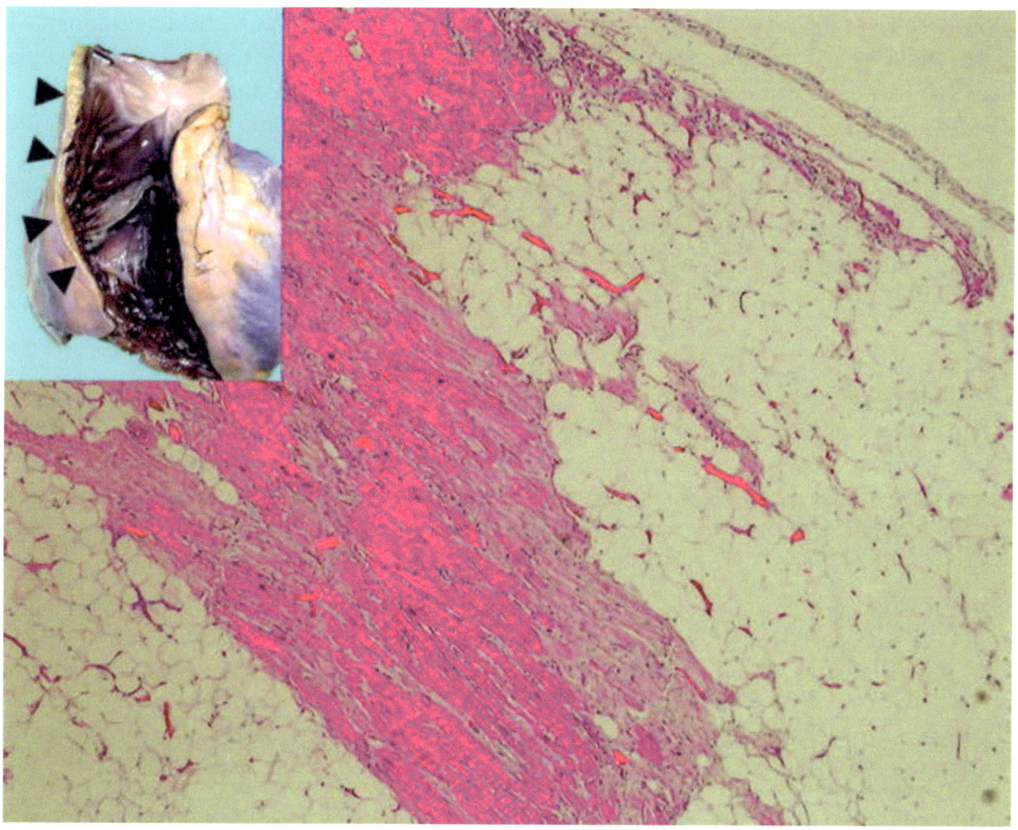

Figure 3. Fibroadipose infiltration of the right ventricle, seen in the inset macroscopically top right, arrowed. Histology shows the adipose and fibrous tissue replacement of the myocyte architecture (hematoxylin & eosin). **Adapted with**

permission from chapter 'Cardiomyopathy' by Sian Hughes from the book 'Cardiac Pathololgy: A Guide to Current Practice' eds' S. Kim Suvarna ISBN: 978-1-4471-2406-1 (Print) 978-1-4471-2407-8 (Online) (Springer).

3.4. Dilated cardiomyopathy

Dilated cardiomyopathy is characterized by loss of myocardial cells with interstitial, perivascular and replacement fibrosis, which provide an arrhythmogenic substrate (figure 4). [24], [25] Frequently the reentry circuits of these arrhythmias exit on the epicardial aspect of the myocardium, as distinct from ischemic cardiomyopathy where endocardial circuits are the rule. [25] This is related to the differences in the pathogenetic mechanism of scar formation in the two groups of patients, patients with ischemic cardiomyopathy having predisposition to endocardial scar due to subendocardial ischemia and acute coronary events, while patients with dilated cardiomyopathy having epicardial scar more often than ischemic cardiomyopathy. This also has implications on therapeutic approach as patients with nonischemic cardiomyopathy with VT frequently require epicardial approach for catheter ablation. [26] Arrhythmic events occurring in patients with idiopathic dilated cardiomyopathy are nonsustained and sustained VT and ventricular fibrillation in addition to isolated ventricular ectopy. [27], [28] Bundle branch reentry VT is relatively commoner form of VT in patients with dilated cardiomyopathy, constituting 6-11% of patients referred for catheter mapping of monomorphic VT. [26], [29] Spontaneous sustained VT is rare in DCM and this diagnosis should raise the suspicion of other types of cardiomyopathies that do commonly cause scar related ventricular arrhythmias, including sarcoidosis, Chagas disease and left dominant arrhythmogenic cardiomyopathy. Spontaneous sustained VTs are caused by scar-related related reentry or bundle branch reentry. [25], [29] Neurohumoral activation, myocardial stretch secondary to mechanical overload and electrolyte disturbance all can contribute to arrhythmogenesis by a non-reentrant mechanism facilitating focal mechanisms of arrhythmogenesis like triggered activity and focal automaticity. [28]

3.5. Left Ventricular noncompaction

Left ventricular noncompaction is a recently recognized form of cardiomyopathy. Also referred to as left ventricular hypertrabeculation, LV myocardium in these patients shows increased trabeculation, unlike normal compact structure of the LV. Imaging with echocardiography or cardiac MRI, showing thick endocardial noncompact layer of myocardium and relatively thin epicardial compact myocardium, usually makes the diagnosis. Apart from heart failure and thromboembolic events, patients with ventricular noncompaction are known to be at an increased risk of sudden cardiac death due to ventricular arrhythmias. Life-threatening ventricular tachycardias are reported in almost one fifth of the patient. The arrhythmogenic substrate is in the form of subdendocardial fibrosis due to microcirculatory dysfunction (figure 5). [30], [31]

3.6. Other cardiomyopathies

Sarcoidosis frequently involves the myocardium, causing infiltration and scarring. Although at least 25% of patients with sarcoidosis have cardiac involvement based on autopsy data, only 5% have cardiac symptoms. Patients with sarcoid cardiomyopathy are at an increased risk of

http://dx.doi.org/10.5772/55636

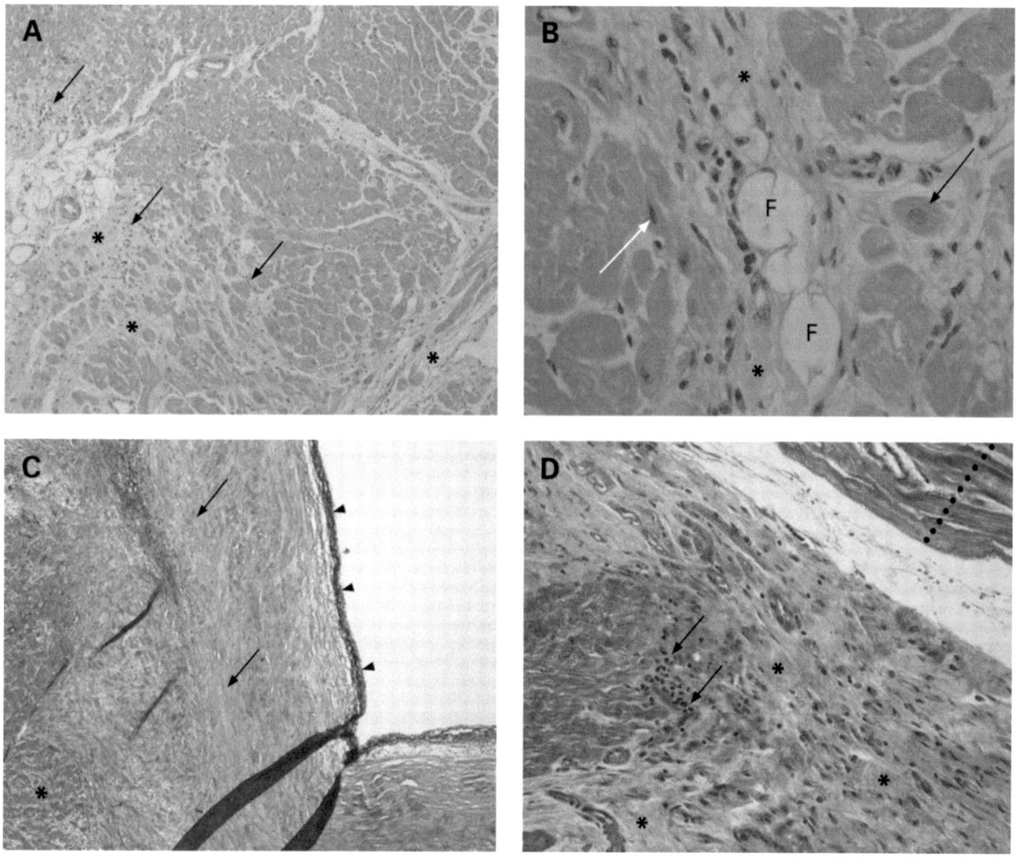

Figure 4. Photomicrographs of the myocardium from a 35-year-old female. (A) Shows evidence of myofibre hypertrophy, interstitial fibrosis (*) and areas of lymphocytic infiltration (arrows) consistent with resolving myocarditis (H&E). (B) While some myocytes are hypertrophied with enlarged nuclei (black arrow), others are thinned and elongated with nuclei that occupy almost the entire width of the myocyte (white arrow). Some myocytes appear "empty"; likely due to diminished numbers of myofibrils. Areas of interstitial fibrosis (*) and fat infiltration (F) can also be seen (H&E). (C) Photomicropgraph showing evidence of interstitial fibrosis (*), subendocardial fibrosis (arrows) and endocardial fibroelastic changes (arrowheads) (H&E). (D) Microphotograph of myocardium showing degenerative changes in the left bundle (dotted line). These changes may appear as a bundle branch block on ECG. Areas of interstitial fibrosis (*) and lymphocytic infiltration (arrows) are also seen (elastic trichrome stain). **Adapted with permission from Luk et al, Dilated cardiomypathy : a review. J Clin Pathol 2009;62:219-225.**

developing a conduction system abnormality due to involvement of basal part of the interventricular septum and this may result in complete heart block [32], [33] and potentially sudden cardiac death. Ventricular arrhythmia is another mechanism of sudden cardiac death in patients with cardiac sarcoidosis. Resolving inflammation and resulting scarring of the myocardium provides substrate for reentrant ventricular arrhythmias. [34], [35]

Cardiac amyloid infiltration is another disorder associated with increased risk of sudden cardiac death. Amyloid infiltration with perivascular fibrosis and small vessel ischemia [36] is instrumental in pathology of cardiac conduction system and myocardium. These pathological changes lead to the electrophysiological abnormalities responsible for sudden cardiac

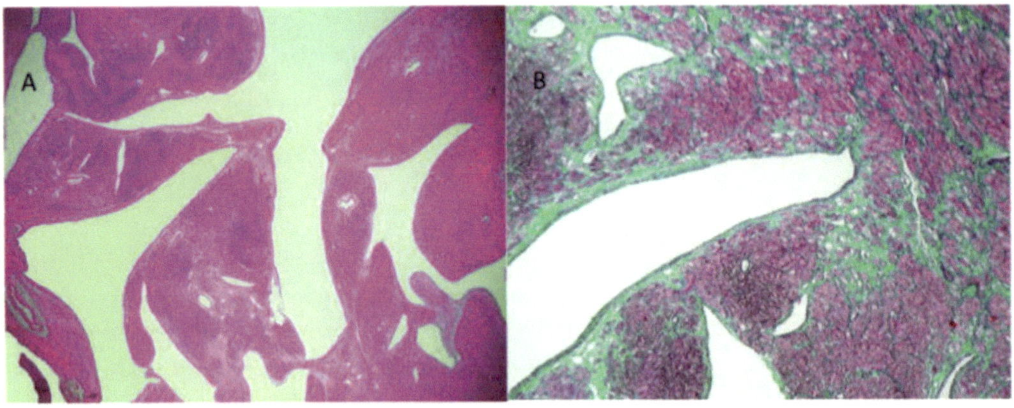

Figure 5. Photomicrographs of myocardium from a patient with LV noncompaction. Panel A shows low-power hematoxylin- and eosin-stained photograph from noncompacted layer shoing 'fingerlike' projections. Panel B has a photomicrograph with Masson's t trichrome stain showing prominent endocardial and subendocardial fibrosis, which is a feature of this disease due to abnormal myocardial microperfusion. **Adapted from chapter 'Cardiomyopathy' by Sian Hughes from the book 'Cardiac Patholoolgy: A Guide to Current Practice' eds' S. Kim Suvarna ISBN: 978-1-4471-2406-1 (Print) 978-1-4471-2407-8 (Online) (Springer).**

death due to bradyarrhythmia or ventricular tachyarrhythmia. [37] Frequently the cause of sudden death in these patients is pulseless electrical activity, presumably resulting from the severe diastolic dysfunction associated with amyloidosis. [38]

Inherited muscular dystrophies like Duchenne and Becker muscular dystrophies have skeletal and cardiac muscle involvement and cardiac pathology essentially manifests as dilated cardiomyopathy with associated heart failure and risk of sudden cardiac death. However, muscular dystrophies like Emery-Dreifuss (X-linked and autosomal variants), limb girdle muscular dystrophy type 1B, entity of DCM with conduction system disease (associated with lamin A/C mutations) and myotonic dystrophy are associated with high risk of sudden cardiac death. In these conditions sudden cardiac death was traditionally thought to be primarily due to conduction system disease and bradyarrhythmia. However, after routine implantation of pacemakers, it has been recognized that ventricular arrhythmias also contribute to sudden cardiac death in these patients. These conditions are associated with cardiomyopathy, with LV dysfunction as a late feature in the natural course of disease; sudden cardiac death is an early feature of cardiac involvement. The molecular pathogenesis of cardiac arrhythmias and conduction system disease in these patients is an area of active research. [39]

4. Risk of sudden cardiac death in cardiomyopathy: Epidemiology and risk stratification

The epidemiologic risk of sudden cardiac death in cardiomyopathy is often difficult to assess because it is frequently impossible to determine the size of the population at risk. Determination of risk is skewed by referral bias. The risk of sudden death has been studied with these

http://dx.doi.org/10.5772/55636

limitations in several groups of patients, most notably in those with ICM but also in hypertrophic cardiomyopathy and arrhythmogenic cardiomyopathy. Attempts to identify features predicting higher risk of sudden cardiac death have helped in management decisions. In this section we will discuss available knowledge about risk of sudden death and risk stratification in patients with cardiomyopathy.

Hypertrophic cardiomyopathy	**Dilated cardiomyopathy**
Major risk factors · Prior cardiac arrest · Spontaneous sustained VT · Family history of 1 or more · instances of SCD · Nonsustained VT (≥3consecutive beats at ≥120 bpm) · Failure of systolic BP to rise by ≥20 mm Hg during maximal upright exercise testing · Unexplained syncope · Maximum LV wall thickness ≥30 mm **Other risk factors** · Resting LV outflow tract · obstruction · Microvascular ischemia · Diffuse late gadolinium · enhancement on cardiovascular · magnetic resonance · Paced electrogram fractionation · analysis · Prior alcohol septal ablation · Burnt out disease · High-risk mutation	· Prior cardiac arrest · Left Ventricular systolic function · History of syncope · Genetic factors · NYHA functional class · Prolongation of QRS · QT dynamicity · QRS fragmentation · Heart rate variability, heart rate turbulence and heart rate recovery, · Baroreflex sensitivity · T-wave alternans · Myocardial fibrosis: serum markers, cardiac MRI
	Ischemic cardiomyopathy
	· Prior cardiac arrest outside the setting of acute coronary syndrome · LV systolic function · NYHA fuctional class · QRS duration · QT interval prolongation
Arrhythmogenic right ventricular cardiomyopathy	· QT dispersion,
· Prior cardiac arrest · History of syncope · RV dilatation/dysfunction · LV involvement · QRS dispersion · Right precordial QRS prolongation and late potentials on SAECG	· T-wave alternans · Abnormal SAECG · Heart rate variability, heart rate turbulence and heart rate recovery, · Baroreflex sensitivity

Table 1. Risk predictors for SCD in cardiomyopathies

4.1. Ischemic cardiomyopathy

Attempts at risk stratification for SCD initially included patient with history of myocardial infarction and LV systolic dysfunction emerged as the strongest predictor of overall mortality and SCD in them. [40]-[45] Many other potential risk factors have been studied, but LVEF remains the strongest and most widely used predictor of SCD risk. ICD trials for prevention of SCD have established the role of LV systolic function as the most important risk predictor. Other important predictors of SCD in these patients include electrocardiographic parameters, functional class, inducibility of ventricular arrhythmia with programmed ventricular stimulation, autonomic and neuro-humoral predictors and disturbances in autonomic innervation of the myocardium.

1. *LV systolic function* emerged from studies in post-MI patients as a predictor of SCD. An analysis of 20 studies found the relative risk of a major arrhythmic event in patients with LVEF≤30% to 40% to be 4.3. [46] The Second Multicenter Automatic Defibrillator Implantation Trial (MADIT-II) and the Sudden Cardiac Death Heart Failure Trial (SCD-HeFT) clearly demonstrated the benefit of ICD implantation in patients with LVEF less than 30% or 35% respectively in preventing sudden death and reducing absolute mortality in patients with history of myocardial infarction. [47], [48]

2. *Functional class* is a surrogate of severity of heart failure and heart failure severity predisposes to arrhythmogenesis by neuro-humoral mechanisms and homeostatic and hemodynamic changes. NYHA class has been used as criterion to enroll patients in the ICD trials and some of these studies have found its predictive value. Subgroup analysis of SCD-HeFT enrolling patients with congestive heart failure with either ischemic or nonischemic cardiomyopathy showed that patients with NYHA class III did not appear to benefit as opposed to patients with NYHA class II. [48] On the other hand in MADIT-II patients, there were no significant differences in the outcomes based on NYHA class. [47] NYHA functional class III was found to be the strongest independent predictor of ICD therapy in the Trigger Of Ventricular Arrhythmia (TOVA) trial. [49]

3. *Programmed ventricular stimulation* with inducible VT/VF has been recognized as a predictor of sudden cardiac death in patients with history of myocardial infarction. MADIT-I study which included patients with inducible VT/VF and LVEF ≤ 35% showed a 26% absolute reduction in mortality at 27 months follow-up. [50] The reduction in mortality was much lower at 6-7% absolute reduction in mortality in patients with MADIT-II trial which enrolled patients with LVEF ≤ 30% and in a mixed population of ischemic and nonischemic cardiomyopathy patients in SCD-HeFT enrolling patients with LVEF ≤ 35% without electrophysiological assessment of inducibility. [47], [48] The Multicenter UnSustained Tachycardia Trial (MUSTT), enrolling patients with LVEF≤40 and inducible VT on invasive assessment showed similarly high absolute reduction in mortality of 31% at five years of follow up. [51]

4. *Ventricular ectopy and NSVT* has been shown to increase the risk of sudden cardiac death in patients with history of MI in multiple studies. In the early observational studies from

1970s and 1980s, VPBs (≥10 per hour) and NSVT in post-MI patients showed increased risk of overall mortality. [40], [42], [52], [53] Similar effect of ventricular ectopy and NSVT in post-MI patients has also been seen in the era of thrombolytic therapy for acute MI. [45], [54]-[57] GISSI-2 trial showed a mortality of 5.5% at six months after MI in patients with more than 10 VPBs per hour compared to 2% in those with less frequent VPBs. [57] Positive predictive value of VPBs in predicting cardiac arrhythmic events is in the range of 5% to 15% with negative predictive value of in the range of 90%. [58] However, when combined with LV ejection fraction, ventricular ectopy becomes a stronger risk predictor of SCD in post-MI patients. In European Myocardial Infarction Amiodarone Trial (EMIAT), post-MI patients with LVEF ≤ 40% had higher mortality in the presence of frequent or complex arrhythmias on ambulatory ECG than in their absence (20% vs. 10%). [59] Moreover, MADIT-I and MUSTT enrolled patients based on the presence of NSVT and showed benefit in terms of reduction in all-cause mortality and SCD with ICD, all these patients had to have inducible ventricular arrhythmia for being enrolled into the study. [50], [51]

5. *Electrocardiographic parameters* have been studied in multiple studies and can be divided into parameters assessing ventricular conduction abnormality and parameters of ventricular repolarization abnormality. Parameters of conduction abnormality including QRS duration, abnormalities on signal averaged ECG, and fractionation of QRS have been studied in many studies. Parameters of repolarization abnormality including QT interval prolongation, QT dispersion, T wave variance, QT dynamics, QT/RR slope and T-wave alternans have all been studies in many studies. Each of these parameters confer a small risk of sudden cardiac death individually. [60]-[62]

6. *Parameters of autonomic function* include heart rate variability, heart rate turbulence, baroreceptor sensitivity and deceleraltion capacity. These again have been found to increase the risk of sudden death in patients history of myocardial infarction with in many small studies. [60]-[62]

7. *Myocardial scar* is instrumental in the pathogenesis of ventricular tachycardia by providing the substrate for reentry circuit. Myocardial scar area assessed by cardiac MRI has been demonstrated to be a predictor of inducible VT on electrophysiological study. [3] Moreover, heterogeneity of scar in the border zone of infarct can be assessed by MRI and has been shown to be a predictor of inducible and spontaneous ventricular arrhythmias. [63], [64]

8. *Cardiac autonomic denervation* has been suggested a potential risk for arrhythmogenesis in post-MI patients. Although denervation of peri-infarct tissue was found to be a risk factor for inducible ventricular arrhythmia in animal model, [65] it failed to show any value in a small clinical study. [66] However, a study in a population of heart failure patients including both ischemic and nonischemic cardiomyopathy, showed increased risk of ventricular arrhythmia with disturbances in myocardial innervation assessed by mIBG scintigraphy. [67]

9. *Combinations of risk factors:* As individual risk factor are not strong enough to predict SCD and probably in isolation do not justify the use of ICD therapy to prevent SCD with the current level of evidence, there has been an attempt to combine multiple risk factors to create a model to enhance the predictability of SCD. Although there are multiple small studies combining various risk factors to achieve the goal of refining the risk stratification strategy, there is a need to assess these risk models in a prospective manner. [61], [68]

Study	Patient population	LVEF of enrolled patients (%)	All-cause mortality (%)		Risk reduction (%)	
Control	**ICD**	**Relative**	**Absolute**			
Primary prevention ICD trials						
AVID	VFib, VT with syncope, VT with EF ≤40%	32	25	18	27	7
CIDS	VFib, out-of-hospital cardiac arrest due to VFib or VT, VT with syncope, VT with symptoms and EF ≤35%, unmonitored syncope with subsequent spontaneous or induced VT	34	21	15	30	6
CASH	VFib, VT	46	44	36	23	8
Primary prevention ICD trials						
MADIT	Prior MI, EF ≤35%, N-S VT, inducible VT non-suppressible with IV procainamide	26	32	13	59	19
CABG Patch	Coronary bypass surgery, EF <36%, SAECG (+)	27	18	18	-	-
MUSTT	CAD (prior MI ~95%), EF ≤40%, N-S VT, inducible VT	30	55	24	58	31
MADIT II	Prior MI (>1 month), EF ≤30%	23	22	16	28	6
DEFINITE	Nonischemic CM, Hx HF, EF ≤35%, ≥10 PVCs/hr or N-S VT	21	14	8	44	6
DINAMIT	Recent MI (6-40 days), EF ≤35%, abnormal HRV or mean 24-hr heart rate >80/min	28	17	19	-	-
SCD-HeFT	Class II-III CHF, EF ≤35%	25	36	29	23	7

Table 2. ICD trials

http://dx.doi.org/10.5772/55636

4.2. Hypertrophic cardiomyopathy

Hypertrophic cardiomyopathy is frequently complicated by sudden cardiac death, and SCD in, for example, athletes is frequently caused by HCM. This being said, early estimates of the gravity of the prognosis of HCM were probably driven by referral bias of difficult cases to specialist centers, and studies of more inclusive cohorts of patients indicate a much more favorable prognosis. [69] A study by Maron et al analyzing a cohort of 774 non-referral-based HCM patients showed an incidence of SCD of 0.7% per year. [70] They showed that although SCDs occur across the age groups in patients with HCM, there are two peaks of SCD risk during life, one in the early childhood and the other later in older age group in seventh and eighth decades of life.

Several risk factors associated with SCD in HCM have been identified and it is important to recognize this high-risk subset of patients for management strategies and prognostication.

1. *History of syncope:* In patients with HCM syncope is an important predictor of SCD. This has been confirmed by multiple survival studies and a systematic review of 11 survival studies. [71] Five of these survival studies showed a significant association between history of syncope and SCD in these patients. [72]-[76] and in the systematic review the hazard ratio was 2.68 (95% CI 0.97-4.38) for SCD. This association is clinically important and a history of syncope in a HCM patient is worrisome and should prompt further intensive investigation.

2. *Non-sustained ventricular tachycardia (NSVT)* with ≥3 consecutive ventricular beats at a rate of 120 beats per minute lasting for <30 seconds has been shown to be significantly associated with SCD in patients with HCM. [73], [77]-[79] The systematic study evaluating the risk of SCD with NSVT showed a hazard ratio of SCD of 2.89 (95%CI 2.2-3.6). [71] The risk of SCD associated with NSVT is lower in patients with older age (31-75 years), whereas younger patient (14-30 years of age) have more than a four-fold increased risk of SCD (HR 4.35, 95% CI1.54-12.28). [77]

3. *Severe left ventricular hypertrophy (LVH)* has been found to be a predictor of sudden cardiac death in multiple studies. [8], [72], [77], [80]-[82]In a recent systematic review the risk of SCD was found to be three-fold (hazard ratio 3.1, 95%CI 1.81-4.4) despite variable definitions. [71] Although most of the studies used a cut off for maximum wall thickness of ≥30 mm, there has been concern about variability in measurement across the studies and lack of data about pattern of LVH. One study used Wigle scores, a semi-quantitative scoring system described earlier, [83] for LVH severity and showed increased risk of SCD with increasing Wigle score. [81]

4. *Family history of SCD and Genetic markers:* Familial association of SCD has been described in patients with HCM in early studies. [84]-[86] A systematic review of survival studies showed an increased risk of SCD in patients with family history of SCD with hazard ratio of 1.27(95%CI 1.16-1.38) [71]Family members tend to share genetic abnormality, and certain specific genetic mutations have been associated with higher risk of SCD. For example, troponin T mutations have been reported to have association with high risk of SCD, often disproportionate to the other phenotypic expression. [87]

5. *Left ventricular outflow tract obstruction (LVOTO):* The severity of the dynamic LVOTO is associated with an increased risk of SCD. The mechanism of this could be reduction of cardiac output and electromechanical dissociation, but myocardial ischemia induced by increased ventricular stress is also of possible etiologic significance. An instantaneous pressure gradient of 50 mmHg across the LVOT is considered to be clinically significant. Five studies have shown significant association between LVOTO and SCD in patients with HCM. [73], [76], [79], [88]

6. *Systolic blood pressure response to exercise* is altered in many patients with HCM probably due to decreased systemic vascular resistance. [89] Sadoul et al demonstrated in 161 HCM patients ≤40 years old that failure of systolic blood pressure to rise ≥20 mmHg during exercise or a fall of >20 from the peak systolic blood pressure was associated with an increased risk of SCD (15% vs 3%, $p<0.009$). [90] However, analysis of multiple survival studies with data from a wider age range did not confirm this association (hazard ratio 1.23, 95%CI 0.64-1.96) [71] but four of these studies did show abnormal systolic blood pressure response to be a risk factor for SCD in subjects ≤40 years old. [73], [76], [77], [80]

7. *Other factors: Atrial fibrillation* and *left atrial size* may reflect the risk of SCD as they reflect the severity of left ventricular pathology. [74], [91] *NYHA functional class* is also a function of diastolic dysfunction, myocardial ischemia, LVOTO, atrial arrhythmias and adverse remodeling, and potentially can be associated with SCD, but studies reporting survival analysis for SCD did not report any significant association. *Late gadolinium enhancement* on MRI, which is suggestive of presence of extracellular myocardial collagen deposition and a potential substrate for ventricular arrhythmias, was not associated with SCD in a recent study, although it was associated with cardiovascular morbidity and mortality. [10] *Increased fractionation* of the paced right ventricular electrogram at invasive electrophysiological study has been found to be associated with SCD in patients with HCM and this is presumably a reflection of myofibrillar disarray. HCM patients with *LV systolic dysfunction* should be considered at a higher risk of SCD similar to other causes of LV systolic dysfunction. *Age* of the patient modifies the risk of SCD in patients with HCM as suggested by multiple studies with higher risk in adolescence and early adulthood. The survival study by Spirito et al showed a significant reduction in SCD risk with increasing age, however, this study did not include other established risk factors in multivariate analysis.[74]

4.3. Arrhythmogenic cardiomyopathy

Ventricular arrhythmia, principally VF is the mode of SCD in patients with arrhythmogenic cardiomyopathy. The absolute risk of SCD in a patient with ARVC has been reported, although inconsistencies between different studies make it hard to establish the degree of risk. The annual risk of SCD in studies from the pre-ICD era in high-risk cohorts was in the range of 1-1.5%. [92]-[94] Sports activity increases the risk of SCD by five fold. [95] Although more recent follow-up studies of patients with ICDs have shown a higher annual rate of ICD intervention, of 5-8%, [96], [97] an ICD intervention may not be a good surrogate for SCD. A follow-up study of patients diagnosed on the basis of aggressive screening of the family members of the probands showed much lower annual incidence of SCD at 0.08% per year. [98] This suggests a strong selection bias of high-risk patients in the previous follow-up studies and with current approach of aggressive screening of the family members of probands; the previous estimates of the degree of risk of SCD may not be applicable. Many studies have tried to establish parameters to predict the risk of sudden death.

1. *History of syncope* has been documented as a precursor of SCD in multiple studies. [93] In a study by Nava et al syncope was the only clinical variable predictive of SCD in probands, while none of the family members of the proband had history of syncope. [98] The Darvin II study and data from the Johns Hopkins arrhythmogenic cardiomyopathy clinic have evaluated the importance of history of syncope in patients receiving ICD. The multi-center Darvin II study showed that syncope is a strong predictor of life-saving device intervention in patients with ICD. In the Johns Hopkins cohort, although 75% of the patients with AC receiving appropriate ICD therapy did not have history of syncope, one half of patients with history of syncope prior to the implantation of ICD received appropriate ICD therapy (9%/year). A recent history of syncope was even stronger predictor of appropriate ICD therapy compared to remote history of syncope. [99]

2. *Prior history of hemodynamically unstable ventricular arrhythmia or cardiac arrest* is a strong predictor of SCD. A history of arrhythmic cardiac arrest or hemodynamically unstable VT, but not a history of hemodynamically stable VT, was found to be independent predictor of life-saving ICD therapy in a study by Corrado et al. [96] In another study by Canu et al with retrospective analysis of 22 patients, previous history of resuscitated VF was present in two out of three patients who died suddenly. [100]

3. *Electrocardiographic parameters* including QRS dispersion, right precordial QRS prolongation and late potentials on signal-averaged ECG (SAECG) have been found to be associated with risk of SCD. Turrini et al demonstrated longer QRS duration in right precordial leads in patients with SCD as compared to those without. [101] QRS dispersion of >40 msec was strong independent predictor of SCD in this study. Late potential on SAECG have not been found to predict arrhythmic risk in these patients. [102]-[104] Although in the study by Turrini et al late potentials were univariate predictors of sustained VT, decreased RV ejection fraction remained the only independent predictor in multivariate analysis. [104]

4. *RV dilatation/dysfunction and LV involvement* are important predictors of poor outcome [105] and SCD [106] in arrhythmogenic cardiomyopathy. RV dysfunction has been associated with increased risk of ICD discharges and sustained VT. [97], [104], [107] It is not clear as yet if LV involvement detected by tissue characterization without LV dilatation or dysfunction increases the risk of SCD.

5. *Other factors:* Most of the *genetic variants* of arrhythmogenic cardiomyopathy have similar risks of SCD. However a very malignant genetic variant with TMEM43 gene mutation significantly increases the risk of SCD. [108] Studies evaluating the significance of *programmed ventricular stimulation* as a predictor of SCD in the patients with arrhythmogenic cardiomyopathy has shown mixed results. The DARVIN studies and the study by

Wichter et al did not show any significant predictive value of programmed ventricular stimulation in predicting ICD discharges. [96], [97], [109] Although the Johns Hopkins study did show some relationship between programmed stimulation of ventricular arrhythmia and later ICD shocks, the association did not confer good positive and negative predictive values (65% and 75% respectively). [99] Hence, withholding ICD therapy on the basis of negative EP study should not be recommended and other parameters for risk stratification should be taken into consideration to make a decision for ICD implantation.

4.4. Dilated cardiomyopathy

SCD in patients with dilated cardiomyopathy is one of the major causes of mortality, constituting nearly one-third of all deaths. Left ventricular systolic function as determined by LVEF and NYHA functional class have become the most extensively used variable to stratify risk of SCD in this group of patients. Other parameters including a history of syncope, genetic factors and programmed ventricular stimulation have been evaluated to stratify the risk of SCD in these patients, and these are summarized below.

1. *Left Ventricular systolic function* is associated with increased overall mortality and SCD in patients with nonischemic dilated cardiomyopathy. [110]-[112] This has been reaffirmed by the reduction in SCD seen with ICD implantation in patients with NIDCM with LV systolic dysfunction in DEFINITE and SCD-HeFT ICD trials. [48], [113]

2. *NYHA functional class* is important determinant of overall survival and SCD in patients with systolic heart failure. [114] However, with worsening NYHA functional class, non-sudden death becomes relatively more important in patients with heart failure compared to SCD. Patients with NYHA class III were significantly more likely to receive ICD therapy for ventricular arrhythmia even after adjusting for LVEF in TOVA study, however, there were very few patients with NYHA class IV in this study. [49] NYHA class IV patients, although at risk of arrhythmic death, are less likely to benefit from ICD due to competing risk of non-sudden heart failure death. Majority of patients in the major ICD trials (SCD-HeFT and DEFINITE) were class II and class III patients, and the reduction in SCD in these groups of patients is well established. [48], [113] However, NYHA class I patients were largely under-represented in majority of the ICD trials with the exception of DEFINITE study which had 21.6% patients in NYHA class I.

3. *History of syncope* increases the risk of SCD in patients with heart failure with dilated cardiomyopathy. In a SCD-HeFT sub-study patients with history of syncope had higher frequency of receiving appropriate ICD therapy compared to those without a history of syncope. Moreover, patients with history of syncope had similarly increased risk of mortality in ICD (HR: 1.54, 95% CI 10.4-2.27), amiodarone (HR: 1.33, 95% CI 0.91-1.93) and placebo (HR: 1.39, 95% CI 0.96-2.02) arms ($p=0.86$ for test of difference between the three arms).

4. *Genetic factors:* There has been a recent recognition of certain genetic mutations associated with increased risk of SCD in patients with dilated cardiomyopathy. For example, dilated

cardiomyopathy associated lamin A/C gene (LMNA), which is also associated with cardiac conduction defects, has been found to have particularly high risk of SCD. A significant proportion of these patients received appropriate ICD therapy even before the development of heart failure. [116], [117] These patients are at a higher risk of sudden death with lower degree of LV systolic dysfunction and a recent study has suggested high risk of malignant ventricular arrhythmia in patients who are male, have dilated LV, have NSVT or LVEF < 45%. [118] SCN5A overlap syndrome with dilated cardiomyopathy are at increased risk of SCD.

5. *NSVTs and PVBs* have not been found to have predictive value in of arrhythmic event in patients with DCM. In medically stabilized patients Zecchin et al failed to show any difference in arrhythmic event between patients with and without NSVTs. [119] NSVT was not evaluated for prediction of SCD in the large primary prevention trial like DEFINITE and SCD-HeFT, [48], [113]

6. *Others factors: Electrocardiographic parameters* have been evaluated to identify the groups of dilated cardiomyopathy patients with risk of SCD. [120], [121] Prolongation of QRS and presence of left bundle branch block are independent predictors of SCD. Parameters of QT dynamicity and QRS fragmentation may be useful in risk stratification of SCD. [122], [123] SAECG, heart rate variability, heart rate turbulence, heart rate recovery, baroreflex sensitivity and T-wave alternans have been evaluated and each individual risk factor has a small effect size. [61], [62] As discussed earlier in the section on ischemic cardiomyopathy, these ECG parameters and parameter of autonomic function have small effect when used individually and may have a stronger risk predictive value in combination. [61], [68] Assessment of myocardial fibrosis by various methods including serum markers of fibrosis and cardiac MRI with late gadolinium enhancement may potentially become a tool in risk stratification for sudden cardiac death in patients with dilated cardiomyopathy. [124]

4.5. Other cardiomyopathies

Left ventricular noncompaction is associated with left ventricular dysfunction and risk of ventricular arrhythmia. Studies to assess the degree of risk and parameters to stratify the risk have not been done in this group of patients, but it is noteworthy that the diagnosis has only recently been recognized. LV systolic dysfunction may be a predictor of SCD in these patients, although concerns have been raised about its value. [125] Any other parameter to stratify the risk is still speculative.

Patients with *cardiac sarcoidosis* have poorer prognosis compared to idiopathic dilated cardiomyopathy with similar degree of LV systolic dysfunction. [126], [127] Patients ventricular tachycardia or atrioventricular block are at a high risk of adverse cardiac events. Presence of AV block in patients with cardiac sarcoidosis younger than 55 years increase the risk of adverse cardiac outcomes over 2 years by ten-fold as compared to patients without cardiac sarcoidosis. [32] Asymptomatic cardiac involvement in sarcoidosis has been largely reported to have benign prognosis, [128]-[130] although one recent report recorded 19% mortality (5 out of 21 patients with MRI diagnosed cardiac sarcoidosis) over a follow-up period of 21 months. [131]

Assessment of SCD risk in *cardiac amyloidosis* is not well defined. Little data is available on risk stratification, and the usual approach in these patients is secondary prophylaxis or extrapolation of risk factors from other types of cardiomyopathies, e.g., LV systolic dysfunction. The degree of myocardial involvement in sarcoidosis may be important in clinical decision-making. Patients with *hereditary dystrophies* behave largely like dilated cardiomyopathy and risk stratification in these patients again conforms to the risk stratification of dilated cardiomyopathy.

5. Management

5.1. Pharmacotherapy and sudden cardiac death prevention

The role of pharmacotherapy in the prevention of SCD is two-fold. First, many neuro-humoral modifiers for the treatment of heart failure result in reverse remodeling of the left ventricle and may therefore reduce the overall mortality, and the risk of SCD. Examples include ACE inhibitors, angiotensin receptor blockers, aldosterone antagonists and beta-blockers. Second, antiarrhythmic medications have been used in patients with cardiomyopathy to reduce the risk of SCD. Examples would be beta-blockers including sotalol, amiodarone and other antiarrhythmic medications.

Amiodarone has been evaluated in large randomized trials in post-MI patients. The Canadian amiodarone myocardial infarction arrhythmia trial (CAMIAT) conducted in 1202 post-MI patients with a mean LVEF of 30% and greater than 10 PVC's per hour demonstrated a small but significant reduction in arrhythmic death (4.5% versus 6.9%, P = 0.016) but no reduction in all-cause mortality in patients on amiodarone. [56] The European Myocardial Infarct Amiodarone Trial (EMIAT) of 1486 similar patients did not show any difference in arrhythmic or all-cause mortality between the two groups of patients. [59] A meta-analysis of 15 randomized controlled trials in a total of 8522 patients that evaluated amiodarone for prevention of SCD showed a small but significant reduction in SCD (7.1% vs 9.7%; OR 0.71, p<0.001) but no important change in overall mortality. [132] In the general population of heart failure patients the SCD-HeFT trial did not show any reduction in all-cause mortality with amiodarone treatment in comparison with placebo. [48]

Sotalol a beta-blocker that is also a class III antiarrhythmic drug (i.e., prolongs QT interval) has been studied for prevention of SCD in patients with post-MI LV systolic dysfunction with mixed results. A study by Julian et al evaluated the role of racemic d,l-sotlol in 1456 patients 5-14 days after MI. Racemic sotalol exhibits both beta blocking properties (the l-isomer) and class III antiarrhythmic effects (the d-isomer), and this combination showed a nonsignificant reduction in mortality over one-year follow up. [133] By contrast, oral d-sotalol, in the SWORD, trial showed increased mortality in 3121 patients with recent (6-42 days) MI or with remote (>42 days) MI with symptomatic CHF with LVEF ≤40%. [134] This lack of benefit or actual harm seen in SWORD trial may be due to lack of beta-blocking property of d-sotalol, which probably led to some benefit seen in the study by Julian et al using racemic sotalol. [135] As a result of the SWORD trial, d-sotalol was abandoned. On the other hand a multicenter placebo

http://dx.doi.org/10.5772/55636

controlled trial in patients with ICD showed a reduction in mortality and ICD shocks in patients receiving d,l-sotalol. Moreover, the mortality benefit in this study did not differ between patients with LVEF <30% and >30%. [136]

Beta-blockers has a proven role in reducing cardiovascular mortality and SCD in patients with heart failure either from non-ischemic cardiomyopathy or ischemic heart disease. [114], [137]-[139] Similarly, ACE inhibitors, ARBs and aldosterone antagonist are used in heart failure patients to reduce all-cause mortality, however, neither ACE inhibitors nor ARB actually reduce SCD in patients with LV systolic dysfunction. [140]-[142] ELITE did show an unexpected reduction of SCD with losartan but this was a non-prespecified endpoint and was never confirmed prospectively. [143]

Class I antiarrhythmic drugs have not been found to reduce SCD in patients with history of MI and LV systolic dysfunction, and in fact most often result in an increase in mortality. The Cardiac Arrhythmia Suppression Trial (CAST) and CAST-II trials, for example, showed increased mortality with the use of class Ic antiarrhythmic drugs in post MI patients. [144] Similarly, propafenone showed increased mortality compared to ICD in Cardiac Arrest Study Hamburg (CASH). [145]

As the data of ICD trials showed reduction in all-cause mortality and SCD in patients with cardiomyopathy as compared to amiodarone, the role of antiarrhythmic drugs in prevention of SCD has become adjunctive, with the goal of reducing ICD shocks. Beta-blockers and other humoral modifiers are generally used in the management of heart failure and improve survival in heart failure patients.

The role of amiodarone for prevention of SCD in HCM is controversial. In a study by McKenna et al, [146] amiodarone found to be effective but it is noteworthy that this study was used historical controls receiving either mexiletine, disopyramide or quinidine. In other studies antiarrhythmic drugs for the prevention of SCD in HCM have not been found to be effective. [147] Similarly, beta-blockers, sotalol and amiodarone have been used to suppress ventricular arrhythmias in ARVC. Efficacy has been variable [148], [149] and, with the increasing practice of use of ICD in the prevention of SCD in these patients, antiarrhythmic drugs are again used to reduce the need for ICD intervention.

5.2. Device therapy: Implantable cardioverter-defibrillator

Implantable cardioverter-defibrillator therapy has emerged as the most important management strategy for prevention of SCD in patients with cardiomyopathy at high risk of sudden cardiac death. The high incidence and high individual risk of SCD in cardiomyopathy patients with impaired left ventricular function, especially in those who had survived a ventricular arrhythmia, and the relative ineffectiveness of antiarrhythmic drugs in these patients led to a series of trials aimed at assessing the role of ICD therapy. This strategy was first tested in trials of patients with highest degree of risk. These were sudden death and ventricular arrhythmia survivors, and the studies are collectively referred to as secondary prevention trials. These trials were followed by trials of increasingly lower risk patients, principally those with heart failure, in primary prevention trials. The major message of these trials is that cost effectiveness is highest in highest risk patients, but that in this group, numerically the number of lives saved by defibrillators is relatively small. Use of defibrillators in lower risk cohorts decreases cost effectiveness, but increases the chance of making a numerical impact of the incidence of SCD in the contemporary US population.

5.3. Secondary prevention ICD trials

Antiarrhythmics versus implantable defibrillators (AVID), Canadian implantable defibrillator study (CIDS) and Cardiac arrest study Hamburg (CASH) trials gave an insight into the benefits of use of ICDs in secondary prevention of SCD after an arrhythmic event. In these studies patients with history of aborted SCD or patients with ventricular arrhythmia in the setting of reduced LV systolic function were enrolled.

The *AVID trial*, which enrolled 1016 patients with history of VF, VT with syncope or VT with LVEF ≤40% and symptoms of hemodynamic compromise (near syncope, congestive heart failure and angina). This study showed reduction in all-cause mortality from 25% to 18% (absolute risk reduction of 7% and relative risk reduction of 27%). The patients had a mean LVEF of 32% in this study. In each arm, 45% of the patients had history of VF and the rest of the patients had history of VT as the inclusion criteria for the study. *CIDS* enrolled 659 patients with VF, out of hospital cardiac arrest due to VF or VT, VT with syncope, VT with symptoms of presyncope or angina and LVEF ≤35%, and unmonitored syncope with subsequent spontaneous or induced VT. The mean LVEF in these patients was 34%. After follow-up of 3 years there was a nonsignificant reduction in all-cause mortality (10.2% per year to 8.3% per year, p=0.142), and of arrhythmic death (4.5% per year to 3.0% per year, p=0.094) in ICD patients. At 2 years there was a reduction in all-cause mortality from 21% to 15% (absolute and relative risk reduction of 30% and 6% respectively).

The *CASH study* was a much smaller study with enrollment of 191 patients with a history of VF or VT without an identified transient reversible cause. In contrast to AVID and CIDS the mean LVEF was 46% making them healthier group of patients. Over a mean follow-up of 57 months the reduction in mortality was from 44% in control to 36% in those receiving ICD (absolute and relative risk reduction of 23% and 8% respectively). Overall survival was higher in the ICD arm, though not statistically significant (hazard ratio 0.766, 97.5% CI upper bound 1.112; p=0.081). There was higher survival free of sudden death in the ICD arm (hazard ratio 0.423, 97.5% upper bound 0.721; p=0.005).

Thus the trials were consistent in their message although CASH and CIDS trials were relatively underpowered to assess the reduction in all-cause mortality. A meta-analysis showed a 28% relative reduction in all cause mortality and a 50% reduction in SCD in patients receiving ICDs. [150] Patients with LVEF < 35% derived the most benefit with hazard ratio for this group of 0.66 (95% CI 0.53-0.83). [150] and overall the number needed to treat to save a life per year of follow-up was 29. [151] When the individual trials are compared it is noteworthy that LVEF was much higher in CASH, and that CIDS included a group of patients with unexplained syncope and VT inducible at EP study. These factors are markers of a lower risk population and reduced that trials' ability to detect the benefit of ICDs in reducing all cause mortality.

http://dx.doi.org/10.5772/55636

Later subgroup analysis of these studies showed that the benefit of ICD therapy was largely restricted to patients with lower LVEF. A subgroup analysis of 396 patients in the AVID trial with LVEF >35% failed to show any survival benefit. In addition a smaller group of 140 patients in this study with LVEF <20% did not show statistically significantly survival benefit. This was in contrast to the 473 patients with LVEF between 20% and 34% who had significantly improved survival. [152] Similarly, in CIDS trial the benefit of ICD therapy was restricted to the patients with higher risk features (age >70 years, LVEF <35% and NYHA class III or IV). [153]

5.4. Primary prevention ICD trials

Primary prevention ICD trials in patients with heart failure due to ischemic and nonischemic cardiomyopathies have provided insights into prevention of SCD in a larger group of patients who are at a high risk of SCD based on epidemiological studies, but are at lower risk than patients who have suffered a ventricular arrhythmia. These studies have played instrumental role in formulation of guidelines for primary prevention of SCDs in patients with cardiomyopathies. The trials include MADIT (I and II), CABG Patch, MUSTT, DINAMIT, DEFINITE and SCD-HeFT.

Multicenter Automatic Defibrillator Implantation Trial (MADIT-I) was the first trial evaluating the efficacy of ICD on survival in patients with history ischemic heart disease. Patients with an LVEF≤35%, non-sustained VT who also sustained VT induced at a ventricular stimulation study and not suppressed by procainamide were randomized to receive best medical therapy or an ICD. 196 of these very high-risk patients were enrolled and mean LVEF was 26%. All cause mortality was reduced from 32% to 13% in the ICD group after 2 years, for a relative risk reduction of 59% [50]

The *Multicenter Unsustained Tachycardia Trial (MUSTT)* trial recruited a lower risk IHD cohort, with NSVT and a LVEF ≤40%. All patients underwent a ventricular stimulation study, and those with inducible sustained ventricular tachycardia were randomized to receive either no specific antiarrhythmic therapy or antiarrhythmic therapy (either an antiarrhythmic drug or an ICD) guided by further ventricular stimulation studies. Patients not inducible into sustained VT were followed in a registry. Among 704 enrolled patients, the median LVEF was 30%. In comparison to controls, patient treated with antiarrhythmic drugs had an increase in overall mortality (from 48% to 55%) whereas patients receiving ICDs all cause mortality improved from 48% in controls to 24% in patients receiving ICD with absolute and relative risk reduction of 24% and 50% in a 5 year analysis (figure 6). [51] Interestingly the cohort of patients not inducible into VT who received no specific antiarrhythmic therapy had a significantly lower mortality than patients who were inducible into sustained VT, but the absolute improvement in mortality predicted by a negative EP study was small (absolute risk reduction and relative risk reduction of 7%,and 25% at 2 years and 4% and 8.3% at 5 years). [154] This study was the first to point out the limited value of ventricular stimulation studies in assessing SCD risk. These studies have now largely been abandoned, and future ICD trials have concentrated on wider, lower risk, patient cohorts.

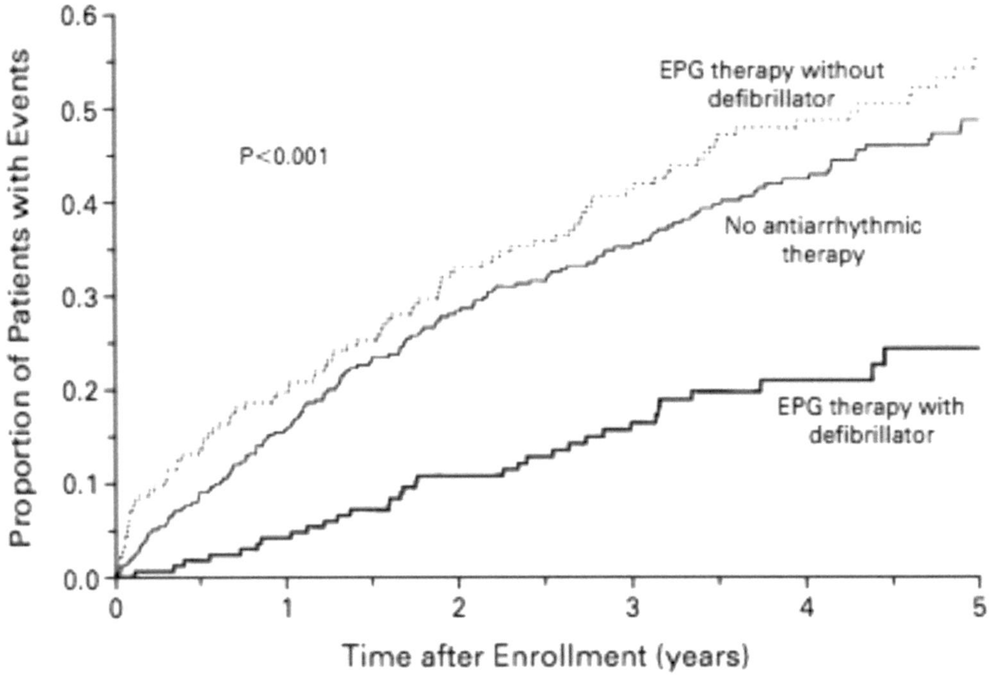

Figure 6. MUSTT: Kaplan–Meier Estimates of the Rates of Overall Mortality According to Whether the Patients Received Treatment with a Defibrillator. The P value refers to two comparisons: between the patients in the group assigned to electrophysiologically guided (EPG) therapy who received treatment with a defibrillator and those who did not receive such treatment, and between the patients assigned to electrophysiologically guided therapy who received treatment with a defibrillator and those assigned to no antiarrhythmic therapy. (From reference 51)

The *MADIT II* trial assessed the effect of an ICD in 1232 patients with prior myocardial infarction (>one month) and LVEF ≤30%. In this study, mainly of long term infarct survivors, mean LVEF was 23% and in the ICD group all-cause mortality was reduced at 16% compared to 22% in the controls after 2-year follow up (absolute and relative risk reduction of 6% and 28% respectively, figure 7). [47] In this cohort of IHD patients without inducible VT the benefit of an ICD was smaller, but the potential population of identified patients who could benefit from ICD therapy is much wider.

Defibrillator use early after acute myocardial infarction trial: The DINAMIT trial evaluated the role of ICD in potentially improving the survival of patients during acute phase of MI (6 to 40 days after MI) with reduced LVEF ≤35% and impaired cardiac autonomic function, assessed as impaired baroreflex sensitivity. During a mean follow-up of $2^1/_2$ years, there was no reduction in overall mortality in these patients. Although there was a reduction in death due to arrhythmia, the benefit was offset by death from non-arrhythmic causes. [155] These data are challenging because the implication is that ICD implantation enhanced the risk for non-arrhythmic death, principally death from heart failure. If the amount of right ventricular pacing in the ICD group accounted for more than 5-10% of heart beats this is a plausi-

http://dx.doi.org/10.5772/55636

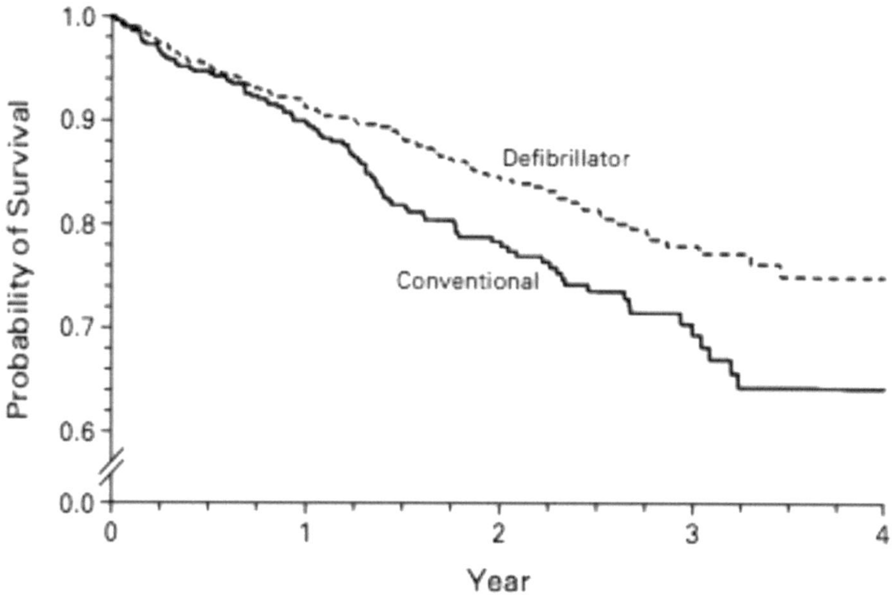

No. at Risk					
Defibrillator	742	503 (0.91)	274 (0.84)	110 (0.78)	9
Conventional	490	329 (0.90)	170 (0.78)	65 (0.69)	3

Figure 7. MADIT II: Kaplan–Meier Estimates of the Probability of Survival in the Group Assigned to Receive an Implantable Defibrillator and the Group Assigned to Receive Conventional Medical Therapy. The difference in survival between the two groups was significant (nominal P=0.007, by the log-rank test). (From reference 47)

ble mechanism because RV pacing in heart failure patients is known to exacerbate heart failure mortality. [156]-[158]

Defibrillators in non-ishchemic cardiomyopathy: The DEFINITE trial investigated the benefit of prophylactic ICD therapy in 458 enrolled patients with non-ischemic cardiomyopathy with LVEF <36% and premature ventricular complexes or NSVT. The patients were mainly symptomatic for heart failure with NYHA functional class of I-III and mean LVEF of the study population was 21%. At two years, the mortality in ICD group was 8% compared to 14% in the standard therapy group (absolute and relative risk reduction of 6% and 44% respectively). However this reduction in overall mortality was not statistically significant with hazard ratio of 0.65 among patients receiving ICD (95% CI 0.40-1.06). This difference reached statistical significance in patients with NYHA class III in subgroup analysis and showed a relative risk of death of 0.37 (95%confidence interval 0.15-0.90). Moreover, the difference in survival was significantly more in males receiving ICD (HR 0.49, 95%CI 0.27-0.90; p=0.018). [113].

Sudden cardiac death in heart failure (SCD-HeFT) trial was conducted in patients with heart failure due to ischemic or nonischemic cardiomyopathy with LVEF≤35% and with NYHA functional class II-III. More than 2500 optimally medically managed patients were equally divided into three groups: ICD, amiodarone and placebo. Mean LVEF was 25%; 52% of the patients had ischemic cardiomyopathy and the remainder were non ischemic. All cause mortality at 5 years in patients receiving ICD was 29% compared to 36% for the control with absolute and relative risk reduction of 7% and 23%. Amiodarone arm did not show any significant reduction in risk of death (HR: 1.06; 97.5% CI 0.86-1.30; p=0.53)(see figure 8). In subgroup analysis by type of cardiomyopathy, reduction in the mortality risk were similar in both ischemic (HR: 0.79, 97.5% CI 0.60-1.04) and nonischemic cardiomyopathy (HR: 0.73, 97.5% CI 0.50-1.07) patients with ICD therapy compared to placebo, although the risk reduction did not reach a statistical significance. NYHA class did affect the effect of amiodarone as well as ICD therapy compared to placebo. Amiodarone was shown to increase the risk of mortality in NYHA class III by 44% (HR: 1.44, 97.5 CI 1.05-1.97), which was not seen in patients with NYHA class II (HR: 0.85, 97.5% CI 0.65-1-11). Similarly, with ICD therapy, patients with NYHA class III did not get mortaliy benefit (HR: 1.16, 97.5% CI 0.84-1.61) as opposed to patients with NYHA class II (HR: 0.54; 97.5% CI 0.40-0.74) [48]

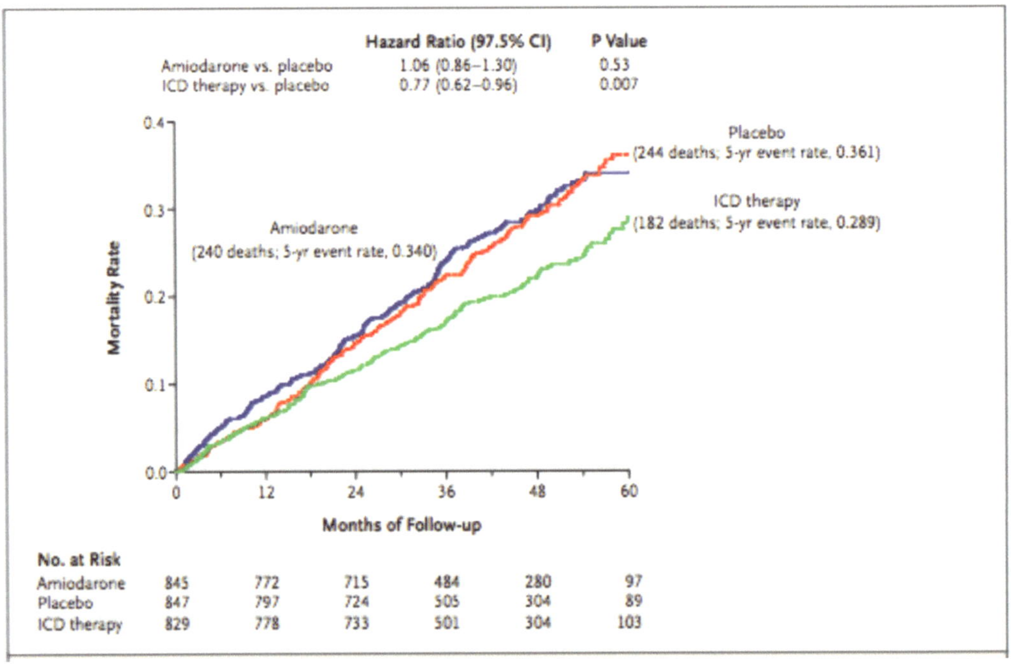

Figure 8. SCD-HeFT: Kaplan–Meier Estimates of Death from Any Cause. (From reference 48)

A meta-analysis of the primary prevention trials in patients with low ejection fraction due to coronary artery disease or dilated cardiomyopathy including eight trials and total of 5343 patients showed reduction of arrhythmic mortality (relative risk: 0.40; 95% CI: 0.27-0.67) and all-cause mortality (relative risk: 0.73; 95% CI: 0.64-0.82). The benefit of ICD therapy was similar in ischemic (relative risk: 0.67; 95% CI: 0.51-0.88) and non-ischemic (RR: 0.74; 95% CI: 0.59-0.93) cardiomyopathies. [159] Another important issue is that the age of the people enrolled in the

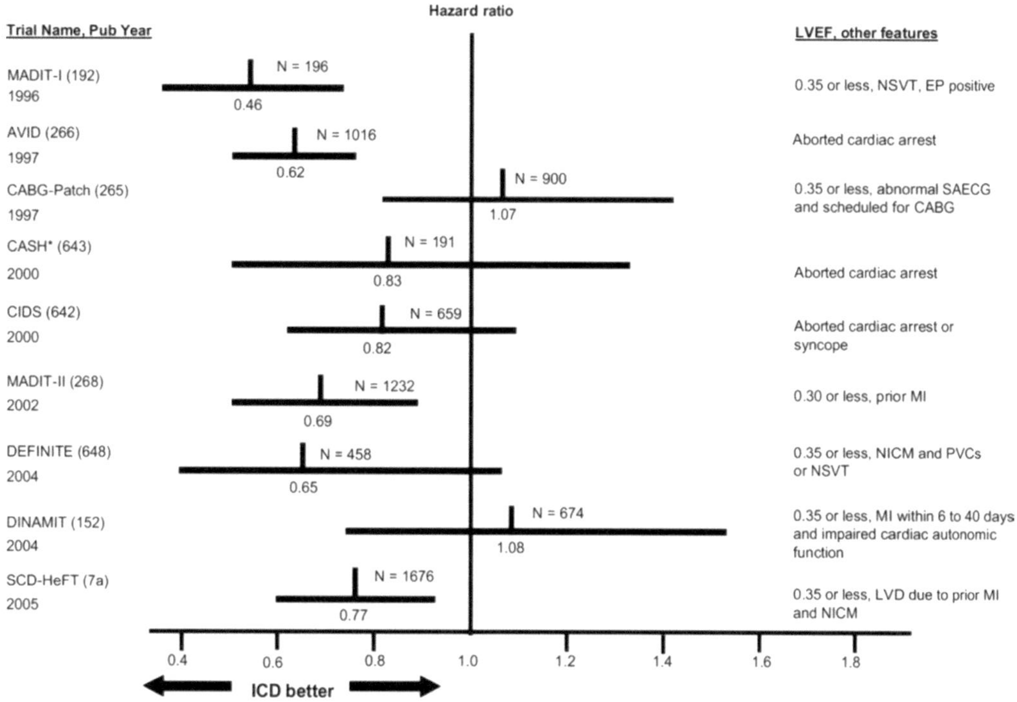

Figure 9. Major implantable cardioverter-defibrillator (ICD) trials. Hazard ratios (vertical line) and 95% confidence intervals (horizontal lines) for death from any cause in the ICD group compared with the non-ICD group. *Includes only ICD and amiodarone patients from CASH. For expansion of trial names, see Appendix 3. CABG: coronary artery bypass graft surgery; EP: electrophysiological study; LVD: left ventricular dysfunction; LVEF: left ventricular ejection fraction; MI: myocardial infarction; N: number of patients; NICM: nonischemic cardiomyopathy; NSVT: nonsustained ventricular tachycardia; PVCs: premature ventricular complexes; SAECG: signal-averaged electrocardiogram. (Adapted with permission from reference 165)

large ICD trials is considerably younger than the people frequently needing ICD implantation in the current clinical practice. This issue has been addressed by two meta-analysis suggesting benefit of ICD therapy in older patients. [160], [161] Another meta-analysis of primary prevention ICD trials showed smaller benefit of ICD in women with dilated cardiomyopathy compared to men. Although overall mortality in both the genders were similar (HR 0.96, 95% CI 0.67-1.39), women received approprite therapy less frequently compared to men (HR 0.63, 95%CI 0.49-0.82) and hence received less benefit from defibrillator therapy. [162] This as well as another meta-analysis of primary prevention ICD trials failed to show significant mortality benefit of ICD in women. [162]

These ICD trials have established the role of ICDs in the primary and secondary prevention of SCD in patients with non-ischemic and ischemic cardiomyopathy (figure 9). Left ventricular ejection fraction has been recognized as the strongest risk stratifier and has been extensively used in all the trials. Based on these studies guidelines have been formulated for the appropriate indications of ICD therapy in these patients. The table 3 summarizes the guidelines for implantation of ICD for prevention of SCD in these patients.

	Indication for ICD	Level of evidence
	Class I	
1	Patients who are survivors of cardiac arrest due to ventricular fibrillation or hemodynamically unstable sustained VT after evaluation to define the cause of the event and to exclude any completely reversible causes.	A
2	**Patients with structural heart disease and spontaneous sustained VT, whether hemodynamically stable or unstable.**	B
3	Patients with syncope of undetermined origin with clinically relevant, hemodynamically significant sustained VT or ventricular fibrillation induced at electrophysiological study.	B
4	**Patients with LVEF less than or equal to 35% due to prior myocardial infarction who are at least 40 days post–myocardial infarction and are in NYHA functional Class II or III.**	A
5	**Patients with nonischemic dilated cardiomyopathy who have an LVEF less than or equal to 35% and who are in NYHA functional Class II or III.**	B
6	**Patients with LV dysfunction due to prior myocardial infarction who are at least 40 days post–myocardial infarction, have an LVEF less than or equal to 30%, and are in NYHA functional Class I.**	A
7	**Patients with nonsustained VT due to prior myocardial infarction, LVEF less than or equal to 40%, and inducible ventricular fibrillation or sustained VT at electrophysiological study.**	B
	Class IIa	
1	**Patients with unexplained syncope, significant LV dysfunction, and nonischemic dilated cardiomyopathy.**	C
2	**Patients with sustained VT and normal or near-normal ventricular function.**	C
3	**Patients with hypertrophic cardiomyopathy who have 1 or more major† risk factor for SCD.**	C
4	**Patients with arrhythmogenic right ventricular dysplasia/cardiomyopathy who have 1 or more risk factor for SCD.**	C
5	Patients with long-QT syndrome who are experiencing syncope and/or VT while receiving beta blockers.	B
6	**Nonhospitalized patients awaiting transplantation.**	C
7	Patients with Brugada syndrome who have had syncope.	C
8	Patients with Brugada syndrome who have documented VT that has not resulted in cardiac arrest.	C
9	Patients with catecholaminergic polymorphic VT who have syncope and/or documented sustained VT while receiving beta blockers.	C
10	**Patients with cardiac sarcoidosis, giant cell myocarditis, or Chagas disease.**	C
	Class IIb	
1	**Patients with nonischemic heart disease who have an LVEF of less than or equal to 35% and who are in NYHA functional Class I.**	C
2	Patients with long-QT syndrome and risk factors for SCD.	B
3	Patients with syncope and advanced structural heart disease in whom thorough invasive and noninvasive investigations have failed to define a cause.	C
4	**Patients with a familial cardiomyopathy associated with sudden death.**	C
5	**Patients with LV noncompaction.**	C
	Class III	
1	**Patients who do not have a reasonable expectation of survival with an acceptable functional status for at least 1 year, even if they meet ICD implantation criteria specified in the Class I, IIa, and IIb recommendations above.**	C
2	**Patients with incessant VT or ventricular fibrillation.**	C

http://dx.doi.org/10.5772/55636

	Indication for ICD	Level of evidence
3	Patients with significant psychiatric illnesses that may be aggravated by device implantation or that may preclude systematic follow-up.	C
4	**NYHA Class IV patients with drug-refractory congestive heart failure who are not candidates for cardiac transplantation or implantation of a CRT device that incorporates both pacing and defibrillation capabilities.**	C
5	Syncope of undetermined cause in a patient without inducible ventricular tachyarrhythmias and without structural heart disease.	C
6	Ventricular fibrillation or VT is amenable to surgical or catheter ablation (e.g., atrial arrhythmias associated with Wolff-Parkinson-White syndrome, right ventricular or LV outflow tract VT, idiopathic VT, or fascicular VT in the absence of structural heart disease).	C
7	Patients with ventricular tachyarrhythmias due to a completely reversible disorder in the absence of structural heart disease (e.g., electrolyte imbalance, drugs, or trauma).	B

Table 3. ACC/AHA/HRS guidelines for implantation of ICDs (2008): indications in bold fonts refer to the indications for various cardiomyopathies.

5.5. Risk stratification of heart failure patients for sudden death prevention

As data has accumulated suggesting that a strategy of wide ranging ICD implantation in patients with impaired left ventricular systolic function will result in improvements in sudden cardiac death mortality, concerns have been raised about the relatively low incidence of life saving therapies in implanted patients. For example in MADIT II 14% of patients received a potentially life saving defibrillator shock, whilst in SCD-HeFT only 21% of patients received appropriate ICD therapy. In addition it has frequently been noted that an appropriate shock does not necessarily represent an aborted sudden death. These considerations have lead to attempts to derive scoring strategies from the data sets in the large prospective trials to try to identify patients at low risk of requiring device therapy – and those in whom device therapy might be futile.

Data from the MADIT II study in chronic IHD suggested that in very high risk (VHR) patients defined as those with a BUN ≥ 50 mg/dl, mortality was high at 50% in two years and was not improved by ICD therapy. ICD implantation in this patient group appears to be unjustified. Among non-VHR patients, SCD risk was to be increased with NYHA functional class >II, a history of atrial fibrillation, QRS duration >120 ms, age >70 years and BUN >26 mg/dl and <50 mg/dl. Patients with none of these risk factors were at low risk of SCD, and had no benefit from ICD therapy. Patients with one to two risk factors derived benefit from an ICD whereas patients with three or more risk factors did not derive as much benefit and behaved like VHR patients. [163] Similarly, analysis of data from the MUSTT study suggested LVEF alone was of limited value to predict the risk of SCD in this patient group. [164] The concern about using a binary cut off of LVEF in deciding on the advisability or otherwise of ICD therapy to reduce the risk of SCD is that SCD risk is a continuous variable and predicted by more than LVEF alone. Multiple factors predict SCD to some extent and hence a risk score based on multiple risk factors may be a better predictor of SCD. However, it should be noted that the mutiple risk models have not been evaluated in a prospective study and are entirely data derived. [68] This being said, it seems inevitable that the guidelines for the implantation of ICDs will be refined in the future and that risk scores will be incorporated.

5.6. ICD in other forms of cardiomyopathies

Implantation of ICD in cardiomyopathy other than ischemic and non-ischemic dilated cardiomyopathy is not supported by evidence from large ICD trials. The majority of patients enrolled in the large ICD trials were post-MI patients with LV dysfunction and patients with dilated non-ischemic cardiomyopathy. In other forms of cardiomyopathies, like hypertrophic cardiomyopathy, arrhythmogenic right ventricular cardiomyopathy, sarcoidosis and other infiltrative cardiomyopathies, secondary prevention of sudden cardiac death with ICD implantation in survivors of SCD and in patients with history of sustained ventricular tachycardia is generally accepted clinical practice. However, implantation of ICD for primary prevention of SCD has remained an unsolved issue in these patients. This has become more of an issue with development of more effective screening of family members, and pre-participation screening of athletes. Risk stratification in them has been attempted for each of these groups.

Primary prevention in patients with *hypertrophic cardiomyopathy* is guided by multiple risk factors for sudden cardiac death as discussed above. These risk factors have been defined as discussed earlier and include (1) a family history of premature HCM-related sudden death; (2) a history of unexplained syncope; (3) multiple and/or prolonged runs of nonsustained VT on serial 24-hour ambulatory ECG monitoring at heart rates ≥120 beats/min; (4) a hypotensive or attenuated blood pressure response to exercise; and (5) massive left ventricular (LV) hypertrophy (maximum wall thickness ≥30 mm). The ACC/AHA/ESC guidelines on sudden cardiac death and ventricular arrhythmia recommend implantation of ICD in patients with one or more of these risk factors, for the primary prevention of SCD. [165]

Primary prevention of SCD in *arrhythmogenic right ventricular cardiomyopathy* is also guided by a set of high risk factors. A multicenter study evaluated the use of ICD for primary prophylaxis of SCD in patients with ARVC with at least one risk factor for SCD. These included syncope, NSVT, a malignant family history, and inducibility of ventricular arrhythmias with programmed ventricular stimulation. Over a mean follow-up of 58 months 25 of 106 patients received appropriate ICD intervention. ACC/AHA/ESC guidelines considers secondary prevention of SCD with AICD to be reasonable (class IIa) in patients with ARVC considered high risk due to LV involvement, one or more affected family member with SCD, or undiagnosed syncope when VT or VF has not been excluded as the cause of syncope, while receiving chronic optimal medical therapy. [165] ACC/AHA/HRS guidelines for device therapy for arrhythmia lists ARVC as reasonable indication for primary implantation of ICD in the presence of one or more risk of SCD. [166]

In patients with left ventricular non-compaction, ICD implantation is generally performed for secondary prevention and for primary prevention in the presence of LV systolic dysfunction. Although patients with normal LV systolic function or mild LV systolic dysfunction may be prone to SCD, [125] lack of data makes the decision ICD implantation in these patients difficult.

In patients with sarcoidosis, cardiac involvement with history of spontaneous VT and/or severe LV systolic dysfunction may warrant ICD therapy despite lack of prospective trials. [165] Implantation of ICD in patients with sarcoidosis in the absence of LV systolic dysfunction or history of ventricular arrhythmias remains controversial. The ACC/AHA/HRS guidelines for device therapy lists cardiac sarcoidosis as reasonable indication for ICD implantation. [166] The use of ICD to prevent SCD in patients with cardiac amyloidosis is not well accepted and may not affect the outcome, although it can be used to bridge the patients to cardiac transplantation. [38], [165] Some of the muscular dystrophies with associated cardiomyopathy are treated in a similar way as dilated non-ischemic cardiomyopathy from other causes.

5.7. Device therapy: Permanent pacemaker

Some cardiomyopathies are prone to cause conduction abnormalities. For example patients with muscular dystrophy due to lamin A/C gene mutation are particularly prone to conduction defect and atrioventricular block. The threshold for pacemaker implantation in these patients is very low to prevent SCD. Similarly, infiltrative myocardial diseases such as sarcoidosis can lead to heart block and SCD as a result of this. Other examples include myotonic muscular dystrophy, where SCD can result both from ventricular arrhythmias and from complete heart block.

6. Future directions

The prevention of sudden cardiac death in patients with cardiomyopathy has evolved dramatically in recent years. With the increasing use of ICDs in conjunction with pharmacotherapy for heart failure, large number patients have benefited from prevention of SCD. However, risk assessment for SCD is still far from accurate and many patients receiving ICDs ultimately will not use them. Although, attempts have been made to refine the risk stratification, the current risk stratification is insufficient at least for many kinds of cardiomyopathies. Data from subgroup analysis do provide some parameters for refining risk stratification, but testing them in a prospective study will be an expensive and time-consuming undertaking. Risk stratification for less common forms of cardiomyopathy has not largely been possible. Some newer parameters like genetic evaluation may help in refining the risk assessment in the future as more data on genetic analysis in various forms of cardiomyopathy comes forth. Finally, newer pharmacotherapy may help in reducing the risk of SCD in these patients.

Author details

Prabhat Kumar and J Paul Mounsey

Department of Medicine, University of North Carolina, Chapel Hill NC, USA

References

[1] Luu M, Stevenson WG, Stevenson LW, Baron K, Walden J: Diverse mechanisms of unexpected cardiac arrest in advanced heart failure. Circulation 1989; 80:1675-1680

[2] Pouleur AC, Barkoudah E, Uno H, Skali H, Finn PV, Zelenkofske SL, Belenkov YN, Mareev V, Velazquez EJ, Rouleau JL, Maggioni AP, Kober L, Califf RM, McMurray JJ, Pfeffer MA, Solomon SD, VALIANT Investigators: Pathogenesis of sudden unexpected death in a clinical trial of patients with myocardial infarction and left ventricular dysfunction, heart failure, or both. Circulation 2010; 122:597-602

[3] Bello D, Fieno DS, Kim RJ, Pereles FS, Passman R, Song G, Kadish AH, Goldberger JJ: Infarct morphology identifies patients with substrate for sustained ventricular tachycardia. J Am Coll Cardiol 2005; 45:1104-1108

[4] Jin H, Lyon AR, Akar FG: Arrhythmia mechanisms in the failing heart. Pacing Clin Electrophysiol 2008; 31:1048-1056

[5] Calkins H, Allman K, Bolling S, Kirsch M, Wieland D, Morady F, Schwaiger M: Correlation between scintigraphic evidence of regional sympathetic neuronal dysfunction and ventricular refractoriness in the human heart. Circulation 1993; 88:172-179

[6] Maron BJ, Spirito P, Shen WK, Haas TS, Formisano F, Link MS, Epstein AE, Almquist AK, Daubert JP, Lawrenz T, Boriani G, Estes NA,3rd, Favale S, Piccininno M, Winters SL, Santini M, Betocchi S, Arribas F, Sherrid MV, Buja G, Semsarian C, Bruzzi P: Implantable cardioverter-defibrillators and prevention of sudden cardiac death in hypertrophic cardiomyopathy. JAMA 2007; 298:405-412

[7] Begley DA, Mohiddin SA, Tripodi D, Winkler JB, Fananapazir L: Efficacy of implantable cardioverter defibrillator therapy for primary and secondary prevention of sudden cardiac death in hypertrophic cardiomyopathy. Pacing Clin Electrophysiol 2003; 26:1887-1896

[8] Spirito P, Bellone P, Harris KM, Bernabo P, Bruzzi P, Maron BJ: Magnitude of left ventricular hypertrophy and risk of sudden death in hypertrophic cardiomyopathy. N Engl J Med 2000; 342:1778-1785

[9] Varnava AM, Elliott PM, Baboonian C, Davison F, Davies MJ, McKenna WJ: Hypertrophic cardiomyopathy: histopathological features of sudden death in cardiac troponin T disease. Circulation 2001; 104:1380-1384

[10] O'Hanlon R, Grasso A, Roughton M, Moon JC, Clark S, Wage R, Webb J, Kulkarni M, Dawson D, Sulaibeekh L, Chandrasekaran B, Bucciarelli-Ducci C, Pasquale F, Cowie MR, McKenna WJ, Sheppard MN, Elliott PM, Pennell DJ, Prasad SK: Prognostic significance of myocardial fibrosis in hypertrophic cardiomyopathy. J Am Coll Cardiol 2010; 56:867-874

[11] Frey N, McKinsey TA, Olson EN: Decoding calcium signals involved in cardiac growth and function. Nat Med 2000; 6:1221-1227

[12] Wehrens XH, Marks AR: Novel therapeutic approaches for heart failure by normalizing calcium cycling. Nat Rev Drug Discov 2004; 3:565-573

[13] Bottinelli R, Coviello DA, Redwood CS, Pellegrino MA, Maron BJ, Spirito P, Watkins H, Reggiani C: A mutant tropomyosin that causes hypertrophic cardiomyopathy is expressed in vivo and associated with an increased calcium sensitivity. Circ Res 1998; 82:106-115

[14] Knollmann BC, Kirchhof P, Sirenko SG, Degen H, Greene AE, Schober T, Mackow JC, Fabritz L, Potter JD, Morad M: Familial hypertrophic cardiomyopathy-linked mutant troponin T causes stress-induced ventricular tachycardia and Ca2+-dependent action potential remodeling. Circ Res 2003; 92:428-436

[15] Sweeney HL, Feng HS, Yang Z, Watkins H: Functional analyses of troponin T mutations that cause hypertrophic cardiomyopathy: insights into disease pathogenesis and troponin function. Proc Natl Acad Sci U S A 1998; 95:14406-14410

[16] Ashrafian H, Redwood C, Blair E, Watkins H: Hypertrophic cardiomyopathy:a paradigm for myocardial energy depletion. Trends Genet 2003; 19:263-268

[17] Cecchi F, Sgalambro A, Baldi M, Sotgia B, Antoniucci D, Camici PG, Sciagra R, Olivotto I: Microvascular dysfunction, myocardial ischemia, and progression to heart failure in patients with hypertrophic cardiomyopathy. J Cardiovasc Transl Res 2009; 2:452-461

[18] Petersen SE, Jerosch-Herold M, Hudsmith LE, Robson MD, Francis JM, Doll HA, Selvanayagam JB, Neubauer S, Watkins H: Evidence for microvascular dysfunction in hypertrophic cardiomyopathy: new insights from multiparametric magnetic resonance imaging. Circulation 2007; 115:2418-2425

[19] Noseworthy PA, Rosenberg MA, Fifer MA, Palacios IF, Lowry PA, Ruskin JN, Sanborn DM, Picard MH, Vlahakes GJ, Mela T, Das S: Ventricular arrhythmia following alcohol septal ablation for obstructive hypertrophic cardiomyopathy. Am J Cardiol 2009; 104:128-132

[20] ten Cate FJ, Soliman OI, Michels M, Theuns DA, de Jong PL, Geleijnse ML, Serruys PW: Long-term outcome of alcohol septal ablation in patients with obstructive hypertrophic cardiomyopathy: a word of caution. Circ Heart Fail 2010; 3:362-369

[21] Cuoco FA, Spencer WH,3rd, Fernandes VL, Nielsen CD, Nagueh S, Sturdivant JL, Leman RB, Wharton JM, Gold MR: Implantable cardioverter-defibrillator therapy for primary prevention of sudden death after alcohol septal ablation of hypertrophic cardiomyopathy. J Am Coll Cardiol 2008; 52:1718-1723

[22] Ellison KE, Friedman PL, Ganz LI, Stevenson WG: Entrainment mapping and radiofrequency catheter ablation of ventricular tachycardia in right ventricular dysplasia. J Am Coll Cardiol 1998; 32:724-728

[23] Kaplan SR, Gard JJ, Protonotarios N, Tsatsopoulou A, Spiliopoulou C, Anastasakis A, Squarcioni CP, McKenna WJ, Thiene G, Basso C, Brousse N, Fontaine G, Saffitz JE: Remodeling of myocyte gap junctions in arrhythmogenic right ventricular cardiomyopathy due to a deletion in plakoglobin (Naxos disease). Heart Rhythm 2004; 1:3-11

[24] Wu TJ, Ong JJ, Hwang C, Lee JJ, Fishbein MC, Czer L, Trento A, Blanche C, Kass RM, Mandel WJ, Karagueuzian HS, Chen PS: Characteristics of wave fronts during ventricular fibrillation in human hearts with dilated cardiomyopathy: role of increased fibrosis in the generation of reentry. J Am Coll Cardiol 1998; 32:187-196

[25] Soejima K, Stevenson WG, Sapp JL, Selwyn AP, Couper G, Epstein LM: Endocardial and epicardial radiofrequency ablation of ventricular tachycardia associated with dilated cardiomyopathy: the importance of low-voltage scars. J Am Coll Cardiol 2004; 43:1834-1842

[26] Soejima K, Stevenson WG, Sapp JL, Selwyn AP, Couper G, Epstein LM: Endocardial and epicardial radiofrequency ablation of ventricular tachycardia associated with dilated cardiomyopathy: the importance of low-voltage scars. J Am Coll Cardiol 2004; 43:1834-1842

[27] Streitner F, Kuschyk J, Dietrich C, Mahl E, Streitner I, Doesch C, Veltmann C, Schimpf R, Wolpert C, Borggrefe M: Comparison of ventricular tachyarrhythmia characteristics in patients with idiopathic dilated or ischemic cardiomyopathy and defibrillators implanted for primary prevention. Clin Cardiol 2011; 34:604-609

[28] Pogwizd SM, McKenzie JP, Cain ME: Mechanisms underlying spontaneous and induced ventricular arrhythmias in patients with idiopathic dilated cardiomyopathy. Circulation 1998; 98:2404-2414

[29] 29. Lopera G, Stevenson WG, Soejima K, Maisel WH, Koplan B, Sapp JL, Satti SD, Epstein LM: Identification and ablation of three types of ventricular tachycardia involving the his-purkinje system in patients with heart disease. J Cardiovasc Electrophysiol 2004; 15:52-58

[30] Jenni R, Wyss CA, Oechslin EN, Kaufmann PA: Isolated ventricular noncompaction is associated with coronary microcirculatory dysfunction. J Am Coll Cardiol 2002; 39:450-454

[31] Burke A, Mont E, Kutys R, Virmani R: Left ventricular noncompaction: a pathological study of 14 cases. Hum Pathol 2005; 36:403-411

[32] Kandolin R, Lehtonen J, Kupari M: Cardiac sarcoidosis and giant cell myocarditis as causes of atrioventricular block in young and middle-aged adults. Circ Arrhythm Electrophysiol 2011; 4:303-309

[33] Yoshida Y, Morimoto S, Hiramitsu S, Tsuboi N, Hirayama H, Itoh T: Incidence of cardiac sarcoidosis in Japanese patients with high-degree atrioventricular block. Am Heart J 1997; 134:382-386

[34] Furushima H, Chinushi M, Sugiura H, Kasai H, Washizuka T, Aizawa Y: Ventricular tachyarrhythmia associated with cardiac sarcoidosis: its mechanisms and outcome. Clin Cardiol 2004; 27:217-222

[35] Banba K, Kusano KF, Nakamura K, Morita H, Ogawa A, Ohtsuka F, Ogo KO, Nishii N, Watanabe A, Nagase S, Sakuragi S, Ohe T: Relationship between arrhythmogenesis and disease activity in cardiac sarcoidosis. Heart Rhythm 2007; 4:1292-1299

[36] Smith TJ, Kyle RA, Lie JT: Clinical significance of histopathologic patterns of cardiac amyloidosis. Mayo Clin Proc 1984; 59:547-555

[37] Reisinger J, Dubrey SW, Lavalley M, Skinner M, Falk RH: Electrophysiologic abnormalities in AL (primary) amyloidosis with cardiac involvement. J Am Coll Cardiol 1997; 30:1046-1051

[38] Kristen AV, Dengler TJ, Hegenbart U, Schonland SO, Goldschmidt H, Sack FU, Voss F, Becker R, Katus HA, Bauer A: Prophylactic implantation of cardioverter-defibrillator in patients with severe cardiac amyloidosis and high risk for sudden cardiac death. Heart Rhythm 2008; 5:235-240

[39] Sen-Chowdhry S, McKenna WJ: Sudden death from genetic and acquired cardiomyopathies. Circulation 2012; 125:1563-1576

[40] Bigger JT,Jr, Fleiss JL, Kleiger R, Miller JP, Rolnitzky LM: The relationships among ventricular arrhythmias, left ventricular dysfunction, and mortality in the 2 years after myocardial infarction. Circulation 1984; 69:250-258

[41] Sanz G, Castaner A, Betriu A, Magrina J, Roig E, Coll S, Pare JC, Navarro-Lopez F: Determinants of prognosis in survivors of myocardial infarction: a prospective clinical angiographic study. N Engl J Med 1982; 306:1065-1070

[42] Risk stratification and survival after myocardial infarction. N Engl J Med 1983; 309:331-336

[43] Volpi A, De Vita C, Franzosi MG, Geraci E, Maggioni AP, Mauri F, Negri E, Santoro E, Tavazzi L, Tognoni G: Determinants of 6-month mortality in survivors of myocardial infarction after thrombolysis. Results of the GISSI-2 data base. The Ad hoc Working Group of the Gruppo Italiano per lo Studio della Sopravvivenza nell'Infarto Miocardico (GISSI)-2 Data Base. Circulation 1993; 88:416-429

[44] Huikuri HV, Tapanainen JM, Lindgren K, Raatikainen P, Makikallio TH, Juhani Airaksinen KE, Myerburg RJ: Prediction of sudden cardiac death after myocardial infarction in the beta-blocking era. J Am Coll Cardiol 2003; 42:652-658

[45] McClements BM, Adgey AA: Value of signal-averaged electrocardiography, radionuclide ventriculography, Holter monitoring and clinical variables for prediction of ar-

rhythmic events in survivors of acute myocardial infarction in the thrombolytic era. J Am Coll Cardiol 1993; 21:1419-1427

[46] Bailey JJ, Berson AS, Handelsman H, Hodges M: Utility of current risk stratification tests for predicting major arrhythmic events after myocardial infarction. J Am Coll Cardiol 2001; 38:1902-1911

[47] Moss AJ, Zareba W, Hall WJ, Klein H, Wilber DJ, Cannom DS, Daubert JP, Higgins SL, Brown MW, Andrews ML, Multicenter Automatic Defibrillator Implantation Trial II Investigators: Prophylactic implantation of a defibrillator in patients with myocardial infarction and reduced ejection fraction. N Engl J Med 2002; 346:877-883

[48] Bardy GH, Lee KL, Mark DB, Poole JE, Packer DL, Boineau R, Domanski M, Troutman C, Anderson J, Johnson G, McNulty SE, Clapp-Channing N, Davidson-Ray LD, Fraulo ES, Fishbein DP, Luceri RM, Ip JH, Sudden Cardiac Death in Heart Failure Trial (SCD-HeFT) Investigators: Amiodarone or an implantable cardioverter-defibrillator for congestive heart failure. N Engl J Med 2005; 352:225-237

[49] Whang W, Mittleman MA, Rich DQ, Wang PJ, Ruskin JN, Tofler GH, Muller JE, Albert CM, TOVA Investigators: Heart failure and the risk of shocks in patients with implantable cardioverter defibrillators: results from the Triggers Of Ventricular Arrhythmias (TOVA) study. Circulation 2004; 109:1386-1391

[50] Moss AJ, Hall WJ, Cannom DS, Daubert JP, Higgins SL, Klein H, Levine JH, Saksena S, Waldo AL, Wilber D, Brown MW, Heo M: Improved survival with an implanted defibrillator in patients with coronary disease at high risk for ventricular arrhythmia. Multicenter Automatic Defibrillator Implantation Trial Investigators. N Engl J Med 1996; 335:1933-1940

[51] Buxton AE, Lee KL, Fisher JD, Josephson ME, Prystowsky EN, Hafley G: A randomized study of the prevention of sudden death in patients with coronary artery disease. Multicenter Unsustained Tachycardia Trial Investigators. N Engl J Med 1999; 341:1882-1890

[52] Kotler MN, Tabatznik B, Mower MM, Tominaga S: Prognostic significance of ventricular ectopic beats with respect to sudden death in the late postinfarction period. Circulation 1973; 47:959-966

[53] Holmes J, Kubo SH, Cody RJ, Kligfield P: Arrhythmias in ischemic and nonischemic dilated cardiomyopathy: prediction of mortality by ambulatory electrocardiography. Am J Cardiol 1985; 55:146-151

[54] Denes P, Gillis AM, Pawitan Y, Kammerling JM, Wilhelmsen L, Salerno DM: Prevalence, characteristics and significance of ventricular premature complexes and ventricular tachycardia detected by 24-hour continuous electrocardiographic recording in the Cardiac Arrhythmia Suppression Trial. CAST Investigators. Am J Cardiol 1991; 68:887-896

http://dx.doi.org/10.5772/55636

[55] Hohnloser SH, Franck P, Klingenheben T, Zabel M, Just H: Open infarct artery, late potentials, and other prognostic factors in patients after acute myocardial infarction in the thrombolytic era. A prospective trial. Circulation 1994; 90:1747-1756

[56] Cairns JA, Connolly SJ, Roberts R, Gent M: Randomised trial of outcome after myocardial infarction in patients with frequent or repetitive ventricular premature depolarisations: CAMIAT. Canadian Amiodarone Myocardial Infarction Arrhythmia Trial Investigators. Lancet 1997; 349:675-682

[57] Maggioni AP, Zuanetti G, Franzosi MG, Rovelli F, Santoro E, Staszewsky L, Tavazzi L, Tognoni G: Prevalence and prognostic significance of ventricular arrhythmias after acute myocardial infarction in the fibrinolytic era. GISSI-2 results. Circulation 1993; 87:312-322

[58] Crawford MH, Bernstein SJ, Deedwania PC, DiMarco JP, Ferrick KJ, Garson A,Jr, Green LA, Greene HL, Silka MJ, Stone PH, Tracy CM, Gibbons RJ, Alpert JS, Eagle KA, Gardner TJ, Gregoratos G, Russell RO, Ryan TH, Smith SC,Jr: ACC/AHA Guidelines for Ambulatory Electrocardiography. A report of the American College of Cardiology/American Heart Association Task Force on Practice Guidelines (Committee to Revise the Guidelines for Ambulatory Electrocardiography). Developed in collaboration with the North American Society for Pacing and Electrophysiology. J Am Coll Cardiol 1999; 34:912-948

[59] Julian DG, Camm AJ, Frangin G, Janse MJ, Munoz A, Schwartz PJ, Simon P: Randomised trial of effect of amiodarone on mortality in patients with left-ventricular dysfunction after recent myocardial infarction: EMIAT. European Myocardial Infarct Amiodarone Trial Investigators. Lancet 1997; 349:667-674

[60] Buxton AE: Risk stratification for sudden death in patients with coronary artery disease. Heart Rhythm 2009; 6:836-847

[61] Exner D: Noninvasive risk stratification after myocardial infarction: rationale, current evidence and the need for definitive trials. Can J Cardiol 2009; 25 Suppl A:21A-27A

[62] Goldberger JJ, Cain ME, Hohnloser SH, Kadish AH, Knight BP, Lauer MS, Maron BJ, Page RL, Passman RS, Siscovick D, Siscovick D, Stevenson WG, Zipes DP, American Heart Association, American College of Cardiology Foundation, Heart Rhythm Society: American Heart Association/American College of Cardiology Foundation/Heart Rhythm Society scientific statement on noninvasive risk stratification techniques for identifying patients at risk for sudden cardiac death: a scientific statement from the American Heart Association Council on Clinical Cardiology Committee on Electrocardiography and Arrhythmias and Council on Epidemiology and Prevention. Circulation 2008; 118:1497-1518

[63] Schmidt A, Azevedo CF, Cheng A, Gupta SN, Bluemke DA, Foo TK, Gerstenblith G, Weiss RG, Marban E, Tomaselli GF, Lima JA, Wu KC: Infarct tissue heterogeneity by

magnetic resonance imaging identifies enhanced cardiac arrhythmia susceptibility in patients with left ventricular dysfunction. Circulation 2007; 115:2006-2014

[64] Roes SD, Borleffs CJ, van der Geest RJ, Westenberg JJ, Marsan NA, Kaandorp TA, Reiber JH, Zeppenfeld K, Lamb HJ, de Roos A, Schalij MJ, Bax JJ: Infarct tissue heterogeneity assessed with contrast-enhanced MRI predicts spontaneous ventricular arrhythmia in patients with ischemic cardiomyopathy and implantable cardioverter-defibrillator. Circ Cardiovasc Imaging 2009; 2:183-190

[65] Sasano T, Abraham MR, Chang KC, Ashikaga H, Mills KJ, Holt DP, Hilton J, Nekolla SG, Dong J, Lardo AC, Halperin H, Dannals RF, Marban E, Bengel FM: Abnormal sympathetic innervation of viable myocardium and the substrate of ventricular tachycardia after myocardial infarction. J Am Coll Cardiol 2008; 51:2266-2275

[66] Bax JJ, Kraft O, Buxton AE, Fjeld JG, Parizek P, Agostini D, Knuuti J, Flotats A, Arrighi J, Muxi A, Alibelli MJ, Banerjee G, Jacobson AF: 123 I-mIBG scintigraphy to predict inducibility of ventricular arrhythmias on cardiac electrophysiology testing: a prospective multicenter pilot study. Circ Cardiovasc Imaging 2008; 1:131-140

[67] Jacobson AF, Senior R, Cerqueira MD, Wong ND, Thomas GS, Lopez VA, Agostini D, Weiland F, Chandna H, Narula J, ADMIRE-HF Investigators: Myocardial iodine-123 meta-iodobenzylguanidine imaging and cardiac events in heart failure. Results of the prospective ADMIRE-HF (AdreView Myocardial Imaging for Risk Evaluation in Heart Failure) study. J Am Coll Cardiol 2010; 55:2212-2221

[68] Goldberger JJ, Buxton AE, Cain M, Costantini O, Exner DV, Knight BP, Lloyd-Jones D, Kadish AH, Lee B, Moss A, Myerburg R, Olgin J, Passman R, Rosenbaum D, Stevenson W, Zareba W, Zipes DP: Risk stratification for arrhythmic sudden cardiac death: identifying the roadblocks. Circulation 2011; 123:2423-2430

[69] Elliott PM, Gimeno JR, Thaman R, Shah J, Ward D, Dickie S, Tome Esteban MT, McKenna WJ: Historical trends in reported survival rates in patients with hypertrophic cardiomyopathy. Heart 2006; 92:785-791

[70] Maron BJ, Olivotto I, Spirito P, Casey SA, Bellone P, Gohman TE, Graham KJ, Burton DA, Cecchi F: Epidemiology of hypertrophic cardiomyopathy-related death: revisited in a large non-referral-based patient population. Circulation 2000; 102:858-864

[71] Christiaans I, van Engelen K, van Langen IM, Birnie E, Bonsel GJ, Elliott PM, Wilde AA: Risk stratification for sudden cardiac death in hypertrophic cardiomyopathy: systematic review of clinical risk markers. Europace 2010; 12:313-321

[72] Efthimiadis GK, Parcharidou DG, Giannakoulas G, Pagourelias ED, Charalampidis P, Savvopoulos G, Ziakas A, Karvounis H, Styliadis IH, Parcharidis GE: Left ventricular outflow tract obstruction as a risk factor for sudden cardiac death in hypertrophic cardiomyopathy. Am J Cardiol 2009; 104:695-699

[73] Elliott PM, Gimeno JR, Tome MT, Shah J, Ward D, Thaman R, Mogensen J, McKenna WJ: Left ventricular outflow tract obstruction and sudden death risk in patients with hypertrophic cardiomyopathy. Eur Heart J 2006; 27:1933-1941

[74] Spirito P, Autore C, Rapezzi C, Bernabo P, Badagliacca R, Maron MS, Bongioanni S, Coccolo F, Estes NA, Barilla CS, Biagini E, Quarta G, Conte MR, Bruzzi P, Maron BJ: Syncope and risk of sudden death in hypertrophic cardiomyopathy. Circulation 2009; 119:1703-1710

[75] Kofflard MJ, Ten Cate FJ, van der Lee C, van Domburg RT: Hypertrophic cardiomyopathy in a large community-based population: clinical outcome and identification of risk factors for sudden cardiac death and clinical deterioration. J Am Coll Cardiol 2003; 41:987-993

[76] Gimeno JR, Tome-Esteban M, Lofiego C, Hurtado J, Pantazis A, Mist B, Lambiase P, McKenna WJ, Elliott PM: Exercise-induced ventricular arrhythmias and risk of sudden cardiac death in patients with hypertrophic cardiomyopathy. Eur Heart J 2009; 30:2599-2605

[77] Monserrat L, Elliott PM, Gimeno JR, Sharma S, Penas-Lado M, McKenna WJ: Nonsustained ventricular tachycardia in hypertrophic cardiomyopathy: an independent marker of sudden death risk in young patients. J Am Coll Cardiol 2003; 42:873-879

[78] Olivotto I, Gistri R, Petrone P, Pedemonte E, Vargiu D, Cecchi F: Maximum left ventricular thickness and risk of sudden death in patients with hypertrophic cardiomyopathy. J Am Coll Cardiol 2003; 41:315-321

[79] Maron MS, Olivotto I, Betocchi S, Casey SA, Lesser JR, Losi MA, Cecchi F, Maron BJ: Effect of left ventricular outflow tract obstruction on clinical outcome in hypertrophic cardiomyopathy. N Engl J Med 2003; 348:295-303

[80] Elliott PM, Poloniecki J, Dickie S, Sharma S, Monserrat L, Varnava A, Mahon NG, McKenna WJ: Sudden death in hypertrophic cardiomyopathy: identification of high risk patients. J Am Coll Cardiol 2000; 36:2212-2218

[81] Elliott PM, Gimeno Blanes JR, Mahon NG, Poloniecki JD, McKenna WJ: Relation between severity of left-ventricular hypertrophy and prognosis in patients with hypertrophic cardiomyopathy. Lancet 2001; 357:420-424

[82] Autore C, Bernabo P, Barilla CS, Bruzzi P, Spirito P: The prognostic importance of left ventricular outflow obstruction in hypertrophic cardiomyopathy varies in relation to the severity of symptoms. J Am Coll Cardiol 2005; 45:1076-1080

[83] Wigle ED, Sasson Z, Henderson MA, Ruddy TD, Fulop J, Rakowski H, Williams WG: Hypertrophic cardiomyopathy. The importance of the site and the extent of hypertrophy. A review. Prog Cardiovasc Dis 1985; 28:1-83

[84] TEARE D: Asymmetrical hypertrophy of the heart in young adults. Br Heart J 1958; 20:1-8

[85] Maron BJ, Lipson LC, Roberts WC, Savage DD, Epstein SE: "Malignant" hypertrophic cardiomyopathy: identification of a subgroup of families with unusually frequent premature death. Am J Cardiol 1978; 41:1133-1140

[86] McKenna W, Deanfield J, Faruqui A, England D, Oakley C, Goodwin J: Prognosis in hypertrophic cardiomyopathy: role of age and clinical, electrocardiographic and hemodynamic features. Am J Cardiol 1981; 47:532-538

[87] Watkins H, McKenna WJ, Thierfelder L, Suk HJ, Anan R, O'Donoghue A, Spirito P, Matsumori A, Moravec CS, Seidman JG: Mutations in the genes for cardiac troponin T and alpha-tropomyosin in hypertrophic cardiomyopathy. N Engl J Med 1995; 332:1058-1064

[88] Maki S, Ikeda H, Muro A, Yoshida N, Shibata A, Koga Y, Imaizumi T: Predictors of sudden cardiac death in hypertrophic cardiomyopathy. Am J Cardiol 1998; 82:774-778

[89] Frenneaux MP, Counihan PJ, Caforio AL, Chikamori T, McKenna WJ: Abnormal blood pressure response during exercise in hypertrophic cardiomyopathy. Circulation 1990; 82:1995-2002

[90] Sadoul N, Prasad K, Elliott PM, Bannerjee S, Frenneaux MP, McKenna WJ: Prospective prognostic assessment of blood pressure response during exercise in patients with hypertrophic cardiomyopathy. Circulation 1997; 96:2987-2991

[91] Sorajja P, Ommen SR, Nishimura RA, Gersh BJ, Berger PB, Tajik AJ: Adverse prognosis of patients with hypertrophic cardiomyopathy who have epicardial coronary artery disease. Circulation 2003; 108:2342-2348

[92] Blomstrom-Lundqvist C, Sabel KG, Olsson SB: A long term follow up of 15 patients with arrhythmogenic right ventricular dysplasia. Br Heart J 1987; 58:477-488

[93] Marcus FI, Fontaine GH, Frank R, Gallagher JJ, Reiter MJ: Long-term follow-up in patients with arrhythmogenic right ventricular disease. Eur Heart J 1989; 10 Suppl D: 68-73

[94] Leclercq JF, Coumel P: Characteristics, prognosis and treatment of the ventricular arrhythmias of right ventricular dysplasia. Eur Heart J 1989; 10 Suppl D:61-67

[95] Corrado D, Basso C, Rizzoli G, Schiavon M, Thiene G: Does sports activity enhance the risk of sudden death in adolescents and young adults?. J Am Coll Cardiol 2003; 42:1959-1963

[96] Corrado D, Leoni L, Link MS, Della Bella P, Gaita F, Curnis A, Salerno JU, Igidbashian D, Raviele A, Disertori M, Zanotto G, Verlato R, Vergara G, Delise P, Turrini P, Basso C, Naccarella F, Maddalena F, Estes NA,3rd, Buja G, Thiene G: Implantable cardioverter-defibrillator therapy for prevention of sudden death in patients with arrhythmogenic right ventricular cardiomyopathy/dysplasia. Circulation 2003; 108:3084-3091

[97] Wichter T, Paul M, Wollmann C, Acil T, Gerdes P, Ashraf O, Tjan TD, Soeparwata R, Block M, Borggrefe M, Scheld HH, Breithardt G, Bocker D: Implantable cardioverter/defibrillator therapy in arrhythmogenic right ventricular cardiomyopathy: single-center experience of long-term follow-up and complications in 60 patients. Circulation 2004; 109:1503-1508

[98] Nava A, Bauce B, Basso C, Muriago M, Rampazzo A, Villanova C, Daliento L, Buja G, Corrado D, Danieli GA, Thiene G: Clinical profile and long-term follow-up of 37 families with arrhythmogenic right ventricular cardiomyopathy. J Am Coll Cardiol 2000; 36:2226-2233

[99] Bhonsale A, James CA, Tichnell C, Murray B, Gagarin D, Philips B, Dalal D, Tedford R, Russell SD, Abraham T, Tandri H, Judge DP, Calkins H: Incidence and predictors of implantable cardioverter-defibrillator therapy in patients with arrhythmogenic right ventricular dysplasia/cardiomyopathy undergoing implantable cardioverter-defibrillator implantation for primary prevention. J Am Coll Cardiol 2011; 58:1485-1496

[100] Canu G, Atallah G, Claudel JP, Champagnac D, Desseigne D, Chevalier P, de Zuloaga C, Moncada E, Kirkorian G, Touboul P: Prognosis and long-term development of arrhythmogenic dysplasia of the right ventricle. Arch Mal Coeur Vaiss 1993; 86:41-48

[101] Turrini P, Corrado D, Basso C, Nava A, Bauce B, Thiene G: Dispersion of ventricular depolarization-repolarization: a noninvasive marker for risk stratification in arrhythmogenic right ventricular cardiomyopathy. Circulation 2001; 103:3075-3080

[102] Blomstrom-Lundqvist C, Olsson SB, Edvardsson N: Follow-up by repeated signal-averaged surface QRS in patients with the syndrome of arrhythmogenic right ventricular dysplasia. Eur Heart J 1989; 10 Suppl D:54-60

[103] Leclercq JF, Coumel P: Late potentials in arrhythmogenic right ventricular dysplasia. Prevalence, diagnostic and prognostic values. Eur Heart J 1993; 14 Suppl E:80-83

[104] Turrini P, Angelini A, Thiene G, Buja G, Daliento L, Rizzoli G, Nava A: Late potentials and ventricular arrhythmias in arrhythmogenic right ventricular cardiomyopathy. Am J Cardiol 1999; 83:1214-1219

[105] Hulot JS, Jouven X, Empana JP, Frank R, Fontaine G: Natural history and risk stratification of arrhythmogenic right ventricular dysplasia/cardiomyopathy. Circulation 2004; 110:1879-1884

[106] Peters S: Long-term follow-up and risk assessment of arrhythmogenic right ventricular dysplasia/cardiomyopathy: personal experience from different primary and tertiary centres. J Cardiovasc Med (Hagerstown) 2007; 8:521-526

[107] Roguin A, Bomma CS, Nasir K, Tandri H, Tichnell C, James C, Rutberg J, Crosson J, Spevak PJ, Berger RD, Halperin HR, Calkins H: Implantable cardioverter-defibrilla-

tors in patients with arrhythmogenic right ventricular dysplasia/cardiomyopathy. J Am Coll Cardiol 2004; 43:1843-1852

[108] Hodgkinson KA, Parfrey PS, Bassett AS, Kupprion C, Drenckhahn J, Norman MW, Thierfelder L, Stuckless SN, Dicks EL, McKenna WJ, Connors SP: The impact of implantable cardioverter-defibrillator therapy on survival in autosomal-dominant arrhythmogenic right ventricular cardiomyopathy (ARVD5). J Am Coll Cardiol 2005; 45:400-408

[109] Corrado D, Calkins H, Link MS, Leoni L, Favale S, Bevilacqua M, Basso C, Ward D, Boriani G, Ricci R, Piccini JP, Dalal D, Santini M, Buja G, Iliceto S, Estes NA,3rd, Wichter T, McKenna WJ, Thiene G, Marcus FI: Prophylactic implantable defibrillator in patients with arrhythmogenic right ventricular cardiomyopathy/dysplasia and no prior ventricular fibrillation or sustained ventricular tachycardia. Circulation 2010; 122:1144-1152

[110] Borleffs CJ, van Welsenes GH, van Bommel RJ, van der Velde ET, Bax JJ, van Erven L, Putter H, van der Bom JG, Rosendaal FR, Schalij MJ: Mortality risk score in primary prevention implantable cardioverter defibrillator recipients with non-ischaemic or ischaemic heart disease. Eur Heart J 2010; 31:712-718

[111] Dec GW, Fuster V: Idiopathic dilated cardiomyopathy. N Engl J Med 1994; 331:1564-1575

[112] Nelson SD, Sparks EA, Graber HL, Boudoulas H, Mehdirad AA, Baker P, Wooley C: Clinical characteristics of sudden death victims in heritable (chromosome 1p1-1q1) conduction and myocardial disease. J Am Coll Cardiol 1998; 32:1717-1723

[113] Kadish A, Dyer A, Daubert JP, Quigg R, Estes NA, Anderson KP, Calkins H, Hoch D, Goldberger J, Shalaby A, Sanders WE, Schaechter A, Levine JH, Defibrillators in Non-Ischemic Cardiomyopathy Treatment Evaluation (DEFINITE) Investigators: Prophylactic defibrillator implantation in patients with nonischemic dilated cardiomyopathy. N Engl J Med 2004; 350:2151-2158

[114] Effect of metoprolol CR/XL in chronic heart failure: Metoprolol CR/XL Randomised Intervention Trial in Congestive Heart Failure (MERIT-HF). Lancet 1999; 353:2001-2007

[115] Olshansky B, Poole JE, Johnson G, Anderson J, Hellkamp AS, Packer D, Mark DB, Lee KL, Bardy GH, SCD-HeFT Investigators: Syncope predicts the outcome of cardiomyopathy patients: analysis of the SCD-HeFT study. J Am Coll Cardiol 2008; 51:1277-1282

[116] Meune C, Van Berlo JH, Anselme F, Bonne G, Pinto YM, Duboc D: Primary prevention of sudden death in patients with lamin A/C gene mutations. N Engl J Med 2006; 354:209-210

[117] Pasotti M, Klersy C, Pilotto A, Marziliano N, Rapezzi C, Serio A, Mannarino S, Gambarin F, Favalli V, Grasso M, Agozzino M, Campana C, Gavazzi A, Febo O, Marini

M, Landolina M, Mortara A, Piccolo G, Vigano M, Tavazzi L, Arbustini E: Long-term outcome and risk stratification in dilated cardiolaminopathies. J Am Coll Cardiol 2008; 52:1250-1260

[118] van Rijsingen IA, Arbustini E, Elliott PM, Mogensen J, Hermans-van Ast JF, van der Kooi AJ, van Tintelen JP, van den Berg MP, Pilotto A, Pasotti M, Jenkins S, Rowland C, Aslam U, Wilde AA, Perrot A, Pankuweit S, Zwinderman AH, Charron P, Pinto YM: Risk factors for malignant ventricular arrhythmias in lamin a/c mutation carriers a European cohort study. J Am Coll Cardiol 2012; 59:493-500

[119] Zecchin M, Di Lenarda A, Gregori D, Merlo M, Pivetta A, Vitrella G, Sabbadini G, Mestroni L, Sinagra G: Are nonsustained ventricular tachycardias predictive of major arrhythmias in patients with dilated cardiomyopathy on optimal medical treatment?. Pacing Clin Electrophysiol 2008; 31:290-299

[120] Baldasseroni S, Opasich C, Gorini M, Lucci D, Marchionni N, Marini M, Campana C, Perini G, Deorsola A, Masotti G, Tavazzi L, Maggioni AP, Italian Network on Congestive Heart Failure Investigators: Left bundle-branch block is associated with increased 1-year sudden and total mortality rate in 5517 outpatients with congestive heart failure: a report from the Italian network on congestive heart failure. Am Heart J 2002; 143:398-405

[121] Iuliano S, Fisher SG, Karasik PE, Fletcher RD, Singh SN, Department of Veterans Affairs Survival Trial of Antiarrhythmic Therapy in Congestive Heart Failure: QRS duration and mortality in patients with congestive heart failure. Am Heart J 2002; 143:1085-1091

[122] Iacoviello M, Forleo C, Guida P, Romito R, Sorgente A, Sorrentino S, Catucci S, Mastropasqua F, Pitzalis M: Ventricular repolarization dynamicity provides independent prognostic information toward major arrhythmic events in patients with idiopathic dilated cardiomyopathy. J Am Coll Cardiol 2007; 50:225-231

[123] Das MK, Maskoun W, Shen C, Michael MA, Suradi H, Desai M, Subbarao R, Bhakta D: Fragmented QRS on twelve-lead electrocardiogram predicts arrhythmic events in patients with ischemic and nonischemic cardiomyopathy. Heart Rhythm 2010; 7:74-80

[124] Koutalas E, Kanoupakis E, Vardas P: Sudden cardiac death in non-ischemic dilated cardiomyopathy: A critical appraisal of existing and potential risk stratification tools. Int J Cardiol 2012

[125] Fazio G, Corrado G, Zachara E, Rapezzi C, Sulafa AK, Sutera L, Pizzuto C, Stollberger C, Sormani L, Finsterer J, Benatar A, Di Gesaro G, Cascio C, Cangemi D, Cavusoglu Y, Baumhakel M, Drago F, Carerj S, Pipitone S, Novo S: Ventricular tachycardia in non-compaction of left ventricle: is this a frequent complication?. Pacing Clin Electrophysiol 2007; 30:544-546

[126] Yazaki Y, Isobe M, Hiramitsu S, Morimoto S, Hiroe M, Omichi C, Nakano T, Saeki M, Izumi T, Sekiguchi M: Comparison of clinical features and prognosis of cardiac sarcoidosis and idiopathic dilated cardiomyopathy. Am J Cardiol 1998; 82:537-540

[127] Ardehali H, Howard DL, Hariri A, Qasim A, Hare JM, Baughman KL, Kasper EK: A positive endomyocardial biopsy result for sarcoid is associated with poor prognosis in patients with initially unexplained cardiomyopathy. Am Heart J 2005; 150:459-463

[128] Dhote R, Vignaux O, Blanche P, Duboc D, Dusser D, Brezin A, Devaux JY, Christoforov B, Legmann P: Value of MRI for the diagnosis of cardiac involvement in sarcoidosis. Rev Med Interne 2003; 24:151-157

[129] Vignaux O, Dhote R, Duboc D, Blanche P, Devaux JY, Weber S, Legmann P: Detection of myocardial involvement in patients with sarcoidosis applying T2-weighted, contrast-enhanced, and cine magnetic resonance imaging: initial results of a prospective study. J Comput Assist Tomogr 2002; 26:762-767

[130] Smedema JP, Snoep G, van Kroonenburgh MP, van Geuns RJ, Dassen WR, Gorgels AP, Crijns HJ: Cardiac involvement in patients with pulmonary sarcoidosis assessed at two university medical centers in the Netherlands. Chest 2005; 128:30-35

[131] Patel MR, Cawley PJ, Heitner JF, Klem I, Parker MA, Jaroudi WA, Meine TJ, White JB, Elliott MD, Kim HW, Judd RM, Kim RJ: Detection of myocardial damage in patients with sarcoidosis. Circulation 2009; 120:1969-1977

[132] Piccini JP, Berger JS, O'Connor CM: Amiodarone for the prevention of sudden cardiac death: a meta-analysis of randomized controlled trials. Eur Heart J 2009; 30:1245-1253

[133] Julian DG, Prescott RJ, Jackson FS, Szekely P: Controlled trial of sotalol for one year after myocardial infarction. Lancet 1982; 1:1142-1147

[134] Waldo AL, Camm AJ, deRuyter H, Friedman PL, MacNeil DJ, Pauls JF, Pitt B, Pratt CM, Schwartz PJ, Veltri EP: Effect of d-sotalol on mortality in patients with left ventricular dysfunction after recent and remote myocardial infarction. The SWORD Investigators. Survival With Oral d-Sotalol. Lancet 1996; 348:7-12

[135] Pratt CM, Camm AJ, Cooper W, Friedman PL, MacNeil DJ, Moulton KM, Pitt B, Schwartz PJ, Veltri EP, Waldo AL: Mortality in the Survival With ORal D-sotalol (SWORD) trial: why did patients die?. Am J Cardiol 1998; 81:869-876

[136] Pacifico A, Hohnloser SH, Williams JH, Tao B, Saksena S, Henry PD, Prystowsky EN: Prevention of implantable-defibrillator shocks by treatment with sotalol. d,l-Sotalol Implantable Cardioverter-Defibrillator Study Group. N Engl J Med 1999; 340:1855-1862

[137] The Cardiac Insufficiency Bisoprolol Study II (CIBIS-II): a randomised trial. Lancet 1999; 353:9-13

[138] Packer M, Coats AJ, Fowler MB, Katus HA, Krum H, Mohacsi P, Rouleau JL, Tendera M, Castaigne A, Roecker EB, Schultz MK, DeMets DL, Carvedilol Prospective Randomized Cumulative Survival Study Group: Effect of carvedilol on survival in severe chronic heart failure. N Engl J Med 2001; 344:1651-1658

[139] Dargie HJ: Effect of carvedilol on outcome after myocardial infarction in patients with left-ventricular dysfunction: the CAPRICORN randomised trial. Lancet 2001; 357:1385-1390

[140] Effects of enalapril on mortality in severe congestive heart failure. Results of the Co-operative North Scandinavian Enalapril Survival Study (CONSENSUS). The CONSENSUS Trial Study Group. N Engl J Med 1987; 316:1429-1435

[141] Effect of enalapril on mortality and the development of heart failure in asymptomatic patients with reduced left ventricular ejection fractions. The SOLVD Investigattors. N Engl J Med 1992; 327:685-691

[142] Cohn JN, Tognoni G, Valsartan Heart Failure Trial Investigators: A randomized trial of the angiotensin-receptor blocker valsartan in chronic heart failure. N Engl J Med 2001; 345:1667-1675

[143] Pitt B, Segal R, Martinez FA, Meurers G, Cowley AJ, Thomas I, Deedwania PC, Ney DE, Snavely DB, Chang PI: Randomised trial of losartan versus captopril in patients over 65 with heart failure (Evaluation of Losartan in the Elderly Study, ELITE). Lancet 1997; 349:747-752

[144] Effect of the antiarrhythmic agent moricizine on survival after myocardial infarction. The Cardiac Arrhythmia Suppression Trial II Investigators. N Engl J Med 1992; 327:227-233

[145] Kuck KH, Cappato R, Siebels J, Ruppel R: Randomized comparison of antiarrhythmic drug therapy with implantable defibrillators in patients resuscitated from cardiac arrest : the Cardiac Arrest Study Hamburg (CASH). Circulation 2000; 102:748-754

[146] McKenna WJ, Oakley CM, Krikler DM, Goodwin JF: Improved survival with amiodarone in patients with hypertrophic cardiomyopathy and ventricular tachycardia. Br Heart J 1985; 53:412-416

[147] Melacini P, Maron BJ, Bobbo F, Basso C, Tokajuk B, Zucchetto M, Thiene G, Iliceto S: Evidence that pharmacological strategies lack efficacy for the prevention of sudden death in hypertrophic cardiomyopathy. Heart 2007; 93:708-710

[148] Wichter T, Borggrefe M, Haverkamp W, Chen X, Breithardt G: Efficacy of antiarrhythmic drugs in patients with arrhythmogenic right ventricular disease. Results in patients with inducible and noninducible ventricular tachycardia. Circulation 1992; 86:29-37

[149] Marcus GM, Glidden DV, Polonsky B, Zareba W, Smith LM, Cannom DS, Estes NA, 3rd, Marcus F, Scheinman MM, Multidisciplinary Study of Right Ventricular Dyspla-

sia Investigators: Efficacy of antiarrhythmic drugs in arrhythmogenic right ventricular cardiomyopathy: a report from the North American ARVC Registry. J Am Coll Cardiol 2009; 54:609-615

[150] Connolly SJ, Hallstrom AP, Cappato R, Schron EB, Kuck KH, Zipes DP, Greene HL, Boczor S, Domanski M, Follmann D, Gent M, Roberts RS: Meta-analysis of the implantable cardioverter defibrillator secondary prevention trials. AVID, CASH and CIDS studies. Antiarrhythmics vs Implantable Defibrillator study. Cardiac Arrest Study Hamburg . Canadian Implantable Defibrillator Study. Eur Heart J 2000; 21:2071-2078

[151] Oseroff O, Retyk E, Bochoeyer A: Subanalyses of secondary prevention implantable cardioverter-defibrillator trials: antiarrhythmics versus implantable defibrillators (AVID), Canadian Implantable Defibrillator Study (CIDS), and Cardiac Arrest Study Hamburg (CASH). Curr Opin Cardiol 2004; 19:26-30

[152] Domanski MJ, Sakseena S, Epstein AE, Hallstrom AP, Brodsky MA, Kim S, Lancaster S, Schron E: Relative effectiveness of the implantable cardioverter-defibrillator and antiarrhythmic drugs in patients with varying degrees of left ventricular dysfunction who have survived malignant ventricular arrhythmias. AVID Investigators. Antiarrhythmics Versus Implantable Defibrillators. J Am Coll Cardiol 1999; 34:1090-1095

[153] Sheldon R, Connolly S, Krahn A, Roberts R, Gent M, Gardner M: Identification of patients most likely to benefit from implantable cardioverter-defibrillator therapy: the Canadian Implantable Defibrillator Study. Circulation 2000; 101:1660-1664

[154] Thomas KE, Josephson ME: The role of electrophysiology study in risk stratification of sudden cardiac death. Prog Cardiovasc Dis 2008; 51:97-105

[155] Hohnloser SH, Kuck KH, Dorian P, Roberts RS, Hampton JR, Hatala R, Fain E, Gent M, Connolly SJ, DINAMIT Investigators: Prophylactic use of an implantable cardioverter-defibrillator after acute myocardial infarction. N Engl J Med 2004; 351:2481-2488

[156] Wilkoff BL, Cook JR, Epstein AE, Greene HL, Hallstrom AP, Hsia H, Kutalek SP, Sharma A, Dual Chamber and VVI Implantable Defibrillator Trial Investigators: Dual-chamber pacing or ventricular backup pacing in patients with an implantable defibrillator: the Dual Chamber and VVI Implantable Defibrillator (DAVID) Trial. JAMA 2002; 288:3115-3123

[157] Olshansky B, Day JD, Moore S, Gering L, Rosenbaum M, McGuire M, Brown S, Lerew DR: Is dual-chamber programming inferior to single-chamber programming in an implantable cardioverter-defibrillator? Results of the INTRINSIC RV (Inhibition of Unnecessary RV Pacing With AVSH in ICDs) study. Circulation 2007; 115:9-16

[158] Sharma AD, Rizo-Patron C, Hallstrom AP, O'Neill GP, Rothbart S, Martins JB, Roelke M, Steinberg JS, Greene HL, DAVID Investigators: Percent right ventricular pacing predicts outcomes in the DAVID trial. Heart Rhythm 2005; 2:830-834

http://dx.doi.org/10.5772/55636

[159] Theuns DA, Smith T, Hunink MG, Bardy GH, Jordaens L: Effectiveness of prophylactic implantation of cardioverter-defibrillators without cardiac resynchronization therapy in patients with ischaemic or non-ischaemic heart disease: a systematic review and meta-analysis. Europace 2010; 12:1564-1570

[160] Kong MH, Al-Khatib SM, Sanders GD, Hasselblad V, Peterson ED: Use of implantable cardioverter-defibrillators for primary prevention in older patients: a systematic literature review and meta-analysis. Cardiol J 2011; 18:503-514

[161] Santangeli P, Di Biase L, Dello Russo A, Casella M, Bartoletti S, Santarelli P, Pelargonio G, Natale A: Meta-analysis: age and effectiveness of prophylactic implantable cardioverter-defibrillators. Ann Intern Med 2010; 153:592-599

[162] Santangeli P, Pelargonio G, Dello Russo A, Casella M, Bisceglia C, Bartoletti S, Santarelli P, Di Biase L, Natale A: Gender differences in clinical outcome and primary prevention defibrillator benefit in patients with severe left ventricular dysfunction: a systematic review and meta-analysis. Heart Rhythm 2010; 7:876-882

[163] Goldenberg I, Vyas AK, Hall WJ, Moss AJ, Wang H, He H, Zareba W, McNitt S, Andrews ML, MADIT-II Investigators: Risk stratification for primary implantation of a cardioverter-defibrillator in patients with ischemic left ventricular dysfunction. J Am Coll Cardiol 2008; 51:288-296

[164] Buxton AE, Lee KL, Hafley GE, Pires LA, Fisher JD, Gold MR, Josephson ME, Lehmann MH, Prystowsky EN, MUSTT Investigators: Limitations of ejection fraction for prediction of sudden death risk in patients with coronary artery disease: lessons from the MUSTT study. J Am Coll Cardiol 2007; 50:1150-1157

[165] European Heart Rhythm Association, Heart Rhythm Society, Zipes DP, Camm AJ, Borggrefe M, Buxton AE, Chaitman B, Fromer M, Gregoratos G, Klein G, Moss AJ, Myerburg RJ, Priori SG, Quinones MA, Roden DM, Silka MJ, Tracy C, Smith SC,Jr, Jacobs AK, Adams CD, Antman EM, Anderson JL, Hunt SA, Halperin JL, Nishimura R, Ornato JP, Page RL, Riegel B, Priori SG, Blanc JJ, Budaj A, Camm AJ, Dean V, Deckers JW, Despres C, Dickstein K, Lekakis J, McGregor K, Metra M, Morais J, Osterspey A, Tamargo JL, Zamorano JL, American College of Cardiology, American Heart Association Task Force, European Society of Cardiology Committee for Practice Guidelines: ACC/AHA/ESC 2006 guidelines for management of patients with ventricular arrhythmias and the prevention of sudden cardiac death: a report of the American College of Cardiology/American Heart Association Task Force and the European Society of Cardiology Committee for Practice Guidelines (Writing Committee to Develop Guidelines for Management of Patients With Ventricular Arrhythmias and the Prevention of Sudden Cardiac Death). J Am Coll Cardiol 2006; 48:e247-346

[166] Epstein AE, Dimarco JP, Ellenbogen KA, Estes NA,3rd, Freedman RA, Gettes LS, Gillinov AM, Gregoratos G, Hammill SC, Hayes DL, Hlatky MA, Newby LK, Page RL, Schoenfeld MH, Silka MJ, Stevenson LW, Sweeney MO, American College of Cardiology, American Heart Association Task Force on Practice Guidelines, American As-

sociation for Thoracic Surgery, Society of Thoracic Surgeons: ACC/AHA/HRS 2008 Guidelines for device-based therapy of cardiac rhythm abnormalities. Heart Rhythm 2008; 5:e1-62

Chapter 10

Role of Traditional Heart Failure Medications on Sudden Cardiac Death Prevention in Patients with Cardiomyopathy

Ann M. Anderson and M. Obadah Al Chekakie

Additional information is available at the end of the chapter

http://dx.doi.org/10.5772/55008

1. Introduction

Sudden cardiac death (SCD) remains a major public health issue with an estimated annual incidence of 300,000 cases per year. The ACC/AHA/ESC 2006 guidelines define SCD as "death from an unexpected circulatory arrest, usually due to a cardiac arrhythmia occurring within an hour of the onset of symptoms" [1]. Trials on traditional antiarrhythmic drugs have failed to show any mortality benefit even when compared to placebo or implantable cardiovertor defibrillators (ICDs) [2]. Most of the patients experiencing sudden cardiac arrest have left ventricular ejection fraction (LVEF) > 50%, with the majority of these patients having a history of coronary artery disease (CAD). Majority of Sudden Cardiac Arrests (85-90%) are the first arrhythmic event a patient experiences[3].Beta blocker therapy, Angiotensin enzymes inhibitors (ACE-I) as well as aldosterone antagonists have been shown to decrease the risk of sudden cardiac death especially in post myocardial infarction (MI) patients and in patients with congestive heart failure. This chapter will review the data on the effects of traditional heart failure medications, especially beta blockers, Renin Angiotensin system blockers, as well as Statin therapy on sudden cardiac death in post MI patients and in patients with cardiomyopathy.

2. β-blockers and sudden cardiac death prevention

2.1. Potential mechanisms of β-blockers on sudden cardiac death prevention

Multiple studies have suggested that the major mechanisms responsible for the cardiac arrhythmias associated with sudden cardiac death are ventricular tachycardia (VT) and ventricular fibrillation (VF). For these arrhythmias to occur, an interaction between substrate (ventricular enlargement and/or hypertrophy, myocardial scar due to ischemic or non-ischemic injury) and triggers (electrolyte abnormalities, changes in the sympathetic and parasympathetic activity, neuro-humeral factors, and premature ventricular contractions) is necessary to initiate reentry leading to ventricular tachycardia and ventricular fibrillation (Figure 1).

Many anatomic or functional substrates such as coronary artery disease, cardiomyopathy or primary electrophysiological disease can lead to sudden cardiac death. Progression of these disease states leads to sympathetic activation. At the cellular level, sympathetic and vagal denervation caused by myocardial ischemia leads to an increase in interstitial potassium and intracellular calcium concentrations [3]. This results in slowed conduction and induces spontaneous electrical activity. All these factors contribute to reentry; which is the most common mechanism of ventricular tachycardia in patients with ischemic heart disease [4].

As myocardial ischemia progresses the neurohumoral system exerts further stimulation of the sympathetic system and the renin-angiotensin-aldosterone system (RAAS). This neurohumoral cascade leads to increasing levels of norepinephrine, angiotensin II, aldosterone, endothelin and vasopressin. Increased norepinephrine levels lead to increased preload and after-load, which in turn increases myocardial oxygen demand. Furthermore, the activation of these systems promotes fibrosis and necrosis [5-7], which over time will lead to cardiac remodeling, left ventricular dilatation, fibrosis and progression into heart failure [8].

Three types of β-receptors are known, designated β_1, β_2 and β_3 receptors. β_1 receptors are located mainly in the heart and in the kidneys and are down regulated in heart failure due to chronically elevated norepinephrine levels. β_2 receptors are located mainly in the lungs, gastrointestinal tract, liver, uterus, vascular smooth muscle, and skeletal muscle. β_3 receptors are located in fat cells. $\beta_1$and $\beta_2$receptors activate cyclic adenosine mono-phosphate (cAMP), which acts as a second messenger and leads to increased contractility (inotropy), increased heart rate (which increases myocardial oxygen demand), increased conduction velocity (which may promote reentry) and have a positive lusitropic effect, which improves active relaxation [9]. $\beta_2$receptors promote the release of renin, which in turn activates angiotensin II and aldosterone, both of which elevate the blood pressure, increase after-load, promote potassium wasting and activate fibroblasts leading to fibrosis.

β-blockers exert their protective effect on the heart via different mechanisms. β-blockers reduce ischemia by decreasing the heart rate, which is the major determinant of myocardial oxygen demand[10]. At the cellular level, β-blockers decrease electrical excitability by limiting calcium entry via catecholamine-dependent channels [9]. All this helps decrease left ventricular mass and volume, decrease LV end diastolic pressure and improve LV function [11]. β-blockers are also considered a class II antiarrhythmic medications. They decrease spontaneous depolarization, prolong the sinus node cycle length, atrioventricular conduction times and atrioventricular refractory periods. They also increase the excitable gap, which prevents reentry and increases the success of anti-tachycardia pacing [12].

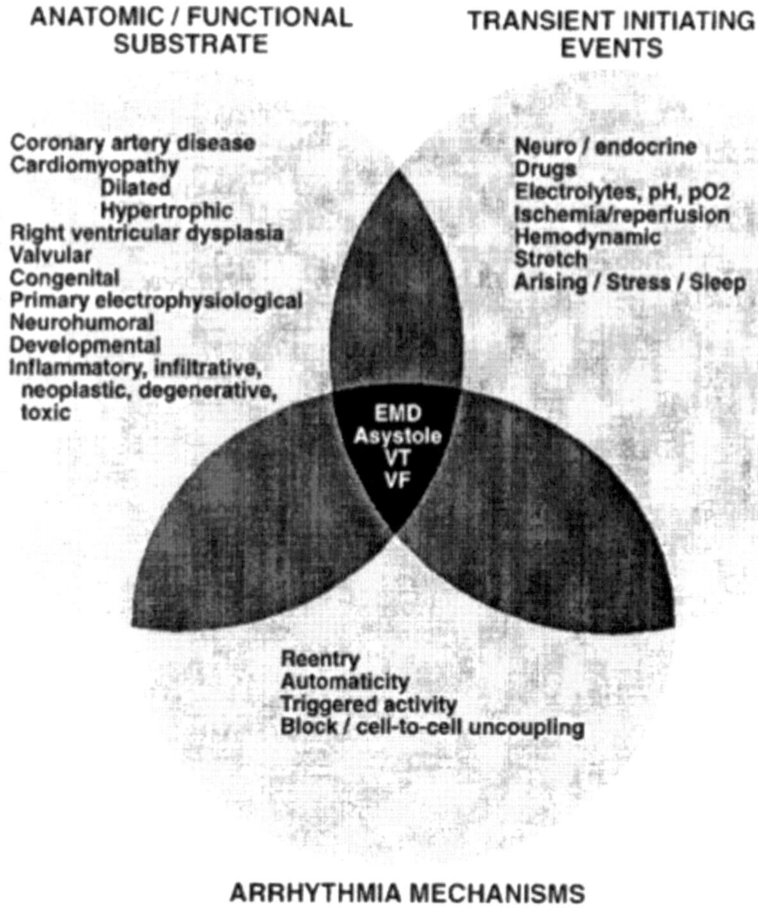

Figure 1. Venn diagram showing interaction of various anatomic/functional and transient factors that modulate potential arrhythmogenic mechanisms capable of causing sudden cardiac death (From Douglas P. Zipes and Hein J. J. Wellens "Sudden Cardiac Death" Circulation. 1998; 98:2334-2351, With Permission)

2.2. Effect of β-blockers on sudden cardiac death prevention in post myocardial infarction patients

β-blockers therapy has been studied in the post myocardial infarction (MI) patients since 1965 when propranolol was found to reduce mortality after acute MI[13]. Pivotal trials such as the *Norwegian Multicenter Study Group* (utilizing Timolol at a starting dose of 5 mgs/day with target of 20 mgs/day), *β-blocker Heart Attack Trial* (*BHAT*, utilizing propranolol at a dose of 180 to 240 mgs/day) in the 1980s showed reduction in total mortality and sudden cardiac death [14, 15]. As therapies post- MI evolved and ACE-I inhibitors were introduced several other trials, including the *Survival and Ventricular Enlargement (SAVE)* and *Acute Infarction Ramipril Efficacy (AIRE)* trials demonstrated that β-blockers provided additional reduction in cardiovascular mortality independent of the use of ACE-I inhibitors[16, 17].

A meta-analysis evaluated several randomized clinical trials looking at the benefits of β-blockers treatment post MI. This analysis revealed a significant reduction in mortality with β-blocker therapy (HR= 0.77, 95% confidence interval: 0.69 to 0.85)[18]. Secondary to lack of physician prescription of β-blocker therapy despite evidence of its benefit the Cooperative Cardiovascular Project was undertaken. This was an observational report that evaluated the care of 200,000 Medicare patients with the diagnosis of MI. Only 34% of the patients were given β-blockers. The mortality reduction for patients who were prescribed beta- blockers at the time of discharge from the hospital was 40% [19].

A sub-analysis of *BHAT* trial showed that propranolol decreased mortality and sudden cardiac death in the subset of patients with depressed LVEF [20]. But it was not until the *Carvedilol Post-Infarct Survival Control in Left Ventricular Dysfunction trial (CAPRICORN)* was a focus also placed on AMI patient with left ventricular (LV) dysfunction. *CAPRICORN* was a multinational prospective, randomized trial recruiting patients with recent acute MI (3-21 days) and left ventricular (LV) dysfunction with ejection fraction (EF) ≤ 40%. A total of 984 patients were placed on placebo and 975 patients were allocated to Carvedilol therapy post MI with an average follow up of 1.3 years. The initial starting dose was 6.25 mgs orally twice daily with target dose of 25 mgs orally twice daily. All-cause mortality was lower in the carvedilol group than in the placebo group (Hazard Ratio of 0.77, 95% CI of 0.60—0.98, p=0.03) [21]. Several secondary prevention trials had demonstrated significant reductions in ventricular arrhythmias but it was not until *CAPRICORN* that patients with substantial left ventricular dysfunction also demonstrated a significant reduction in malignant ventricular arrhythmias (HR of 0.37 (95% CI 0.24 to 0.58; p < 0.0001)[22]. It is important to emphasise that in this trial that 98% of the patients were treated with an ACE-I inhibitor. The effect of ACE-I inhibitors on reduction of ventricular arrhythmias will be discussed in a later section.

2.3. Effect of β-blockers on sudden cardiac death prevention in patients with congestive heart failure

β-blockers were initially thought to be contra-indicated in patients with heart failure due to their negative inotropic effects in the short term. However, later studies showed they consistently improve morbidity and mortality in patients with heart failure; they also lead to a 40% reduction in hospitalization. Currently, there are 3 medications available in the United States that have shown mortality benefits in patients with heart failure. Carvedilol is a non-selective β_1, $\beta_2$and α_1 blocker that was tested in two trials and was shown to improve mortality. The first is the *US Carvedilol trial* which enrolled 1094 patients with congestive heart failure (CHF) and left ventricular ejection fraction (LVEF) of ≤ 35%. Patients were assigned to four treatment protocols based on exercise capacity. Within each protocol patients were assigned to either placebo (n=398) or Carvedilol (n=696). Although this trial was not designed as mortality trial, itdemonstrated a 65% decrease in the risk of death with Carvedilol compared to placebo (p<0.001). Sudden death was reduced from 3.8% in the placebo group to 1.7% in the Carvedilol group [23].

The Carvedilol Prospective Randomized Cumulative Survival (COPERNICUS) trial examined the effect of Carvedilol in 2289 patients with severe CHF, defined as dyspnea at rest and LVEF ≤ 25%. This trial validated the mortality benefit of Carvedilol in patients with severe heart failure with a 50% reduction in all-cause mortality (HR 0.50, 95% CI of 0.10-0.63) [24]. Unfortunately this trial did not have data available on the impact of Carvedilol on sudden death.

The Cardiac Insufficiency Bisoprolol Study (CIBIS) II was a multicenter, double-blind, randomized, placebo-controlled trial that evaluated the efficacy of Bisoprolol in reducing the incidence of all-cause mortality in heart failure. Bisoprolol is a $\beta_1$receptor blocker, and the target dose was 10 mgs daily. All patients enrolled received standard therapy with diuretics and ACE-I inhibitors. A total of2647 patients with New York Heart Association (NYHA) class III or IV with LVEF of ≤ 35% were randomized to either Bisoprolol (n=1327) or placebo (n=1320). This study was stopped prematurely because Bisoprolol showed a significant mortality benefit. Death from any cause in the Bisoprolol group was 11.8% versus 17.3% in the placebo group (HR, 0.66, 95% CI, 0.54-0.80). Sudden death was also reduced in the Bisoprolol group by 42% compared to the placebo group [25].

The Metoprolol CR/XL Randomized Intervention Trial in CHF (MERIT-HF) was a double-blind randomized controlled study which included 3991 patients with CHF, NYHA class II-IV with an LVEF of ≤40%. These patients were stable on optimal medical therapy. This trial evaluated whether controlled release/extended release formulation of Metoprolol taken daily would reduce mortality in this patient population. The starting dose was 12.5 mgs once daily with target dose of 200 mgs orally once daily. Patients were randomized to Metoprolol CR/XL (n=1990) up-titrated to 200 mg daily over and eight week period of time or placebo (n=2001). The trial demonstrated a 34% relative risk reduction in all-cause mortality with controlled release/extended release formulation of Metoprolol. Similar, to CIBIS II, MERIT–HF showed a 41% relative risk reduction of sudden death [26].

2.4. Effect of β-blockers on sudden cardiac death prevention in patients who survived a cardiac arrest

In patients who have implantable cardioverter defibrillators (ICDs), β-blockers have been shown to decrease the frequency of ICD shocks [27]. In an analysis of the Antiarrhythmics Versus Implantable Defibrillators Registry (*AVID registry*), β-blockers therapy was associated with lower mortality in patients with sustained ventricular tachycardia [28]. β-Blockers increase the time to first ICD shock in patients implanted for secondary prevention of sudden death[29].

Furthermore, the higher the dose of β-blockers used, the less patients experience VT and the more likely the therapies are successful. In a study of 282 patients with left ventricular dysfunction (EF < 50%) with standard indications for ICD without cardiac resynchronization therapy, the higher the dose of β-blockers

3. Renin-Angiotensin-aldosterone system and sudden cardiac death prevention

3.1. Potential mechanisms of Renin-Angiotensin-aldosterone system inhibitors/blockers on sudden cardiac death prevention

The Renin-Angiotensin-aldosterone system (RAAS) is activated during many disease states, but especially during myocardial ischemia and heart failure. Renin activates the angiotensin converting enzyme, which converts Angtiotensin I to Angiotensin II. Angiotensin II is a potent vasoconstrictor; it activates fibroblasts promoting interstitial fibrosis and scar formation. Furthermore, Angiotensin II also activates the secretion of Aldosterone and Norepinephrine. All of these factors also increase after-load, which increases myocardial oxygen demand. At the cellular level, angiotensin II decreases the effective refractory period of the cardiac myocyte and enhances conduction [30].Furthermore, Aldosterone promotes sodium retention, increases potassium secretion in the urine and activates fibroblasts leading to myocardial and vascular fibrosis. This promotes remodeling, LV dilatation and creates the substrate for reentry [31]. ACE-I inhibitors decrease preload and after-load, which decreases myocardial oxygen demand and LV end diastolic pressure. They also block Angiotensin II production and inhibit the breakdown of bradykinin [23]. Blocking angiotensin II prevents the progression of ventricular remodeling, reduces ventricular dilatation and fibrosis. ACE-I inhibitors result in a reduction in potassium depletion and have several effects on the autonomic nervous system via enhanced baroreflex sensitivity and hemodynamics which can lead to reduced sympathetic and parasympathetic tone and circulating catecholamines. Angiotensin II could persist despite treatment with ACE-I inhibitors since it can be formulated by non-ACE-I-dependent pathways. ARBs can also block the angiotensin II receptor without an increase in bradykinin levels [32].

Even with the utilization of ACE-I inhibitors or Angiotensin-Receptor blockers (ARBs) there is not full suppression of Aldosterone synthesis. Aldosterone receptor blockers prevent sudden cardiac death by controlling potassium loss, blocking aldosterone effect on the formation of collagen and by increasing the myocardial uptake of norepinephrine, which decreases sympathetic activation [32, 33]. Myocardial fibrosis may increase the risk of ventricular arrhythmias by causing variations in the ventricular conduction times. Spirinolactone decreases the level of serum markers of collagen synthesis at 6 months, which correlates with survival benefit [33].

3.2. Effect of ACE-I on sudden cardiac death prevention in post myocardial infarction patients and in patients with heart failure

Three post myocardial infarction trials; Survival and Ventricular Enlargement (SAVE), Trandolapril Cardiac Evaluation (TRACE-I) and Acute Infarction Ramipril Efficacy (AIRE) specifically investigated the impact of ACE-I inhibitors on mortality and morbidity in post MI patients who have LV dysfunction.

Survival and Ventricular Enlargement (SAVE) was a randomized double-blind placebo controlled trial that evaluated the use of captopril (n=1115) versus placebo (n= 1116) in post MI patients with LVEF ≤ 40%. Randomization was done 3-16 days post MI. During an average of 42 months, there was an 18% RRR in all-cause mortality with captopril compared to placebo. However, there was a non-significant trend towards lower SCD in patients taking captopril (odds ratio 0.83, 95% CI 0.63-1.8)[34].

Trandolapril Cardiac Evaluation (TRACE-I) was designed to examine whether patients with a recent MI and LV dysfunction would benefit from long term ACE-I inhibitor therapy. A total of 1749 patients 3-7 days post MI with echocardiographic evidence of LV dysfunction (EF≤ 35%) were randomized to Trandolapril (n=876) or placebo (n=873). During follow up the relative risk for death from any cause in the Trandolapril group versus the placebo group was 0.78 (95 percent confidence interval, 0.67 to 0.91). The Trandolapril group also showed a significant reduction in sudden death versus the placebo group (HR 0.76, 95% CI 0.59-.98, p=0.03) [35]. TRACE-I was the first placebo-controlled trial to show a significant reduction in sudden death with the use of the ACE-I inhibitors.

The Acute Infarction Ramipril Efficacy (AIRE) Trial once again looked at the use of ACE-I inhibitors in the post MI patient who had clinical or radiological evidence of congestive heart failure (CHF) to receive Ramipril (n=1014) versus placebo (n=992). After 15 months of follow up,there was a 27% reduction in the risk of death with Ramipril compared to placebo. In this study Ramipril also reduced the risk for sudden death by approximately 30% compared to placebo (p=0.011)[36].

A further Meta-analysis looked at 15 trials including SAVE, TRACE-I and AIRE to evaluate the effect of ACE-I inhibitors on sudden death post MI. This meta-analysis revealed a significant reduction in the risk for sudden death an odds ratio of 0.80 (95% CI 0.70-0.92)[37].

Currently only three trials have reported results for sudden cardiac death in heart failure patients taking ACE-I. *The Cooperative North Scandinavian Enalapril Survival (CONSENSUS)* Study was designed to evaluate the effect of Enalapril compared to placebo on mortality in patients with severe heart failure (class IV). This study randomized 253 patients to either Enalapril (n=127) or placebo (n=126) in addition to conventional therapy. CONSENSUS showed a 40% reduction in mortality after 6 months of treatment and a 27% reduction at the end of the study. The greatest reduction in mortality was in death caused by progression of pump failure[38].

*The Studies of Left Ventricular Dysfunction (SOLVD)-Prevention trial*was designed to determine whether and ACE-I inhibitor, Enalapril, could reduce mortality, the incidence of heart failure and the rate of hospitalizations in patients with EF ≤ 35% with mild to moderate heart failure (class II or III). Following randomization, patients received double-blind treatment with either placebo (n=1284) or Enalapril (n=1285). There was noted a reduction in mortality due to progression of heart failure with a risk reduction of 16% but no clear reduction in sudden cardiac death was noted[39].

The V-HeFT-II trial was the first trial to suggest an effect of ACE-I inhibitors on sudden death in patients with heart failure. This trial compared the effects of Enalapril with hydralazine and isosorbide dinitrate on mortality in patients with NYHA class II-III. After randomization, double blind treatment was instituted with Enalapril (n= 403) versus hydralazine/isosorbide dinitrate (n=401). Interestingly the mortality curves of the treatment arms separate early after randomization. There was a 28% relative risk reduction with Enalapril compared to hydralazine and isosorbide dinitrate (p=0.16).The overall reduction in mortality associated with Enalapril was due to a reduction in the incidence of sudden death [40].

3.3. Effect of Angiotensin-Receptor Blockers (ARBs) on sudden cardiac death prevention in patients with congestive heart failure

The Evaluation of Losartan in the Elderly Study (ELITE) is the only ARB trial to demonstrate a reduction in sudden death. This prospective, double-blind, randomized, parallel group controlled clinical trial compared the safety and efficacy in the treatment of CHF with the use of Losartan vs Captopril. Patients were randomly assigned to losartan (n=352) versus captopril (n=370). Follow up at 48 weeks showed a 45% reduction in all-cause mortality with a relative risk reduction of 36% in the incidence of sudden cardiac death [41].

ELITE II was designed to compare the effects of losartan and captopril on all-cause mortality and sudden death or resuscitated cardiac arrest. Similar to ELITE patients were randomly assigned to losartan (n=1578) or captopril (n=1574). After 1.5 years of follow there was no statistically difference in all-cause mortality, sudden death or resuscitated cardiac arrest (losartan 9% versus captopril 7.3%, p= 0.08) between the two groups[42].

3.4. Effect of Aldosterone antagonists on sudden cardiac death prevention in post MI patients and in patients with congestive heart failure

The Randomized Aldactone Evaluation Study (RALES) was a randomized double-blind placebo controlled trial. This trial hypothesized that daily treatment with Spirinolactone would reduce the risk of death from all causes among patients who had severe heart failure. Patients enrolled had class III or IV heart failure and were being treated with an ACE-I inhibitor, loop diuretic and had an EF $\leq$ 35%. They were randomly assigned to either Spirinolactone (n=822) or placebo (n=841). This trial was ended prematurely when analysis found that Spirinolactone demonstrated a 31% reduction in cardiac death. This reduction was due to a 36% in death related to progressive heart failure and a 29% reduction in sudden cardiac death [43].

The Eplerone Post Myocardial Heart Failure Efficacy and Survival Study (EPHESUS) was conducted to evaluate the effect of aldosterone blocker, Eplerenone on morbidity and mortality among patients with acute myocardial infarction complicated by left ventricular dysfunction and heart failure. In this double-blind, placebo-controlled study patients were randomly assigned to Eplerenone (n=3313) versus placebo (n=3319) in addition to optimal medical therapy. Eplerenone demonstrated a reduction in death from cardiovascular causes or hospitalization for cardiovascular events (relative risk, 0.83; 95% CI, 0.72-0.94; p=0.005). There was also a reduction in sudden death from cardiac causes (relative risk, 0.79; 95% CI 0.64-0.97; p=0.03) [44].

http://dx.doi.org/10.5772/55008

4. Statins (3 hydroxy-3-methylglutaryl coenzyme-A reductase inhibitors) and sudden cardiac death prevention

4.1. Potential mechanisms of 3 hydroxy-3-methylglutaryl coenzyme A reductase inhibitors on sudden cardiac death prevention

Statins (3 Hydroxy-3-Methylglutaryl Coenzyme-A Reductase inhibitors) have been shown to decrease cardiovascular morbidity and mortality in both primary and secondary prevention trials. Statins are known to stabilize the plaque and to even promote plaque regression[45].This stabilization improves myocardial perfusion, oxidative stress and reduces the risk of plaque rupture[46]. This leads to decreased ischemic events and arrhythmic events, since even small areas of ischemia can promote reentry, induce ventricular arrhythmias and lead to sudden cardiac death. Statins improve endothelial function by increasing nitric oxide production from endothelial cells and they reduce ischemia mediated oxidative stress and intracellular calcium overload [47, 48]. They also have anti-inflammatory actions and reduce C-reactive protein, and they decrease endothelin-1 secretion [49]. All these effects will decrease myocardial ischemia, limit myocardial injury and prevent myocyte hypertrophy [50, 51].

4.2. Effect of statin therapy on shock burden and sudden cardiac death in post MI patients and in patients with congestive heart failure

Statins are widely accepted as preventing coronary heart disease death and MI; however their effect on sudden cardiac death prevention is unclear.

Randomized trial in post myocardial infarction patients showed the benefits of statins on overall mortality but failed to show benefit on sudden cardiac death prevention [52-54]. However, observational data from hospitalized patients with myocardial infarction showed that early statin administration (within 24 hours) of an acute MI led to a decrease in the incidence of VT/VF [55].

Furthermore, statins appear to decrease appropriate shocks in patients who have ICDs whether or not they received them for primary or secondary prevention of sudden cardiac death. In a subanalysis of AVID trial, a secondary prevention trial which compared anti-arrhythmic drugs to ICDs in patients who survived a cardiac arrest, patients who received statins had a lower risk of ventricular arrhythmias compared to those who are not on statins [56]. This was also demonstrated in the Multicenter Automatic Defibrillator Implantation Trial-II (MADIT-II). Post hoc analysis of MADIT-II showed that patients receiving statin therapy > 90% of the time had a significantly reduced cumulative rate of ICD therapy for VT/VF or cardiac death[57].

Subsequently, an analysis of SCD-HeFT trial data was undertaken to evaluate the impact of statin use in heart failure. SCD-HeFT studied 2521 functional class II and III heart failure patients with left ventricular ejection fractions ≤ 35%. The cause of CHF was ischemic in 52% of the study patients. Statin use was reported in 965 (38%) of 2521 patients at baseline and 1187 (47%) at last follow-up with the median time to follow up of 45.5 months. This analysis revealed that mortality reduction related to statin therapy (HR= 0.70, 95% CI: 0.58-0.83] was identical in both ischemic and non-ischemic cardiomyopathy (HR 0.69 vs 0.67 respectively) [58].

5. Conclusions and future directions

Sudden cardiac death remains a challenge for health providers and policy makers. Whether more stringent guidelines for prevention and screening will be applied is balanced by the enormous costs. In order to identify the groups at risk for sudden cardiac death there must first be a standardization of the definition. The worldly variation in this definition of sudden cardiac death of 1 hour from onset of symptoms to 24 hours, not only effects epidemiological data but also alters clinical trial outcomes when evaluating the effectiveness of treatment options.

Currently, antiarrhythmic medications have failed to show any benefit of sudden cardiac death prevention, while traditional heart failure medications have been shown to decrease total mortality, sudden cardiac death and defibrillator shocks. They are only used in a small subset of patients that present in sudden cardiac death, since most of the patients who have sudden cardiac death have it as a first presentation and do not have congestive heart failure or history of coronary artery disease. This poses a diagnostic and therapeutic challenge for the clinician. Taking statins as an example, most of the primary prevention algorithms used to start lipid lowering agents usually leads to delayed intervention, especially since coronary atherosclerosis has been shown to start at a young age. The cost of starting this treatment is also enormous, especially if it is started on a global scale at a young age and it is not without side effects. Genetic studies to identify patients at risk for coronary atherosclerosis are still under development. Preventing sudden cardiac death is definitely a challenge for the 21st century clinician and might remain so for the near future.

Author details

Ann M. Anderson[1] and M. Obadah Al Chekakie[2]

1 Cheyenne Regional Medical Center, Cheyenne, WY, USA

2 University of Colorado, Cheyenne Regional Medical Center, Cheyenne, Wyoming,, USA

References

[1] Zipes DP, Camm AJ, Borggrefe M, Buxton AE, Chaitman B, Fromer M, et al. ACC/AHA/ESC 2006 guidelines for management of patients with ventricular arrhythmias and the prevention of sudden cardiac death: a report of the American College of Cardiology/American Heart Association Task Force and the European Society of Cardiology Committee for Practice Guidelines (Writing Committee to Develop Guidelines for Management of Patients With Ventricular Arrhythmias and the Prevention of Sudden Cardiac Death). J Am Coll Cardiol. 2006;48(5):e247-346.

[2] Bardy GH, Lee KL, Mark DB, Poole JE, Packer DL, Boineau R, et al. Amiodarone or an implantable cardioverter-defibrillator for congestive heart failure. N Engl J Med. 2005;352(3):225-237.

[3] Cabassi A, Vinci S, Calzolari M, Bruschi G, Borghetti A. Regional sympathetic activity in pre-hypertensive phase of spontaneously hypertensive rats. Life Sci. 1998;62(12):1111-1118.

[4] Huikuri HV, Castellanos A, Myerburg RJ. Sudden death due to cardiac arrhythmias. N Engl J Med. 2001;345(20):1473-1482.

[5] Mann DL. Basic mechanisms of disease progression in the failing heart: the role of excessive adrenergic drive. Prog Cardiovasc Dis. 1998;41(1 Suppl 1):1-8.

[6] Chidsey CA, Sonnenblick EH, Morrow AG, Braunwald E. Norepinephrine stores and contractile force of papillary muscle from the failing human heart. Circulation. 1966;33(1):43-51.

[7] Hasegawa K, Iwai-Kanai E, Sasayama S. Neurohormonal regulation of myocardial cell apoptosis during the development of heart failure. J Cell Physiol. 2001;186(1): 11-18.

[8] Francis GS, Benedict C, Johnstone DE, Kirlin PC, Nicklas J, Liang CS, et al. Comparison of neuroendocrine activation in patients with left ventricular dysfunction with and without congestive heart failure. A substudy of the Studies of Left Ventricular Dysfunction (SOLVD). Circulation. 1990;82(5):1724-1729.

[9] Gorre F, Vandekerckhove H. Beta-blockers: focus on mechanism of action. Which beta-blocker, when and why? Acta Cardiol.65(5):565-570.

[10] Swedberg K, Viquerat C, Rouleau JL, Roizen M, Atherton B, Parmley WW, et al. Comparison of myocardial catecholamine balance in chronic congestive heart failure and in angina pectoris without failure. Am J Cardiol. 1984;54(7):783-786.

[11] Gilbert EM, Abraham WT, Olsen S, Hattler B, White M, Mealy P, et al. Comparative hemodynamic, left ventricular functional, and antiadrenergic effects of chronic treatment with metoprolol versus carvedilol in the failing heart. Circulation. 1996;94(11): 2817-2825.

[12] Jimenez-Candil J, Hernandez J, Martin A, Ruiz-Olgado M, Herrero J, Ledesma C, et al. Influence of beta-blocker therapy on antitachycardia pacing effectiveness for monomorphic ventricular tachycardias occurring in implantable cardioverter-defibrillator patients: a dose-dependent effect. Europace.12(9):1231-1238.

[13] Snow PJ. Effect of propranolol in myocardial infarction. Lancet. 1965;2(7412):551-553.

[14] Timolol-induced reduction in mortality and reinfarction in patients surviving acute myocardial infarction. N Engl J Med. 1981;304(14):801-807.

[15] A randomized trial of propranolol in patients with acute myocardial infarction. II. Morbidity results. JAMA. 1983;250(20):2814-2819.

[16] Vantrimpont P, Rouleau JL, Wun CC, Ciampi A, Klein M, Sussex B, et al. Additive beneficial effects of beta-blockers to angiotensin-converting enzyme inhibitors in the Survival and Ventricular Enlargement (SAVE) Study. SAVE Investigators. J Am Coll Cardiol. 1997;29(2):229-236.

[17] Spargias KS, Hall AS, Greenwood DC, Ball SG. beta blocker treatment and other prognostic variables in patients with clinical evidence of heart failure after acute myocardial infarction: evidence from the AIRE study. Heart. 1999;81(1):25-32.

[18] Freemantle N, Cleland J, Young P, Mason J, Harrison J. beta Blockade after myocardial infarction: systematic review and meta regression analysis. BMJ. 1999;318(7200): 1730-1737.

[19] Gottlieb SS, McCarter RJ, Vogel RA. Effect of beta-blockade on mortality among high-risk and low-risk patients after myocardial infarction. N Engl J Med. 1998;339(8):489-497.

[20] Chadda K, Goldstein S, Byington R, Curb JD. Effect of propranolol after acute myocardial infarction in patients with congestive heart failure. Circulation. 1986;73(3): 503-510.

[21] Dargie HJ. Effect of carvedilol on outcome after myocardial infarction in patients with left-ventricular dysfunction: the CAPRICORN randomised trial. Lancet. 2001;357(9266):1385-1390.

[22] McMurray J, Kober L, Robertson M, Dargie H, Colucci W, Lopez-Sendon J, et al. Antiarrhythmic effect of carvedilol after acute myocardial infarction: results of the Carvedilol Post-Infarct Survival Control in Left Ventricular Dysfunction (CAPRICORN) trial. J Am Coll Cardiol. 2005;45(4):525-530.

[23] Packer M, Bristow MR, Cohn JN, Colucci WS, Fowler MB, Gilbert EM, et al. The effect of carvedilol on morbidity and mortality in patients with chronic heart failure. U.S. Carvedilol Heart Failure Study Group. N Engl J Med. 1996;334(21):1349-1355.

[24] Packer M, Coats AJ, Fowler MB, Katus HA, Krum H, Mohacsi P, et al. Effect of carvedilol on survival in severe chronic heart failure. N Engl J Med. 2001;344(22): 1651-1658.

[25] The Cardiac Insufficiency Bisoprolol Study II (CIBIS-II): a randomised trial. Lancet. 1999;353(9146):9-13.

[26] Hjalmarson A, Goldstein S, Fagerberg B, Wedel H, Waagstein F, Kjekshus J, et al. Effects of controlled-release metoprolol on total mortality, hospitalizations, and well-being in patients with heart failure: the Metoprolol CR/XL Randomized Intervention Trial in congestive heart failure (MERIT-HF). MERIT-HF Study Group. JAMA. 2000;283(10):1295-1302.

[27] Seidl K, Hauer B, Schwick NG, Zahn R, Senges J. Comparison of metoprolol and sotalol in preventing ventricular tachyarrhythmias after the implantation of a cardioverter/defibrillator. Am J Cardiol. 1998;82(6):744-748.

[28] Anderson JL, Hallstrom AP, Epstein AE, Pinski SL, Rosenberg Y, Nora MO, et al. Design and results of the antiarrhythmics vs implantable defibrillators (AVID) registry. The AVID Investigators. Circulation. 1999;99(13):1692-1699.

[29] Hreybe H, Bedi M, Ezzeddine R, Barrington W, Jain S, Ngwu O, et al. Indications for internal cardioverter defibrillator implantation predict time to first shock and the modulating effect of beta-blockers. Am Heart J. 2005;150(5):1064.

[30] Schrier RW, Abraham WT. Hormones and hemodynamics in heart failure. N Engl J Med. 1999;341(8):577-585.

[31] Zannad F, Dousset B, Alla F. Treatment of congestive heart failure: interfering the aldosterone-cardiac extracellular matrix relationship. Hypertension. 2001;38(5): 1227-1232.

[32] Minisi AJ, Thames MD. Distribution of left ventricular sympathetic afferents demonstrated by reflex responses to transmural myocardial ischemia and to intracoronary and epicardial bradykinin. Circulation. 1993;87(1):240-246.

[33] Zannad F, Alla F, Dousset B, Perez A, Pitt B. Limitation of excessive extracellular matrix turnover may contribute to survival benefit of spironolactone therapy in patients with congestive heart failure: insights from the randomized aldactone evaluation study (RALES). Rales Investigators. Circulation. 2000;102(22):2700-2706.

[34] Rutherford JD, Pfeffer MA, Moye LA, Davis BR, Flaker GC, Kowey PR, et al. Effects of captopril on ischemic events after myocardial infarction. Results of the Survival and Ventricular Enlargement trial. SAVE Investigators. Circulation. 1994;90(4): 1731-1738.

[35] Kober L, Torp-Pedersen C, Carlsen JE, Bagger H, Eliasen P, Lyngborg K, et al. A clinical trial of the angiotensin-converting-enzyme inhibitor trandolapril in patients with left ventricular dysfunction after myocardial infarction. Trandolapril Cardiac Evaluation (TRACE) Study Group. N Engl J Med. 1995;333(25):1670-1676.

[36] Cleland JG, Erhardt L, Murray G, Hall AS, Ball SG. Effect of ramipril on morbidity and mode of death among survivors of acute myocardial infarction with clinical evidence of heart failure. A report from the AIRE Study Investigators. Eur Heart J. 1997;18(1):41-51.

[37] Domanski MJ, Exner DV, Borkowf CB, Geller NL, Rosenberg Y, Pfeffer MA. Effect of angiotensin converting enzyme inhibition on sudden cardiac death in patients following acute myocardial infarction. A meta-analysis of randomized clinical trials. J Am Coll Cardiol. 1999;33(3):598-604.

[38] Effects of enalapril on mortality in severe congestive heart failure. Results of the Cooperative North Scandinavian Enalapril Survival Study (CONSENSUS). The CONSENSUS Trial Study Group. N Engl J Med. 1987;316(23):1429-1435.

[39] Effect of enalapril on mortality and the development of heart failure in asymptomatic patients with reduced left ventricular ejection fractions. The SOLVD Investigattors. N Engl J Med. 1992;327(10):685-691.

[40] Cohn JN, Johnson G, Ziesche S, Cobb F, Francis G, Tristani F, et al. A comparison of enalapril with hydralazine-isosorbide dinitrate in the treatment of chronic congestive heart failure. N Engl J Med. 1991;325(5):303-310.

[41] Pitt B, Segal R, Martinez FA, Meurers G, Cowley AJ, Thomas I, et al. Randomised trial of losartan versus captopril in patients over 65 with heart failure (Evaluation of Losartan in the Elderly Study, ELITE). Lancet. 1997;349(9054):747-752.

[42] Pitt B, Poole-Wilson PA, Segal R, Martinez FA, Dickstein K, Camm AJ, et al. Effect of losartan compared with captopril on mortality in patients with symptomatic heart failure: randomised trial--the Losartan Heart Failure Survival Study ELITE II. Lancet. 2000;355(9215):1582-1587.

[43] Pitt B, Zannad F, Remme WJ, Cody R, Castaigne A, Perez A, et al. The effect of spironolactone on morbidity and mortality in patients with severe heart failure. Randomized Aldactone Evaluation Study Investigators. N Engl J Med. 1999;341(10):709-717.

[44] Pitt B, Remme W, Zannad F, Neaton J, Martinez F, Roniker B, et al. Eplerenone, a selective aldosterone blocker, in patients with left ventricular dysfunction after myocardial infarction. N Engl J Med. 2003;348(14):1309-1321.

[45] Nissen SE, Nicholls SJ, Sipahi I, Libby P, Raichlen JS, Ballantyne CM, et al. Effect of very high-intensity statin therapy on regression of coronary atherosclerosis: the ASTEROID trial. JAMA. 2006;295(13):1556-1565.

[46] Cascio WE. Myocardial ischemia: what factors determine arrhythmogenesis? J Cardiovasc Electrophysiol. 2001;12(6):726-729.

[47] Laufs U, La Fata V, Plutzky J, Liao JK. Upregulation of endothelial nitric oxide synthase by HMG CoA reductase inhibitors. Circulation. 1998;97(12):1129-1135.

[48] Rikitake Y, Kawashima S, Takeshita S, Yamashita T, Azumi H, Yasuhara M, et al. Anti-oxidative properties of fluvastatin, an HMG-CoA reductase inhibitor, contribute to prevention of atherosclerosis in cholesterol-fed rabbits. Atherosclerosis. 2001;154(1): 87-96.

[49] Ridker PM, Rifai N, Pfeffer MA, Sacks FM, Moye LA, Goldman S, et al. Inflammation, pravastatin, and the risk of coronary events after myocardial infarction in patients with average cholesterol levels. Cholesterol and Recurrent Events (CARE) Investigators. Circulation. 1998;98(9):839-844.

[50] Weber KT, Anversa P, Armstrong PW, Brilla CG, Burnett JC, Jr., Cruickshank JM, et al. Remodeling and reparation of the cardiovascular system. J Am Coll Cardiol. 1992;20(1):3-16.

[51] Lee TM, Chou TF, Tsai CH. Effects of pravastatin on cardiomyocyte hypertrophy and ventricular vulnerability in normolipidemic rats after myocardial infarction. J Mol Cell Cardiol. 2003;35(12):1449-1459.

[52] Randomised trial of cholesterol lowering in 4444 patients with coronary heart disease: the Scandinavian Simvastatin Survival Study (4S). Lancet. 1994;344(8934): 1383-1389.

[53] Pedersen TR, Faergeman O, Kastelein JJ, Olsson AG, Tikkanen MJ, Holme I, et al. High-dose atorvastatin vs usual-dose simvastatin for secondary prevention after myocardial infarction: the IDEAL study: a randomized controlled trial. JAMA. 2005;294(19):2437-2445.

[54] LaRosa JC, Grundy SM, Waters DD, Shear C, Barter P, Fruchart JC, et al. Intensive lipid lowering with atorvastatin in patients with stable coronary disease. N Engl J Med. 2005;352(14):1425-1435.

[55] Fonarow GC, Wright RS, Spencer FA, Fredrick PD, Dong W, Every N, et al. Effect of statin use within the first 24 hours of admission for acute myocardial infarction on early morbidity and mortality. Am J Cardiol. 2005;96(5):611-616.

[56] Mitchell LB, Powell JL, Gillis AM, Kehl V, Hallstrom AP. Are lipid-lowering drugs also antiarrhythmic drugs? An analysis of the Antiarrhythmics versus Implantable Defibrillators (AVID) trial. J Am Coll Cardiol. 2003;42(1):81-87.

[57] Vyas AK, Guo H, Moss AJ, Olshansky B, McNitt SA, Hall WJ, et al. Reduction in ventricular tachyarrhythmias with statins in the Multicenter Automatic Defibrillator Implantation Trial (MADIT)-II. J Am Coll Cardiol. 2006;47(4):769-773.

[58] Dickinson MG, Ip JH, Olshansky B, Hellkamp AS, Anderson J, Poole JE, et al. Statin use was associated with reduced mortality in both ischemic and nonischemic cardiomyopathy and in patients with implantable defibrillators: mortality data and mechanistic insights from the Sudden Cardiac Death in Heart Failure Trial (SCD-HeFT). Am Heart J. 2007;153(4):573-578.

Chapter 11

Risk Stratification of Sudden Cardiac Death by Evaluating Myocardial Sympathetic Nerve Activity Using Iodine-123 Metaiodobenzylguanidine Scintigraphy in Patients with Chronic Heart Failure and Dilated Cardiomyopathy

Yoshikazu Yazaki, Toshimasa Seki, Atsushi Izawa,
Minoru Hongo and Uichi Ikeda

Additional information is available at the end of the chapter

http://dx.doi.org/10.5772/55615

1. Introduction

A Sudden Cardiac Death in Heart Failure Trial (SCD-HeFT) has proven the efficacy of prophylactic implantable cardioverter defibrillator (ICD) use for chronic heart failure patients without sustained ventricular tachycardia (SVT) and a history of ventricular fibrillation, not restricted in those with myocardial infarction [1]. Since ICD is an expensive device, risk stratification is required to identify heart failure patients at high risk for sudden death without SVT.

Iodine-123 Metaiodobenzylguanidine (^{123}I-MIBG) is an analogue that metabolizes in a manner similar to that of norepinephrine (NE) [2]. ^{123}I-MIBG is used to assess myocardial sympathetic nervous activity, and a decrease in myocardial ^{123}I-MIBG uptake and an increase in spillover have been observed in patients with heart failure and are related to disease severity [3-5]. An increase in sympathetic tone is associated with ventricular tachyarrhythmia and sudden cardiac death [6, 7].

Therefore, the purpose of this study was to test our hypothesis that ^{123}I-MIBG scintigraphy may be useful in the prediction of future sudden death in heart failure patients without SVT and a history of ventricular fibrillation.

2. Methods

2.1. Patients

We retrospectively examined 120 consecutive heart failure patients with a left ventricular ejection fraction (LVEF) of less than 50 % who underwent ^{123}I-MIBG scintigraphy between April 1998 and December 2004. There were 84 men and 36 women with a mean age of 57±14 years ranging from 22 to 95 years. New York Heart Association (NYHA) functional class assessment at the time of the scintigraphy showed 23 patients in class I, 66 in class II and 31 in class III. All patients underwent cross sectional and M-mode echocardiography as well as coronary angiography. The study population included non-ischemic dilated cardiomyopathy in 73 patients, ischemic cardiomyopathy in 21 and others in 26 which systolic dysfunction might be caused by valvular diseases, hypertension and/or congenital heart disease. All patients showed stable clinical condition for at least 3 months on conventional medications with angiotensin-converting enzyme inhibitor and diuretics. Fifty-nine patients were on β–blocker drugs.

2.2. ^{123}I-MIBG data acquisition

^{123}I-MIBG is an analogue of guanethidine that is metabolized in a qualitatively similar manner to norepinephrine at the synaptic nerve terminal. After ^{123}I-MIBG uptakes through the uptake-1 mechanism and storages in the synaptic nerve ending, it releases according to the sympathetic activity. Since the myocardium of patients with chronic heart failure is characterized by a significant reduction of pre-synaptic norepinephrine uptake and post-synaptic beta-adrenoreceptor density, uptake-1 function and beta–receptor downregulation can be evaluated by ^{123}I-MIBG imaging [8]. Under resting and fasting condition, patients were injected intravenously with 111MBq of commercially available ^{123}I-MIBG (Daiichi Radioisotopes Labs, Tokyo, Japan). Anterior planar images were acquired 15 minutes and 3 hours after the injection and stored in a 64 x 64 matrix by means of a scintillation camera (model ZLC 7500; Siemens, Solana, Sweden) equipped with a long-energy, general purpose collimator interfaced to a minicomputer (SCINTIPAC 7000; Shimazu, Kyoto, Japan), with a 20% window centered on the 159keV photopeak of Iodine-123. Regions of interest (ROI) were manually drawn over the heart and upper mediastinum by a nuclear cardiologist without knowledge of the patient's data (Figure 1). The total number of counts of each ROI was determined, and a geometric mean was calculated as counts per pixel. We determined the heart to mediastinum activity ratio (H/M) for all early and delayed images. ^{123}I-MIBG washout rate from the heart was calculated from the difference between early and delayed images according to the formula shown in figure 1.

Demonstrable two cases are shown in figure 1. A case with NYHA class III shows lower H/M ratio and higher washout rate as compared to a case with NYHA class I.

2.3. Follow-up information and end-point

Medical records of all patients were carefully reviewed. The primary end-point of this study was the occurrence of cardiac death including death due to congestive heart failure and sudden

http://dx.doi.org/10.5772/55615

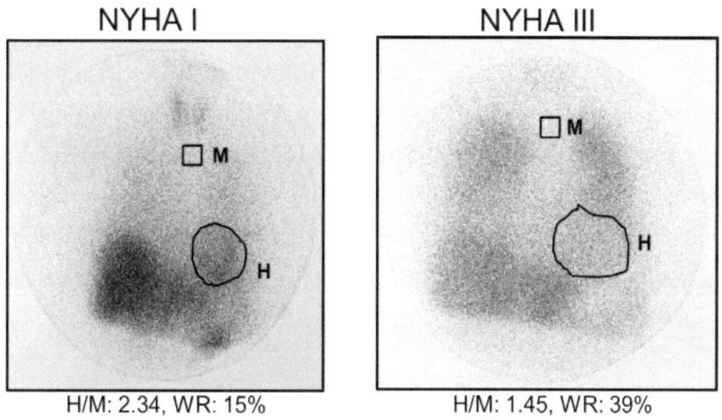

$$\underline{\text{Washout Rate}} = \frac{\text{Early}\,(H - M) - \text{Delayed}\,(H - M)}{\text{Early}\,(H - M)} \times 100$$

H: heart; M:mediastinum; H/M: heart to mediastinum activity ratio; 123I-MIBG: Iodine-123 Metaiodobenzylguanidine; NYHA: New York Heart Association.

Figure 1. ^{123}I-MIBG imaging. (A) A case of NYHA functional class I status. (B) A case of NYHA functional class III status.

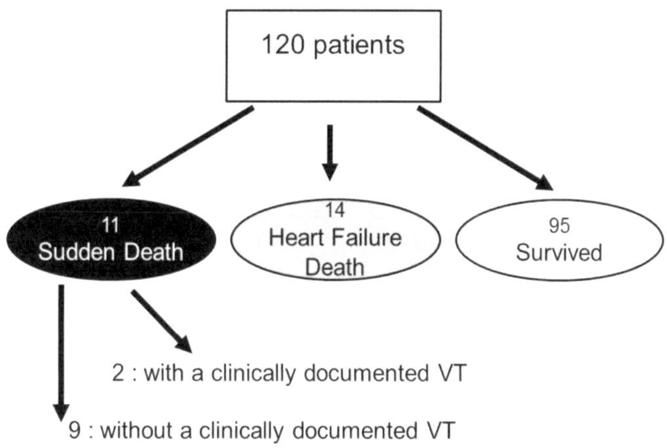

VT: ventricular tachycardia

Figure 2. Clinical course of all patients.

cardiac death. Sudden cardiac death was defined as death within 1 hour after the acute onset of symptom, death during sleep or unwitnessed death. Clinical course of the 120 patients are summarized in figure 2. During a mean follow-up of 57±24 months, 14 patients died of refractory heart failure and 11 died suddenly including 9 without clinical VT. Echocardiagraphic and hemodynamic variables ware compared among the three groups. Plasma norepinephrin concentration of 40 patients and brain natriuretic polypeptide (BNP) of 64 patients were measured close to the time of scintigraphic examination.

2.4. Statistical analysis

Student's *t*-test was used to compare all continuous variables expressed as mean ± SD of the two groups. Incidence was compared by means of χ^2 tests. Receiver operating characteristic analysis was used to select the most appropriate indicator of ^{123}I-MIBG. Survival rates were estimated with the Kaplan-Meier method, and differences in survival assessed with the log-rank test. Univariate and multivariate analyses of the event risks associated with selected clinical variables used the Cox proportional hazard model (SPSS v 9.0, Chicago, IL). A *p* value of < 0.05 was considered statistically significant.

3. Results

3.1. Comparisons of clinical variables among patients stratified by cause of death (table 1)

Patients who died of congestive heart failure were significantly older than those who survived, or died suddenly without SVT. The patients with congestive heart failure death also showed the most deteriorated echocardiographic and hemodynamic conditions among the 3 groups. There were no statistically significant differences in any variables between surviving patients and patients who died suddenly without SVT.

	Sudden death without s-VT	**CHF**	**Survived**
	(N=9)	**(N=14)**	**(N=95)**
Age (yrs.)	56.0±5.8	64.0±8.5*	55.3±14.2
Gender: Female	1 (10)	3 (21)	32(33)
β-blockers	4 (40)	5 (36)	59(63)
LVEDd (mm)	62.5±15.0	67.6±12.1†	62.8±9.8
LVEF (%)	30.8±11.2	22.6±10.3†	36.1±13.2
PCWP (mmHg)	13.1±6.3	21.0±8.7*	11.0±6.1
mPAP (mmHg)	22.8±7.4	30.9±9.0*	18.5±7.2
CI (l/min/mm^2)	2.51±0.73	2.21±0.47	2.61±1.25
BNP (pg/ml)	**219±255**	**697±516†**	**107±110**

* p < 0.05 (for sudden death and survived patients); † p <0.05 (for survived patients)

BNP:brain natreuretic peptide; CI:cardiac index; LVDd:left ventricular end-diastolic diameter; LVEF: left ventricular ejection fraction; PCWP:pulmonary capillary wedge pressure; mPAP:mean pulmonary wedge pressure

Table 1. Clinical Variables among the Patients Stratified by Cause of Death

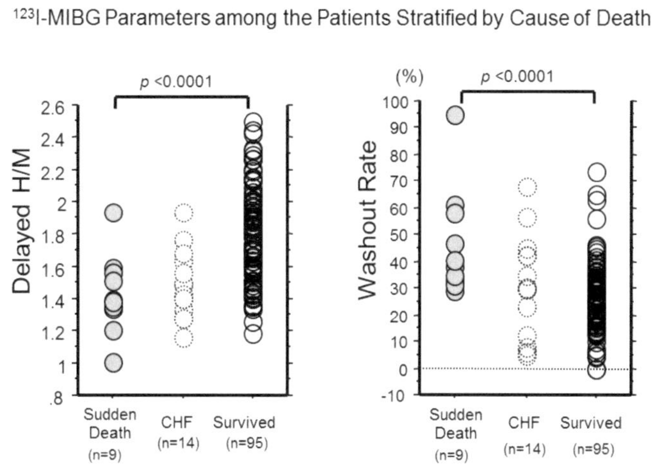

CHF: congestive heart failure; H/M: heart to mediastinum activity ratio; 123I-MIBG: Iodine-123 Metaiodobenzylguanidine

Figure 3. Comparisons of delayed H/M (left panel) and washout rate (right panel) of 123I-MIBG among the patients stratified by cause of death

3.2. Comparisons of ^{123}I-MIBG parameters among patients stratified by cause of death (figure 3)

^{123}I-MIBG parameters were better in surviving patients compared to those in patients with death due to congestive heart failure and with sudden death. There were significant differences in delayed H/M and washout rate of ^{123}I-MIBG between surviving patients and patients who died suddenly, although clinical variables were similar between the two groups.

3.3. Survival

Comparison of Kaplan-Meier survival curve was depicted in figure 4. Receiver operating characteristic analysis indicated that the optimal cut-off point of the delayed heart to mediastinum ratio for all cause of cardiac death was 1.6. Survival of the patients with delayed H/M ratio greater than 1.6 was significantly worse than that less than 1.6. Receiver operating characteristic analysis indicated that the optimal cut-off point of heart ^{123}I-MIBG washout rate for all cause of cardiac death was 38%. Survival of the patients with washout rate greater than 38% was significantly worse than that less than 38%. In the analysis of washout rate, a log-rank statistics of sudden cardiac death in heart failure patients without SVT was greater than that of death due to heart failure, whereas similar in the analysis of the delayed H/M ratio.

3.4. Univariate predictors for heart failure death and sudden death

Univariate predictors for heart failure death are summarized in Table 2. Age, left ventricular end-diastolic diameter, left ventricular ejection fraction (LVEF), pulmonary capillary wedge pressure, mean pulmonary artery pressure, delayed H/M ratio, and heart ^{123}I-MIBG washout

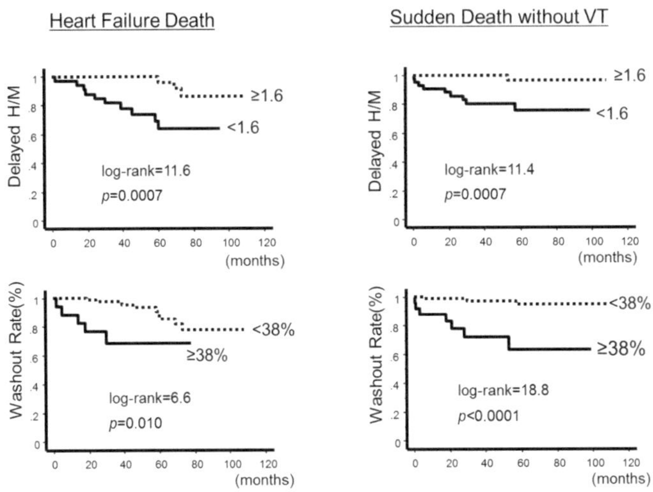

H/M: heart to mediastinum activity ratio; 123I-MIBG: Iodine-123 Metaiodobenzylguanidine; VT: ventricular tachycardia

Figure 4. Comparison of Kaplan-Meier survival curves. Heart failure death (left panel) abd sudden cardiac death (right panel).

rate were associated with death due to heart failure. Univariate predictors for sudden cardiac death are summarized in Table 3. Delayed H/M ratio and heart ^{123}I-MIBG washout rate were associated with sudden cardiac death in heart failure patients without SVT.

	X²	HR	95%CI	*p value*
Age (yrs.)*	4.39	1.07	1.004–1.141	.036
Gender :Male	0.72	0.57	0.153–2.104	.397
on β-blockade	2.25	0.40	0.119–1.327	.134
LVDd (mm)*	2.31	1.04	0.988–1.105	.129
PCWP (mmHg)*	21.3	1.24	1.131–1.357	.0000
mPAP (mmHg)*	20.8	1.19	1.105–1.283	.0000
CI (l/min/mm²)†	5.17	0.19	0.045–0.795	.023
LVEF (%)*	8.90	0.91	0.861–0.969	.003
Delayed H/M*	11.9	0.01	0.001–0.124	.0006
Washout rate (%)*	2.17	1.03	0.991–1.064	.141

Hazard ratio reflects risk with an increase of 1* and 0.1†.

CI:cardiac index; H/M:heart to mediastinum activity ratio; LVDd:left ventricular end-diastolic diameter; LVEF: left ventricular ejection fraction; PCWP:pulmonary capillary wedge pressure; mPAP:mean pulmonary wedge pressure

Table 2. Univariate Predictors for Heart Failure Death

	X^2	HR	95%CI	*p value*
Age (yrs.)*	0.27	0.99	0.953–1.028	.605
Gender :Male	2.96	0.17	0.022–1.282	.085
on β-blockade	1.71	0.47	0.154–1.452	.191
LVDd (mm)*	0.41	1.02	0.965–1.073	.521
PCWP (mmHg)*	0.18	1.02	0.937–1.107	.671
mPAP (mmHg)*	0.87	1.03	0.966–1.104	.350
CI (l/min/mm^2)†	0.02	0.94	0.425–2.086	.881
LVEF (%)*	1.00	0.98	0.934–1.023	.318
Delayed H/M*	12.8	0.01	0.001–0.116	.0004
Washout rate (%)*	14.8	1.06	1.027–1.086	.0001

Hazard ratio reflects risk with an increase of 1* and 0.1†.

CI:cardiac index; H/M:heart to mediastinum activity ratio; LVDd:left ventricular end-diastolic diameter; LVEF: left ventricular ejection fraction; PCWP:pulmonary capillary wedge pressure; mPAP:mean pulmonary wedge pressure; VT:ventricular tachycardia

Table 3. Univariate Predictors for Sudden Death without Sustained VT

3.5. Multivariate analysis

Cox multiple variable logistic regression model with a backward stepwise approach including 10 clinical variables (age, gender, on beta-blockers, left ventricular end-diastolic diameter, pulmonary capillary wedge pressure, mean pulmonary artery pressure, cardiac index, LVEF, delayed H/M ratio, heart ^{123}I-MIBG washout rate) identified pulmonary capillary wedge pressure and delayed H/M ratio as independent predictors of death due to heart failure, and delayed H/M ratio and heart ^{123}I-MIBG washout rate as independent predictors of sudden cardiac death in heart failure patients without SVT (Table 4).

	X^2	HR	95%CI	*p* value
PCWP*	15.3	1.28	1.078–1.409	.0000
Delayed H/M*	6.25	0.01	0.001–0.124	.012

(a) For Heart Failure Death

	X^2	HR	95%CI	*p* value
Washout rate*	5.12	1.05	1.007–1.126	.024
Delayed H/M*	4.29	0.02	0.023–0.346	038

(b) For Sudden Death without Sustained VT

(a) Hazard ratio (HR) reflects risk with an increase of 1*. H/M:heart to mediastinum activity ratio; PCWP:pulmonary capillary wedge pressure

(b) Hazard ratio (HR) reflects risk with an increase of 1*. H/M:heart to mediastinum activity ratio; VT: ventricular tachycardia

Table 4. Multiivariate analysis

4. Discussion

The principal finding of this study is that ^{123}I-MIBG parameters, especially washout rate is useful for the risk stratification of sudden cardiac death in chronic heart failure patients without SVT. To the best of our knowledge, this is the first report to show a relation between sudden cardiac death and cardiac sympathetic nervous function using ^{123}I-MIBG in heart failure patients without documented VT.

4.1. MIBG parameters and heart failure

Reduced pre-synaptic norepinephrine uptake and post-synaptic beta-adrenoreceptor density might contribute to the remodeling process of the left ventricle in the diseased heart [9]. Increased washout and decreased uptake of ^{123}I-MIBG in the myocardium are related to the severity and prognosis of heart failure [10]. A recent meta-analysis including 18 studies with a total of 1755 patients reconfirmed that decreased uptake and increased washout of ^{123}I-MIBG showed a poor prognosis in patients with heart failure. ^{123}I-MIBG also has been used to assess the functioning of the pulmonary capillary endothelium under a variety of experimental or clinical conditions [11, 12]. Mu et al. speculated the increased lung uptake of ^{123}I-MIBG in heart failure patients might be due to the enhanced permeability of the pulmonary endothelial cells [13]. We have demonstrated that the combined assessment of lung and heart ^{123}I-MIBG uptake may help to predict future clinical outcome in patients with idiopathic dilated cardiomyopathy more accurately than myocardial evaluation alone [14].

4.2. Autoantibody against the beta1 adrenoreceptor and heart failure

We previously investigated the relationship between ^{123}I-MIBG parameters and the anti-beta1-adrenoreceptor autoantibody level in chronic heart failure patients [15]. The autoantibodies stimulate the second extracellular domain of the beta1-adrenoreceptor like norepinephrine, and are associated with reduced cardiac function in patients with heart failure [16]. We have demonstrated that the anti-beta1-adrenoreceptor autoantibodies are closely associated with cardiac sympathetic nervous activity assessed by ^{123}I-MIBG and cardiac event in patients with chronic heart failure [15]. Iwata et al. has reported that the autoantibodies predict VT and sudden death in patients with idiopathic dilated cardiomyopathy [17]. These results suggest that sudden cardiac death associated with ventricular tachyarrhythmias might be related to sympathetic nervous activity evaluated by ^{123}I-MIBG scintigraphy.

4.3. Cardiac sympathetic nervous function and sudden cardiac death associated with ventricular tachyarrhythmias

Several electrocardiographic markers such as heart rate variability, single-averaged electrocardiogram, and QT dispersion have been proposed for the prediction of cardiac event in patients with heart failure [18-20]. Heart rate variability is a noninvasive tool for the condition of autonomic nervous activity and has been shown to predict future sudden cardiac death. Tamaki et al. reported a comparison of cardiac ^{123}I-MIBG imaging with other electrocardiographic markers, and concluded that washout rate of ^{123}I-MIBG was the most powerful predictor for sudden cardiac death in patients with mild-to-moderate heart failure [21].

Using ^{123}I-MIBG, the role of impaired cardiac sympathetic innervations has been reported in patients with ventricular tachyarrhythmias. Akutsu et al. reported that impairment of cardiac sympathetic nervous system predicted recurrent ventricular tachyarrhythmic events in patients with a history of VT or fibrillation [22]. A prospective multicenter pilot study demonstrated that only defect severity of ^{123}I-MIBG single photon emission computed tomography (SPECT) was predictive of inducibility of VT or fibrillation, whereas the conventional index such as H/M was not [23].

4.4. ^{123}I-MIBG kinetics and indication for implantable cardioverter defibrillator (ICD)

A recent Sudden Cardiac Death in Heart Failure Trial (SCD-HeFT) [1] has proven the efficacy of prophylactic ICD use for chronic heart failure patients without sustained VT and a history of ventricular fibrillation, not restricted in those with myocardial infarction. Since ICD is an expensive device, risk stratification is required to identify heart failure patients at high risk for sudden death without sustained VT. Based on the several guidelines, prophylactic use of an ICD is recommended in patients with ventricular tachycardia who have severe systolic dysfunction. Nagahara et al. demonstrated that when combined with plasma BNP or cardiac function, impairment of cardiac sympathetic innervations would predict an ICD shock associated with lethal arrhythmias, contributing to identify suitable candidates for prophylactic ICD implantation [24]. Severely reduced left ventricular systolic function is a powerful predictor of sudden cardiac death. They concluded that ^{123}I-MIBG scintigraphic evaluation for cardiac sympathetic innervations may be an option for screening patients at high risk for sudden cardiac death. Furthermore, such abnormality had incremental and additive prognostic power when combined with left ventricular dysfunction.

Those recent reports mentioned above support our present results. Increased neuronal release of norepinephrine and decreased efficiency in the reuptake of norepinephrine through the uptake-1 mechanism contribute to the increased cardiac adrenergic drive, and lead to life threatening ventricular tachyarrhythmias in patients with heart failure.

4.5. Study limitations

There are several limitations in this study. First, because of the retrospective study design, definite conclusions could not be drawn from our present data. BNP which is one of the important prognostic factors should be excluded in our multivariate analysis for prognostic determinants because of imperfect data. Second, the number of cardiac death was relatively small because the follow-up period was not long enough, so that more extensive case studies and longer follow-ups are required to validate the results reported here.

5. Conclusions

We investigated the relationship between ^{123}I-MIBG findings and mode of death in patients with chronic heart failure. Sudden cardiac death in heart failure patients is closely associated with cardiac sympathetic nervous activity assessed by ^{123}I-MIBG scintigraphy. Our data, thus, confirm that increased sympathetic tone in the myocardium play a harmful role on the progression of life-threatening ventricular tachyarrhythmias. Assessment of cardiac sympathetic nervous activity using ^{123}I-MIBG may be helpful for the candidate selection of ICD in heart failure patients without sustained ventricular tachycardia.

Author details

Yoshikazu Yazaki[1*], Toshimasa Seki[1], Atsushi Izawa[2], Minoru Hongo[3] and Uichi Ikeda[1]

*Address all correspondence to: yoshiy@athena.ocn.ne.jp

1 Division of Cardiology, NHO Mastumoto Medical Center, Matsumoto Hospital, Matsumoto, Japan

2 Department of Cardiovascular Medicine, Shinshu University School of Medicine, Matsumoto, Japan

3 Department of Allied Health Science, Shinshu University School of Medicine, Matsumoto, Japan

References

[1] Bardy, G. H, Lee, K. L, Mark, D. B, et al. Sudden Cardiac Death in Heart Failure Trial (SCD-HeFT) Investigators. Amiodarone or an implantable cardioverter-defibrillator for congestive heart failure. N Engl J Med (2005). , 352, 225-37.

[2] Schofer, J, Spielmann, R, Schuchert, A, Weber, K, & Schüter, M. Iodine-123 metaiodobenzylguanidine scintigraphy: a non invasive method to demonstrate myocardial adrenergic disintegrity in patients with idiopathic dilated cardiomyopathy. J Am Coll Cardiol (1988). , 12, 1252-8.

[3] Eisenhofer, G, Friberg, P, Rundqvist, B, et al. Cardiac sympathetic nerve function in congestive heart failure. Circulation (1996). , 93, 1667-1676.

[4] Merlet, P, Pouillart, F, Dubois-randé, J. L, et al. Sympathetic nerve alterations assessed with ^{123}I-MIBG in the failing human heart. J Nucl Med (1999). , 40, 224-31.

[5] Verberne, H. J, Brewster, L. M, & Somsen, G. A. van Eck-Smit BLF. Prognostic value of myocardial ^{123}I metaiodobenzylguanidine (MIBG) parameters in patients with heart failure: a systematic review. Eur Heart J (2008). , 29, 1147-59.

[6] Jeroen, J. Bax, Otakar Kraft, Alfred E. Buxton, et al. 123I-mIBG Scintigraphy to Predict Inducibility of Ventricular Arrhythmias on Cardiac Electrophysiology Testing: A Prospective Multicenter Pilot Study. Circ Cardiovasc Imaging (2008). , 1, 131-40.

[7] Akutsu, Y, Kaneko, K, Kodama, Y, et al. The Significance of Cardiac Sympathetic Nervous System Abnormality in the Long-Term Prognosis of Patients with a History of Ventricular Tachyarrhythmia. J Nucl Med (2009). , 50, 61-7.

[8] Mardon, K, Montaqne, O, Elbaz, N, et al. Uptake-1 carrier downregulates in parallel with the beta-adrenergic receptor desensitization in rat hearts chronically exposed to high levels of circulating norepinephrine: implications for cardiac neuroimaging in human cardiomyopathies. J Nucl Med (2003). , 44, 1459-1466.

[9] Carrio, I, Cowie, M. R, Yamazaki, J, Udelson, J, & Camici, P. D. Cardiac sympathetic imaging with mIBG in heart failure. J Am Coll Cardiol Imag (2010). , 3, 92-100.

[10] Kasama, S, Toyama, T, Sumino, H, et al. M. Prognostic Value of Serial Cardiac 123I-MIBG Imaging in Patients with Stabilized Chronic Heart Failure and Reduced Left Ventricular Ejection Fraction. J Nucl Med (2008). , 49, 907-14.

[11] Richalet, J. P, Merlet, P, Bourguignon, M, Vaysse, J, Larmignat, P, & Boom, A. MIBG scintigraphic assessment of cardiac adrenergic activity in response to altitude hypoxia. J Nucl Med (1990). , 31, 34-7.

[12] Koizumi, T, Kubo, K, Hanaoka, M, et al. Serial scintigraphic assessment of iodine-123 metaiodobenzylguanidine lung uptake in a patient with high-altitude pulmonary edema. Chest (1999). , 116, 1129-31.

[13] Mu, X, Hasegawa, S, Yoshioka, J, et al. Clinical value of lung uptake of iodine-123 metaiodobenzylguanidine (MIBG), a myocardial sympathetic nerve imaging agent, in patients with chronic heart failure. Ann Nucl Med (2001). , 15, 411-416.

[14] Kamiyoshi, Y, Yazaki, Y, Urushibata, K, et al. Risk stratification assessed by combined lung and heart iodine-123 metaiodobenzylguanidine uptake in patients with idiopathic dilated cardiomyopathy. Am J Cardiol (2008). , 101, 1482-6.

[15] Aso, S. I, Yazaki, Y, Kasai, H, et al. Anti- beta1-adrenoreceptor Autoantibodies and Myocardial Sympathetic Nerve Activity in Chronic Heart Failure. Int J Cardiol (2009). , 131, 240-5.

[16] Jahns, R, Boivin, V, Siegmund, C, Inselmann, G, Lohse, M. J, & Boege, F. Autoantibodies activating human β1-adrenergic receptors are associated with reduced cardiac function in chronic heart failure. Circulation (1999). , 99, 649-54.

[17] Iwata, M, Yoshikawa, T, Baba, A, Anzai, T, Mitamura, H, & Ogawa, S. Autoantibodies against the second extracellular loop of beta1-adrenergic receptors predict ven-

tricular tachycardia and sudden death in patients with idiopathic dilated cardiomyopathy. Am Heart J (2006). , 152, 697-704.

[18] La RoverPinna GD, Maestri R, et al. Short-term heart rate variability strongly predicts sudden cardiac death in chronic heart failure patients. Circulation (2003). , 107, 565-70.

[19] Goedel-meinen, L, Hofmann, M, Ryba, S, & Schomig, A. Prognostic value of an abnormal signal-averaged electrocardiogram in patients with nonischemic dilated cardiomyopathy. Am J Cardiol (2001). , 87, 809-12.

[20] Galinier, M, Viallete, J. C, Fourcade, J, et al. QT interval dispersion as a predictor of arrhythmic events in congestive heart failure. Importance of aetiology. Eur Heart J (1998). , 19, 1054-62.

[21] Tamaki, S, Yamada, T, Okuyama, Y, et al. Cardiac Iodine-123 Metaiodobenzylguanidine Imaging redicts Sudden Cardiac Death Independently of LeftVentricular Ejection Fraction in Patients With ChronicHeart Failure and Left Ventricular Systolic Dysfunction: Results From a Comparative Study With Signal-Averaged Electrocardiogram, Heart Rate Variability, and QT Dispersion. J Am Coll Cardiol (2009). , 53, 426-35.

[22] Akutsu, Y, Kaneko, K, Kodama, Y, et al. The significance of cardiac sympathetic nervous system abnormality in the long-term prognosis of patients with a history of ventricular tachyarrhythmia. J Nucl Med (2009). , 50, 61-7.

[23] Bax, J. J, Kraft, O, Buxton, A. E, et al. I-mIBG Scintigraphy to Predict Inducibility of Ventricular Arrhythmias on Cardiac Electrophysiology Testing: A Prospective Multicenter Pilot Study. Circ Cardiovasc Imaging (2008). , 1, 131-40.

[24] Nagahara, D, Nakata, T, Hashimoto, A, et al. Predicting the need for an implantable cardioverter defibrillator using cardiac metaiodobenzylguanidine activity together with plasma natriuretic peptide concentration or left ventricular function. J Nucl Med (2008). , 49, 225-33.

Section 5

Cardiomyopathies in Special Populations

Chapter 12

Potential Target Molecules in Diabetic Cardiomyopathy: Hepatocyte Growth Factor (HGF) and Ryanodine Receptor 2 (RyR2)

Jan Klimas

Additional information is available at the end of the chapter

http://dx.doi.org/10.5772/55780

1. Introduction

Patients with diabetes mellitus have an increased cardiovascular mortality rate and, in particular, cardiovascular complications are the leading cause of diabetes-related morbidity and mortality. Diabetes mellitus is a well-recognized risk factor for developing heart failure and it also can affect cardiac structure and function even in the absence of traditional cardiovascular risk factors. Four decades ago Rubler and colleagues introduced the term 'diabetic cardiomyopathy' describing diabetic patients with congestive heart failure and normal coronary arteries [1]. Since then, many epidemiological and clinical studies have documented the existence of this entity in humans [2].

Individuals with diabetes mellitus (DM), both type 1 DM as well as type 2 DM, have an increased risk of developing end-organ damage. Clinically, the concept of diabetic cardiomyopathy is defined as ventricular dysfunction that occurs independently of coronary artery disease and hypertension, *i.e.* as a distinct primary disease process which develops secondary to a metabolic insult and results in structural and functional abnormalities of the myocardium leading to heart failure. Diabetic cardiomyopathy in humans is predominantly manifested by diastolic dysfunction, which may precede the development of systolic dysfunction [3]. Interestingly, only approximately 30% of type 2 DM and type 1 DM patients develop diabetic nephropathy, in contrast to diabetic cardiomyopathy that is present in 50% type 2 DM patients and diabetic retinopathy diagnosed in more than 90% of type 1 DM patients [4; 5]. This indicates a different time-course of end-organ damage in DM. Consequently, individual cell types are differentially sensitive to high blood glucose-induced damage likely because of different expression or activity of molecular factors responsible for damage activation and progression.

The prevalence of heart failure (HF) in the general population ranges from 1 to 4%, but in diabetic patients it is 12%, rising to 22% in those over the age of 64 years [6; 7]. The Framingham Heart Study reported a 2.4-fold increase in the incidence of HF in diabetic men and a 5.1-fold increase in diabetic women, when compared with age-matched controls [8; 9]. Diabetic patients are also more likely than non-diabetic patients to develop HF following myocardial infarction, despite comparable infarct sizes [10].

Based on the assumption of detrimental effects of hyperglycaemia on various tissues, reduction of blood glucose would reverse (or at least reduce) the development of end-organ damage. However, recent data showed unexpected findings. Castagno and colleagues conducted a meta-analysis of randomized controlled trials comparing strategies of more versus less intensive glucose-lowering that reported HF events. Interestingly, it became evident that tight glycemic control in patients with type 2 DM did not reduce the risk of HF and, additionally, when glucose lowering was achieved with thiazolidinediones, it increased that risk [11]. Additionally, evidence for a direct, causal link between insulin resistance, a hallmark of diabetes, and ventricular dysfunction has not been established [12]. The reason why intensive glucose control does not lead to the reduction in risk of HF predicted by epidemiological studies is uncertain but it may reflect an insufficient duration of treatment or follow-up, a treatment intervention too late in the course of the disease, off-target toxicity of the treatments used, or the possibility that hyperglycemia *per se* does not directly govern the development of HF in diabetic patients. In other words, hyperglycaemia could be a trigger of molecular changes causing end-organ damage, which are later regulated at least partially independently from the systemic glucose changes. These assumptions foster the search for local signalling molecules involved in end-organ damage in DM.

It is widely accepted that the pathogenesis of diabetic cardiomyopathy is multifactorial. Beyond the stereotypical function of metabolism as a provider of ATP, alterations in metabolic flux within the cell create essential signals for the adaptation of the heart to disturbed blood sugar regulation and insulin abnormalities in DM. In general, the prevailing concept of the heart's response to changes in its environment is a complex network of interconnecting signal transduction cascades where the focus is on communication of various cell surface receptors, heterotrimeric G-proteins, protein kinases, and transcription factors [13]. Several hypotheses have been proposed, including autonomic dysfunction, metabolic derangements, abnormalities in ion homeostasis, alteration in structural proteins, and interstitial fibrosis, and increased glycation of interstitial proteins such as collagen, which results in myocardial stiffness and impaired contractility [2]. Collectively, metabolic imbalance induces alterations in downstream transcription factors which result in changes in gene expression, myocardial substrate utilization, myocyte growth, endothelial function and myocardial compliance [14]. Indeed, alterations in gene expression have been observed for a number of key inducer or transducer molecules in diabetic cardiomyopathy. In particular, oxidative stress due to increased production of reactive oxygen species (ROS) by multiple sources, such as the NADPH oxidase or dysfunctional nitric oxide (NO)-signaling cascade, is considered to be a principal mechanism involved in the development of diabetic cardiomyopathy [15; 16; 17]. However, this review focuses on two of them which are currently not in the centre of interest but which might play a role not only in beginning but also in development of diabetic cardiomyopathy. These are (1) hepatocyte growth factor/c-Met signalling cascade, and (2) calcium release system.

2. Hepatocyte growth factor/c-Met signalling

2.1. Structure and function of HGF and c-Met

The hepatocyte growth factor (HGF) is known to be involved in a huge variety of cellular processes playing a major role in the repair and regeneration of various tissues, including the liver, kidney, lung, and stomach. In addition, it is involved in embryogenesis, organ development and also carcinogenesis, and its role in autoimmune diseases has been suggested as well [18; 19].

Liver regeneration has long been a subject of active research, because it has impressive regenerative capacities. Humoral factors that trigger liver cell growth, and so hepatic regeneration, have been detected in the blood circulation of liver-injured animals, and many researchers have tried to isolate these factors ensuring this liver characteristic. One of them, HGF was first recognised as a molecule that stimulates hepatocyte proliferation and so to be a key player in the regulation of liver regeneration. It was originally identified in the plasma of partially hepatectomised rats and initially thought to be a liver-specific mitogen [20; 21; 22]. Actually, HGF is known to be a multifunctional cytokine and such as it has been a subject of immense research efforts during the past decade [23].

Physiologically, HGF is a mesenchyme-derived pleiotropic growth factor which consists of two polypeptide chains, heavy 69-kDa alpha-chain and a light 34-kDa beta-chain which are held together by a disulfide bond. Like plasminogen, HGF is synthesised as pro-HGF, an 82-kDa single-chain inactive precursor, and subsequently transformed in the active heterodimer [24]. HGF is latent in normal states, and is activated specifically at the site of tissue injury, predominantly by HGF activator - HGFA [19; 25; 26]. The domains of HGF are very similar to those of proteases in the blood coagulation and fibrinolytic system, HGF shows the highest similarity to plasminogen (about 40% amino acid similarity). Thus, the HGF system is functionally linked to the blood coagulation and fibrinolytic system.

The HGF receptor c-Met is a transmembrane tyrosine kinase that mediates several biological responses after stimulation by its cognate ligand. c-Met is synthesised as a precursor (170 kDa) and then, it is converted into the active disulphide-linked heterodimer composed of a 50 kDa extracellular alpha-chain and a longer 145 kDa beta-chain with a transmembrane helix and a cytoplasmic portion. The alpha-chain is exposed extracellularly, while the beta-chain is a transmembrane subunit containing an intracellular tyrosine kinase domain [27; 28; 29; 30].

Multiple biological effects of HGF/c-Met system on a wide variety of cells have been documented. HGF is a cytokine regulating cell growth, cell motility and morphogenesis of various types of cells. Additionally, mitogenic, motogenic, chemotactic and anti-apoptotic activities of HGF have been documented on multiple cell type. This cytokine stimulates endothelial proliferation and, consequently, angiogenesis, as well as stimulates growth of other target cells including melanocytes, epithelial cells, and haemopoietic cells. Thus, HGF is considered a humoral mediator of the epithelial-mesenchymal interactions responsible for morphogenic tissue interactions during embryonic development and organogenesis [23; 31]. According to current hypothesis, HGF is an activating ligand of c-Met receptor, whose activity is essential for normal tissue development and organ regeneration but abnormal activation of c-Met has been implicated in growth, invasion, and metastasis of many types of solid tumors. While HGF is produced in various mesenchymal cells mostly in response to tissue injury, its receptor c-Met is expressed on epithelial cells, irrespective of the organ. This ligand-receptor pair (HGF/c-Met) has a role during embryogenesis, organogenesis and carcinogenesis [28; 32; 33; 34; 35] as well as in the homeostasis of adult tissues [27; 28]. The paracrine signalling between HGF and c-Met plays an important role in regulating epithelial–mesenchymal cell interactions.

2.2. HGF/c-Met in cardiovascular pathology

HGF and its receptor c-Met are expressed in several tissues, including the heart although at low levels. Several reports have focused on the role of HGFc-Met in cardiovascular pathophysiology and, comparable to pleiotropic effects in other organs, a huge variety of actions have been described also in cardiovascular system. Animal studies demonstrated that treatment with HGF gene or protein may reduce acute myocardial ischemia and reperfusion injury, decrease infarct size, and improve cardiac perfusion and function in acute myocardial infarction. These beneficial effects are associated with angiogenesis and reduced apoptosis. HGF protects cardiomyocytes against oxidative stress and can counteract the loss of cardiomyocytes usually observed in cardiac diseases [36; 37]. In addition to its beneficial effects on cardiomyocytes under acute stress, recent research has demonstrated that HGF also exerts beneficial effects on cardiac function in animal models of chronic heart diseases, including ischemic cardiomyopathy following old myocardial infarction and hereditary cardiomyopathy. In those cases, the main mechanisms appeared to be a hypertrophic effect on cardiomyocytes as well as angiogenic and antifibrotic actions.

Interestingly, several injuries alter the expression of HGF in cardiac tissue. In the heart, acute myocardial infarction, ischemia reperfusion injury, and congestive heart failure induce expression of HGF [37; 38; 39]. In myocardial ischemia, HGF has been suggested to counteract damage and to mediate a regenerative response (Nakamura et al. 2000). Apparently, there is a time dynamics in HGF production and/or secretion in the diseased myocardium. Although there is an upregulation of cardiac HGF/cMet in the acute phase of myocardial infarction, the cardiac HGF production appears to be downregulated in the late phase of myocardial infarction (MI). HGF quantity measured 24 hours after infarction was confirmed to be higher in the border than in the remote myocardium [40]. Aoki and colleagues observed that the cardiac HGF level was significantly decreased at 14 days after MI [41]. Others supported this time dynamics. In rats, myocardial expression of HGF mRNA and c-Met receptor mRNA are significantly elevated following myocardial ischemia/reperfusion induced by transient coronary ligation or MI induced by permanent coronary ligation. Both levels rapidly increase, peak between 24-72 hours, and remain significantly elevated for at least 5-7 days. Myocardial gene expression of HGF and c-Met remained activated for one month after cardiac ischemia/

http://dx.doi.org/10.5772/55780

reperfusion in rats. The peak in c-Met expression occurs 24 hours after ischemia/reperfusion, whereas HGF gene expression peaks at 72 hours. The peak mRNA levels increase by 4- fold for HGF and 8.3-fold for c-Met. The c-Met mRNA returned to near normal levels by one week, and HGF gene expression is substantially reduced from the peak level by one week and then gradually returns to baseline levels over 15-30 days [42]. Thus increased blood HGF may reflect a defensive reaction and possibly participate in cardioprotection during myocardial infarction [36]. From a mechanistic point of view, HGF exerts anti-apoptotic and angiogenic properties by activating its c-Met receptor and a downstream ERK1/2-mediated signalling pathway in cardiomyocytes and endothelial cells both on the myocardial infarction border zone and in regions of the heart remote from the infarct.

Several experimental studies have shown that HGF can stimulate myocardial regeneration by inducing endogenous cardiac stem cells to migrate, differentiate, and proliferate in situ to replace lost cardiomyocytes. c-Met is expressed on different populations of putative cardiac stem cells and cardiac progenitor cells migration, proliferation and homing are predominantly modulated by the HGF/c-Met receptor system [43; 44]. Thus, HGF/c-Met signalling might play a key role in self-renewal of myocardial tissue.

2.3. HGF as a biomarker of cardiac damage

Currently, the use of HGF as a clinical marker of cardiovascular injury is under intensive debate as several papers reported increased serum HGF in patients with heart failure. Lamblin and colleagues investigated the prognostic value of 2 cytokines, vascular endothelial growth factor (VEGF) and HGF, in patients evaluated for a reduced left ventricular ejection fraction [45]. Vascular endothelial growth factor was shown to have limited prognostic utility. However, increased levels of HGF were strongly associated with markers of congestive heart failure severity such as higher NYHA class and lower left ventricular ejection fraction, as well as clinical outcomes including both cardiac and overall mortality *(see figure 1)*. The association of HGF with adverse outcomes persisted in multivariable analysis that incorporated state-of-the-art risk factors such as BNP and peak oxygen consumption, an important step when assessing a new biologic marker. In detail, HGF levels were higher in patients with a cardiovascular event (1001 [741-1327] pg/mL) than in the patients without it (773 [610-1045] pg/mL, $P < 0.0001$). Similar results were found when overall mortality was considered. HGF levels were higher in the patients who died of any cause (940 [748-1306] pg/mL) than in patients who did not. Importantly, HGF concentrations were strongly associated with age, diabetes mellitus, and all markers of congestive heart failure severity. Consequently, the survival curves indicated a worse outcome for patients with high HGF levels. Similarly, in a small clinical study, Ueno and colleagues found 5.3 times higher serum HGF levels as compared to healthy volunteers in patients with acute exacerbation of congestive heart failure [39]. In another study of Lamblin and colleagues studied patients with a first anterior Q-wave myocardial infarction [46]. They observed that plasma HGF levels were positively associated with left ventricular volumes, wall motion systolic index, early transmitral velocity to mitral annular early diastolic velocity ratio, and BNP levels. High HGF levels were associated with higher C-reactive protein levels. On the other hand, HGF levels were negatively associated with left ventricular ejection fraction. Multivariate analysis showed that both BNP and C-reactive protein were independently associated with HGF levels at 3 and 12 months. Patients who died or were re-hospitalized for HF during follow-up had higher HGF levels at 1 month, 3 months, and 1 year after myocardial infarction. Thus, circulating HGF levels correlate with all markers of LV remodelling after MI and are associated with re-hospitalization for heart failure.

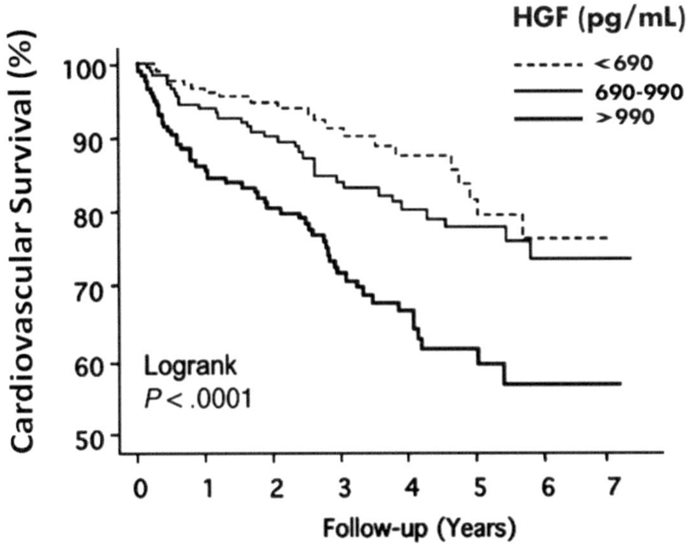

Figure 1. Kaplan-Meier survival curves according to the tertiles of HGF. These survival curves indicates a worse outcome for patients with high HGF levels [45].

Rychli and colleagues assessed the prognostic value of HGF in heart failure in a prospective cohort study [47]. They demonstrated that the risk of all-cause mortality increases with endogenous HGF concentrations in patients with advanced HF with a 3.1-fold higher risk in the third tertile compared with the first tertile. Interestingly, additional subgroup analysis stratifying by the aetiology of HF showed that the prognostic value of HGF was only present in patients with ischaemic HF and not in those with HF of other aetiology. In patients with ischaemic HF they observed a 4.4-fold higher risk in the third tertile compared with the first tertile. The main increase of risk was between the first and the second tertile of HGF. Therefore, it might be speculated that a certain threshold of HGF has to be exceeded to initiate mechanisms linked with a poor survival. Additional analysis evaluating the predictive potential of HGF for the secondary end point cardiovascular mortality yielded similar results as reported for all-cause mortality. In patients with ischaemic HF the adjusted hazard for a cardiovascular death was 6.2-fold higher in the third tertile of HGF compared with the first tertile. The predictive value of HGF was independent of BNP and other potential predictors of outcome in patients with HF. Stratified analyses evaluating the combined risk prediction by HGF and BNP levels showed that high HGF indicates a poor prognosis even in patients with low BNP. This subgroup of patients had a comparable risk to those with elevated BNP, but a low HGF.

As expected, the greatest risk was found when both factors were raised. This additive prognostic value of HGF might help to identify patients at high risk who would benefit from intensive treatment.

Although several figures have been suggested such as 0.26, 0.39, 0.69, and 0.99 ng/ml [45; 48; 49], no practical cutoff values discriminating between normal and abnormal HGF concentrations linked to human cardiovascular pathology have been defined yet. Moreover, although HGF was associated with adverse outcomes in heart failure patients, Wang and colleagues show that its prognostic value for mortality and heart transplant necessity in various forms of cardiomyopathy is poor [50]. In their prospective cohort study, HGF concentrations were measured in patients with Chagas' disease related dilated cardiomyopathy or idiopathic dilated cardiomyopathy. When compared to healthy individuals, no difference was detected for patients with NYHA class I–II but HGF was significantly increased in advanced HF patients (NYHA III–IV) in both groups of patients. In addition, there was a strong correlation between HGF and left ventricular ejection fraction in patients suffering from Chagas' disease but HGF failed to predict mortality and necessity for heart transplant in both groups of patients.

In spite of still controversial findings, HGF might be an attractive biomarker in patients with congestive heart failure because it is increased in the setting of cardiomyocyte apoptosis and active remodeling, thereby identifying individuals who are at increased risk of adverse clinical outcomes. However, based on available evidence, the etiology of cardiac abnormality has to be considered before applying HGF as a biomarker [51].

2.4. HGF as a therapeutic factor

It remains unclear what mechanism is responsible for the cardioprotective effects of HGF but its therapeutic potential is undisputable. In current literature, the focus is stressed on influence of HGF in stem cell mobilization in damaged myocardium. HGF belongs to factors that increase recruitment of progenitor cells to damaged myocardium by its chemotactic effects on cardiac progenitor cells [52]. In other words, HGF attracts cardiac stem cells to start transport and differentiate in infarcted area.

Several methods were developed to affect injured hearts in a variety of animal models. Most of investigators use gene transfections. HGF gene therapy decreases adverse ventricular remodelling and improves cardiac function in various species. In a hamster model of dilated cardiomyopathy, transfection with the HGF gene attenuates the progression of cardiac impairment, including the reduction of myocardial fibrosis and reorganization of the cytoskeletal proteins and these changes lead to an improvement in life expectancy [53; 54; 55]. Li and colleagues studied its chronic effects on post-infarction left ventricular remodeling and heart failure in mice. They applied adenovirus encoding human HGF and observed improved left ventricular remodeling and function and hypertrophied cardiomyocytes near infarcted area at 4 weeks after induction of myocardial infarction. Postinfarction HGF gene therapy improved LV remodeling and dysfunction through hypertrophy of cardiomyocytes, infarct wall thickening, preservation of vessels, and antifibrosis [56]. In rats, HGF gene transfer following a large myocardial infarction results in preservation of ventricular geometry and function, and is associated with enhanced angiogenesis and a reduction in apoptosis (Jayasankar et al. 2003, Jayasankar et al. 2005). Iwasaki and colleagues reported that recombinant human HGF delivered by ultrasound-mediated destruction of microbubbles into the cardiomyopathic hearts prevents cardiac dysfunction in an animal model of doxorubicin-induced cardiomyopathy [57]. In this form of anthracycline induced cardiomyopathy in mice, findings of Esaki and colleagues suggest that HGF gene delivery by adenoviral vector exerts therapeutic antiatrophic/degenerative and antifibrotic effects on myocardium and mitigation of cardiac dysfunction. These beneficial effects appear to be related to HGF-induced MAPK/ERK activation and upregulation of c-Met, GATA-4, and sarcomeric proteins [58]. Okayama et al demonstrated in transegenic mice that HGF reduced cardiac fibrosis by inhibiting endothelial mesenchymal transition and the transformation of fibroblasts into myofibroblasts. The amount of cardiac fibrosis significantly decreased in pressure-overloaded HGF-transgenic mice compared with pressure-overloaded nontransgenic controls, particularly in the perivascular region. This pattern was accompanied by a reduction in the expression levels of fibrosis-related genes and by significant preservation of echocardiographic measurements of cardiac function in the HGF-transgenic mice [59]. In dogs with intracoronary microembolization-induced heart failure, intramyocardial injections of HGF naked DNA plasmid attenuated the expression abnormalities of the SR Ca^{2+}-cycling proteins, improved regional and global left ventricular function and prevented progressive LV remodeling [60]. In a ventricular rapid pacing heart failure canine model, gene transfection of HGF promoted angiogenesis, improved perfusion, decreased fibrosis and apoptosis, promoted recovery from myocyte atrophy, and thereby attenuated cardiac remodeling and improved myocardial function in the failing canine hearts [61]. The gene therapy with hepatocyte growth factor–complementary DNA plasmids reduced coronary artery ligation-induced cardiac impairment in goats (Shirakawa et al. 2005). Taken together, a number of experimental data support the potential therapeutic value of HGF.

Importantly, the concept of gene therapy using HGF has been used in human as well. The intracoronary administration of adenovirus vector encoding the human HGF gene in patients with coronary heart disease resulted in high levels of gene expression of HGF and its receptor c-Met, as well as increased serum concentrations of HGF. Adenovirus vector encoding the human HGF gene effectively induced temporarily high expression of the HGF gene in peripheral blood mononuclear cells and consequently increased serum HGF levels [62]. Nevertheless, the clinical utility of HGF therapy in the myocardium still remains enigmatic. It is still unclear which mechanisms are the most important for the cardioprotective effect of HGF. For a successful translation to clinical application of a protein, a clearly defined primary mode of action and knowledge on pharmacokinetic properties are necessary for the rational development of the protein as a therapeutic [52].

2.5. HGF/c-Met in diabetic cardiomyopathy

The role of HGF/c-Met signalling in cardiac tissue is predominantly linked to ischemic damage and little is known about its role in diabetic cardiomyopathy. Since HGF contributes to the protection or repair of vascular endothelial cells and decreased serum and tissue HGF levels are related to the progression of endothelial cell damage induced by diabetes [63], the same might be true for cardiac tissue. In general, increased HGF is believed to be a marker of complications. However, local HGF production in vascular cells was shown to be markedly suppressed by high D-glucose [64] what suggests that decreased local HGF production may accelerate the progression of atherosclerotic vascular changes as well as cardiomyocytes injury in DM. In turn, an adaptive increase of HGF in advanced DM might support the hypothesis that serum HGF concentrations are elevated in response to various organ injuries.

The results of a clinical study [65] showed for the first time that serum HGF concentrations are increased in type 1 diabetic patients. Interestingly, these results were similar at the diagnosis time point and after more than 10 years duration with or without pathologic albumin excretion. This finding suggests a stable increase of HGF during development and progression of DM 1. In contrary, Nakamura and colleagues [63] found a decrease of serum HGF concentration in DM patients without hypertension but an increase in patients suffering from both DM as well as arterial hypertension. In the latter group, HGF concentration progressively increased with the stage of hypertension and it positively correlated with systolic blood pressure in DM patients. In addition, both animal and clinical data showed that serum HGF concentration were negatively correlated with HbAIc in subjects without any complications, suggesting a loss of this endothelial protection in accordance with the severity of diabetes. In fact, the serum HGF concentration in DM patients may be determined by a balance of stimulating factors (hypertension, atherosclerosis, *etc.*) and suppressing factors (high glucose, TGF-beta, Ang II, *etc.*). Consequently, the elevation of the serum HGF concentration may be considered as an index of the severity of complications in DM. Systemic HGF may work in tissue regeneration as a humoral mediator, although it might be insufficient to promote tissue regeneration, owing to a decrease in local HGF production. In conclusion, the HGF/c-Met signalling might play a crucial role in cardiac damage such as diabetic cardiomyopathy (*see figure 2)* and exact identification of this role may pave new ways towards drug development and to contribute to better management of DM in future.

3. Calcium release and Ryanodine receptor 2

3.1. Regulation of calcium cycle in cardiac cells

One of the long reported general hypotheses of cardiac impairment is based on the calcium overload. Fleckenstein's calcium theory of myocardial cell necrosis from 1970' is widely quoted in literature as a general mechanism of myocardial cell damage [66]. It must be noted that intracellular calcium dysregulation is present in all types of advanced cardiomyopathy and apparently is a late stage event that represents a final common pathway for myocardial cell damage and death. There is now increasing evidence that depression of contractility in heart failure is linked to a malfunction of calcium regulation in cardiomyocytes, in particular to sarcoplasmic reticulum (SR) Ca^{2+} uptake and/or release [67; 68].

Sarcoplasmic reticulum (SR) Ca^{2+} release is maintained by a macromolecular protein complex consisting of the ryanodine receptor (RyR) – a Ca^{2+} release channel, calsequestrin (CSQ), triadin, and junctin that is activated by L-type Ca^{2+} current [69; 70]. Aside from cytosolic Ca^{2+}, RyR activity is also regulated by SR luminal Ca^{2+} [71; 72]. Its storage and release are under the

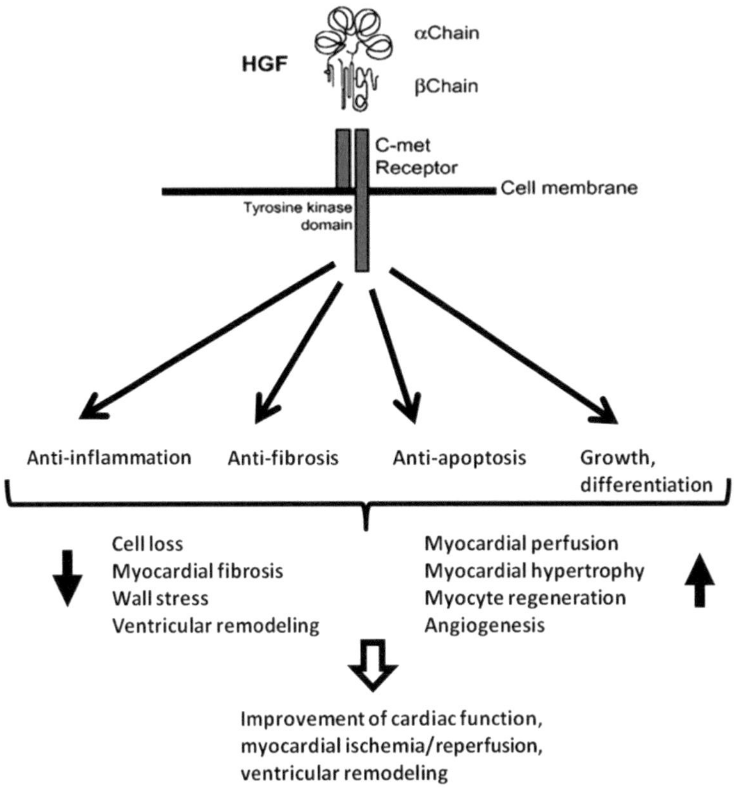

Figure 2. A schematic illustration of potential effects of HGF/c-Met in diabetic cardiomyopathy [24; 42].

control of CSQ [71], whereas triadin and junctin may serve as linker proteins between CSQ and the RyR [70; 73]. The tethering of CSQ to the inner surface of the SR allows it to sequester Ca^{2+} in the vicinity of the RyR during SR Ca^{2+} cycling [74]. CSQ may act as a Ca^{2+} sensor that inhibits the RyR at low SR luminal Ca^{2+} via interaction with triadin/junctin [75]. An increase of SR luminal Ca^{2+} disrupts the inhibition of the RyR because the CSQ Ca^{2+} binding sites become more occupied with Ca^{2+}, resulting in a weakened interaction between CSQ and triadin/junctin and an increased open probability of the channel [76]. Sorcin, a 22-kDa Ca^{2+}-binding protein, also binds to cardiac RyR with high affinity, and its interaction with RyR is facilitated by annexin A7 in a Ca^{2+}-dependent manner. Thus the interaction between these proteins appears to be critical for the regulation of SR Ca^{2+} release. For relaxation to occur, calcium ions must be removed from the cytosol, the majority of which is pumped back into the SR by cardiac specific SERCA2a (sarcoplasmic/endoplasmic reticulum Ca^{2+}-ATPase 2a), while the remainder is ejected out of the cell through the sarcolemmal NCX (Na^{2+}/Ca^{2+} exchange), PMCA (plasma-membrane Ca^{2+}-ATPase) or mitochondrial calcium uniport.

Cardiac specific ryanodine receptor 2 (RyR2), a Ca^{2+}-activated Ca^{2+} channel situated in the SR membrane, plays the dominant role in Ca^{2+} release from the SR in cardiac myocytes. In general, the RyR is a huge tetrameric protein with each monomer constituted of around 5000 amino

http://dx.doi.org/10.5772/55780

acids (Mw: 565 kDa). Three isoforms of RyR have been described in mammalian tissues (RyR1, RyR2 and RyR3) of which RyR2 is predominant in cardiac muscle. The RyR is a tetramer consisting of four subunits and forms a complex with other proteins of which the FK506-binding protein (FKBP), calsequestrin, triadin 1 and junctin were identified in cardiac muscle. FKBPs are known for immunosuppressive properties; however, members of this protein family, FKBP12 and FKBP12.6, also bind to the cytoplasmic part of the RyR in skeletal and cardiac muscle and seem to modulate the gating properties of the RyR. Calsequestrin is a 55-kDa high-capacity calcium binding protein located in the lumen of the cardiac or skeletal junctional SR storing the calcium to be released by the RyR. Both triadin and junctin are transmembrane proteins in the junctional SR which bind directly to the RyR and to calsequestrin suggesting that these proteins attach calsequestrin to the RyR. Initially, two functional cardiac isoforms of triadin with apparent molecular weights of 35 kDa (triadin 1) and 40 kDa (triadin 2) were cloned of which triadin 1 is predominant and representing more than 95% of cardiac triadin. Junctin was first identified as a 26-kDa calsequestrin-binding protein in cardiac and skeletal muscle. Triadin and junctin are encoded on different genes but exhibit structural and amino acid similarities with single membrane spanning domains (62% identity within this domain), short cytoplasmic N-terminal segments and long highly-charged basic C-terminal domains situated in the lumen of the SR [67; 68; 75; 77].

Indeed, several disorders of the SR Ca^{2+} release complex have been identified as causes of heart disease. Hyperphosphorylation of the RyR by PKA and Ca/Calmodulin-dependent protein kinase II (CaMKII) induces a Ca^{2+} leak during diastole, which can cause heart failure and lead to fatal arrhythmias [78; 79; 80; 81]. The forced expression of triadin or junctin in rat myocytes resulted in an increase of the RyR open probability or a depressed contractility, respectively [77; 82]. Consistently, the ablation of junctin was associated with enhanced cardiac function and increased Ca^{2+} cycling parameters in mice [83]. Similarly, overexpression of CSQ induces rapid development of heart failure in transgenic mice [84].

3.2. Calcium regulation abnormalities in diabetic cardiomyopathy

Predominantly, diabetic cardiomyopathy is related to diastolic abnormalities. In both Type 1 and Type 2 rodent models of diabetes, altered expression, activity and function of all transporters involved in excitation–contraction coupling, SERCA2a, NCX, and PMCA, leading to dysfunctional intracellular calcium signalling. In particular, abnormalities of SERCA2a, the major splice variant in the heart have been documented in diabetic cardiomyopathy. Protein, mRNA, and also activity of this protein decreases in response to diabetes [10].

Depressed SERCA activity causes inefficient sequestration of calcium in the SR, resulting in cytosolic calcium overload, impaired relaxation and hence diastolic dysfunction. On the other hand, cardiac overexpression of SERCA improves Ca^{2+} homeostasis and contraction in diabetic models [12; 85; 86; 87; 88; 89]. Because heart muscle from diabetic animals exhibits a diastolic dysfunction, SERCA2a has been considered a major site for contractile dysfunction. Indeed, perfusion of hearts with glucose can lead to lowered SERCA2a mRNA levels [2; 13]. Several factors may alter proteins regulating cardiomyocytes calcium homeostasis. The process of advanced glycation has been related directly to alterations in myocardial calcium handling and hence contractility. The advanced glycation of SERCA2a has been shown to lead to a decrease in its activity and a prolongation of cardiac relaxation [14].

Recently, attention has been focused on abnormalities of calcium release in diabetic conditions. In diabetic subjects, oxidative stress arises from an imbalance between production of reactive oxygen and nitrogen species and capability of the system to readily detoxify reactive intermediates. Importantly, it is now well established that RyR channels are highly susceptible to modification by various endogenous redox agents. Furthermore, RyR channels serve a role as intracellular redox sensors, via redox induced Ca2+ release and they are likely to connect cellular redox state with Ca2+ signaling cascades. Indeed, endogenous redox active molecules enhance RyR2 channel activity and RyR2 is one of the well-characterized redox-sensitive ion channels in heart. In general, oxidizing conditions increase RyR2 activity and so stimulate SR Ca^{2+} and causing Ca^{2+} leak (*see figure 3*). In addition, RyR2 is activated also by reactive nitrogen species and S-nitrosylation increases RyR open probability in cardiac muscle and leads to increased Ca^{2+} leak [14]. Redox reactions by biological oxidants and antioxidants have been shown to alter the kinetics of Ca^{2+}-induced Ca^{2+} release in the heart tissue. Besides several potential phosphorylation sites, the tetrameric RyR2 channel contains ~84 free thiols and is S-nitrosylated in vivo. S-Nitrosylation of up to 12 sites (3 per subunit) led to progressive channel activation that was reversed by denitrosylation. RyR2 is activated also by reactive nitrogen species. For example, nNOS is expressed in SR and can supply NO to RyR2 in the immediate vicinity for S-nitrosylation, which increases RyR2 open probability in cardiac muscle and leads to increased Ca^{2+} release. Thus, sulfydryl-oxidizing agents, hydrogen peroxide and diamide, diminished RyR2-FKBP12.6 binding [90].

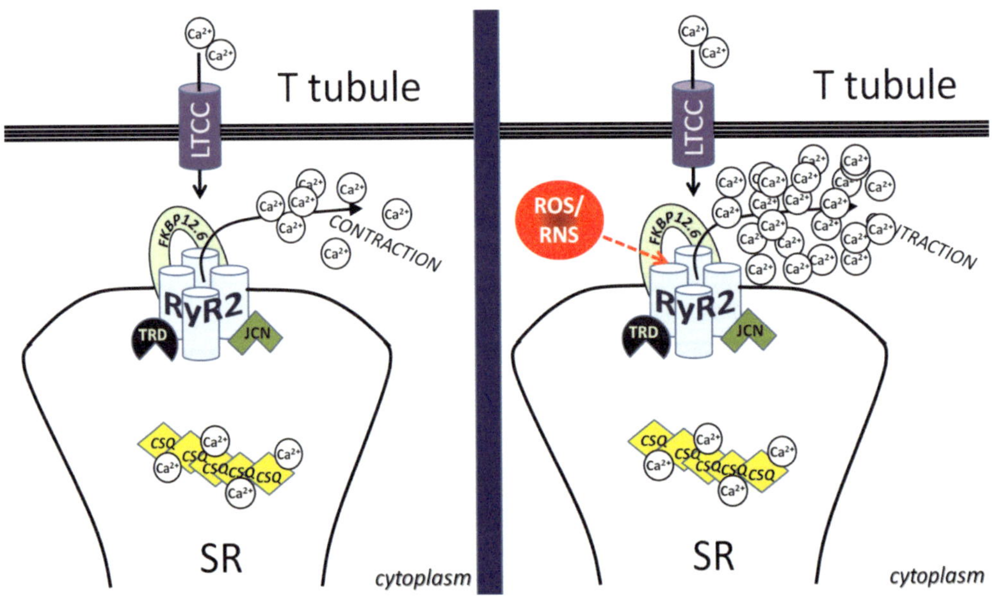

Figure 3. Intracellular calcium regulation and influence of oxidizing molecules (ROS, reactive oxygen species; RNS, reactive nitrogen species) on RyR2 function.

Modulation of cardiomyocyte Ca^{2+} handling by RyR2 is long known to occur by caffeine and tetracaine, which increase RyR2 open probability. More recently, flecainide was reported to prevent catecholamine polymorphic ventricular tachycardia as a result of decreasing RyR2 conductance and RyR2 open time RyR2s from these hearts were S-nitrosylated and depleted of FKBP12.6, resulting in leaky RyR2 channels and a diastolic SR-Ca^{2+} leak. Inhibiting the depletion of calstabin2 from the RyR2 complex with the Ca^{2+} channel stabilizer S107, a novel RyR2-specific benzothiazepine derivative compound, inhibited the SR-Ca^{2+} leak and prevented arrhythmias in vivo. Similarly in skeletal muscle, S107 which binds to RyR1 and recovers the binding of FKBP12.6 to the nitrosylated channel inhibits SR Ca^{2+} leak, improves muscle function, and increases exercise performance in muscular dystrophic-deficient mouse model [90; 91]. Taken together, these data opens new era of new drugs – stabilizers of RyR complex (rycals), in regulation of calcium in various cells what could have an impact also in treatment of diabetic cardiomyopathy in the future.

Acknowledgements

This article was supported by the grant EFSD New Horizons 2012 *The role of HGF/c-Met signalling in diabetic end-organ damage* from the European Foundation for the Study of Diabetes - New Horizons, Collaborative Research Initiative and the grant APVV-0887-11 *Molecular aspects of drug induced heart failure and ventricular arrhythmias* from the Slovak Research and Development Agency.

Author details

Jan Klimas

Department of Pharmacology and Toxicology, Faculty of Pharmacy, Comenius University in Bratislava, Slovak Republic

References

[1] Rubler S, Dlugash J, Yuceoglu YZ, Kumral T, Branwood AW, Grishman A, New type of cardiomyopathy associated with diabetic glomerulosclerosis. Am J Cardiol 30 (1972) 595-602.

[2] Boudina S, Abel ED, Diabetic cardiomyopathy revisited. Circulation 115 (2007) 3213-3223.

[3] Bell DS, Diabetic cardiomyopathy. Diabetes Care 26 (2003) 2949-2951.

[4] Kiencke S, Handschin R, von Dahlen R, Muser J, Brunner-Larocca HP, Schumann J, Felix B, Berneis K, Rickenbacher P, Pre-clinical diabetic cardiomyopathy: prevalence, screening, and outcome. Eur J Heart Fail 12 (2010) 951-957.

[5] Parving HH, Tarnow L, Rossing P, Genetics of diabetic nephropathy. J Am Soc Nephrol 7 (1996) 2509-2517.

[6] Bertoni AG, Hundley WG, Massing MW, Bonds DE, Burke GL, Goff DC, Jr., Heart failure prevalence, incidence, and mortality in the elderly with diabetes. Diabetes Care 27 (2004) 699-703.

[7] Thrainsdottir IS, Aspelund T, Thorgeirsson G, Gudnason V, Hardarson T, Malmberg K, Sigurdsson G, Ryden L, The association between glucose abnormalities and heart failure in the population-based Reykjavik study. Diabetes Care 28 (2005) 612-616.

[8] Kannel WB, Hjortland M, Castelli WP, Role of diabetes in congestive heart failure: the Framingham study. Am J Cardiol 34 (1974) 29-34.

[9] Kannel WB, McGee DL, Diabetes and cardiovascular disease. The Framingham study. JAMA 241 (1979) 2035-2038.

[10] Asghar O, Al-Sunni A, Khavandi K, Khavandi A, Withers S, Greenstein A, Heagerty AM, Malik RA, Diabetic cardiomyopathy. Clin Sci (Lond) 116 (2009) 741-760.

[11] Castagno D, Baird-Gunning J, Jhund PS, Biondi-Zoccai G, MacDonald MR, Petrie MC, Gaita F, McMurray JJ, Intensive glycemic control has no impact on the risk of heart failure in type 2 diabetic patients: evidence from a 37,229 patient meta-analysis. Am Heart J 162 (2011) 938-948 e932.

[12] Battiprolu PK, Gillette TG, Wang ZV, Lavandero S, Hill JA, Diabetic Cardiomyopathy: Mechanisms and Therapeutic Targets. Drug Discov Today Dis Mech 7 (2010) e135-e143.

[13] Young ME, McNulty P, Taegtmeyer H, Adaptation and maladaptation of the heart in diabetes: Part II: potential mechanisms. Circulation 105 (2002) 1861-1870.

[14] Hayat SA, Patel B, Khattar RS, Malik RA, Diabetic cardiomyopathy: mechanisms, diagnosis and treatment. Clin Sci (Lond) 107 (2004) 539-557.

[15] Jankyova S, Kmecova J, Cernecka H, Mesarosova L, Musil P, Brnoliakova Z, Kyselovic J, Babal P, Klimas J, Glucose and blood pressure lowering effects of Pycnogenol(R) are inefficient to prevent prolongation of QT interval in experimental diabetic cardiomyopathy. Pathol Res Pract 208 (2012) 452-457.

[16] Jankyova S, Kucera P, Goldenberg Z, Yaghi D, Navarova J, Kyselova Z, Stolc S, Klimas J, Racanska E, Matyas S, Pycnogenol efficiency on glycaemia, motor nerve conduction velocity and markers of oxidative stress in mild type diabetes in rats. Phytother Res 23 (2009) 1169-1174.

[17] Klimas J, Kmecova J, Jankyova S, Yaghi D, Priesolova E, Kyselova Z, Musil P, Ochodnicky P, Krenek P, Kyselovic J, Matyas S, Pycnogenol improves left ventricular

function in streptozotocin-induced diabetic cardiomyopathy in rats. Phytother Res 24 (2010) 969-974.

[18] Futamatsu H, Suzuki J, Mizuno S, Koga N, Adachi S, Kosuge H, Maejima Y, Hirao K, Nakamura T, Isobe M, Hepatocyte growth factor ameliorates the progression of experimental autoimmune myocarditis: a potential role for induction of T helper 2 cytokines. Circ Res 96 (2005) 823-830.

[19] Miyazawa K, Hepatocyte growth factor activator (HGFA): a serine protease that links tissue injury to activation of hepatocyte growth factor. FEBS J 277 (2010) 2208-2214.

[20] Madonna R, Cevik C, Nasser M, De Caterina R, Hepatocyte growth factor: molecular biomarker and player in cardioprotection and cardiovascular regeneration. Thromb Haemost 107 (2012) 656-661.

[21] Nakamura T, Nawa K, Ichihara A, Partial purification and characterization of hepatocyte growth factor from serum of hepatectomized rats. Biochem Biophys Res Commun 122 (1984) 1450-1459.

[22] Nakamura T, Nishizawa T, Hagiya M, Seki T, Shimonishi M, Sugimura A, Tashiro K, Shimizu S, Molecular cloning and expression of human hepatocyte growth factor. Nature 342 (1989) 440-443.

[23] Boros P, Miller CM, Hepatocyte growth factor: a multifunctional cytokine. Lancet 345 (1995) 293-295.

[24] Isobe M, Futamatsu H, Suzuki J, Hepatocyte growth factor: Effects on immune-mediated heart diseases. Trends Cardiovasc Med 16 (2006) 188-193.

[25] Itoh H, Naganuma S, Takeda N, Miyata S, Uchinokura S, Fukushima T, Uchiyama S, Tanaka H, Nagaike K, Shimomura T, Miyazawa K, Yamada G, Kitamura N, Koono M, Kataoka H, Regeneration of injured intestinal mucosa is impaired in hepatocyte growth factor activator-deficient mice. Gastroenterology 127 (2004) 1423-1435.

[26] Kataoka H, Kawaguchi M, Hepatocyte growth factor activator (HGFA): pathophysiological functions in vivo. FEBS J 277 (2010) 2230-2237.

[27] Birchmeier C, Birchmeier W, Gherardi E, Vande Woude GF, Met, metastasis, motility and more. Nat Rev Mol Cell Biol 4 (2003) 915-925.

[28] Boccaccio C, Comoglio PM, Invasive growth: a MET-driven genetic programme for cancer and stem cells. Nat Rev Cancer 6 (2006) 637-645.

[29] Peschard P, Park M, From Tpr-Met to Met, tumorigenesis and tubes. Oncogene 26 (2007) 1276-1285.

[30] Trusolino L, Comoglio PM, Scatter-factor and semaphorin receptors: cell signalling for invasive growth. Nat Rev Cancer 2 (2002) 289-300.

[31] Funakoshi H, Nakamura T, Hepatocyte growth factor: from diagnosis to clinical applications. Clin Chim Acta 327 (2003) 1-23.

[32] Bladt F, Riethmacher D, Isenmann S, Aguzzi A, Birchmeier C, Essential role for the c-met receptor in the migration of myogenic precursor cells into the limb bud. Nature 376 (1995) 768-771.

[33] Schmidt C, Bladt F, Goedecke S, Brinkmann V, Zschiesche W, Sharpe M, Gherardi E, Birchmeier C, Scatter factor/hepatocyte growth factor is essential for liver development. Nature 373 (1995) 699-702.

[34] Uehara Y, Minowa O, Mori C, Shiota K, Kuno J, Noda T, Kitamura N, Placental defect and embryonic lethality in mice lacking hepatocyte growth factor/scatter factor. Nature 373 (1995) 702-705.

[35] Woolf AS, Kolatsi-Joannou M, Hardman P, Andermarcher E, Moorby C, Fine LG, Jat PS, Noble MD, Gherardi E, Roles of hepatocyte growth factor/scatter factor and the met receptor in the early development of the metanephros. J Cell Biol 128 (1995) 171-184.

[36] Nakamura T, Mizuno S, Matsumoto K, Sawa Y, Matsuda H, Myocardial protection from ischemia/reperfusion injury by endogenous and exogenous HGF. J Clin Invest 106 (2000) 1511-1519.

[37] Ueda H, Nakamura T, Matsumoto K, Sawa Y, Matsuda H, A potential cardioprotective role of hepatocyte growth factor in myocardial infarction in rats. Cardiovasc Res 51 (2001) 41-50.

[38] Ono K, Matsumori A, Shioi T, Furukawa Y, Sasayama S, Enhanced expression of hepatocyte growth factor/c-Met by myocardial ischemia and reperfusion in a rat model. Circulation 95 (1997) 2552-2558.

[39] Ueno S, Ikeda U, Hojo Y, Arakawa H, Nonaka M, Yamamoto K, Shimada K, Serum hepatocyte growth factor levels are increased in patients with congestive heart failure. J Card Fail 7 (2001) 329-334.

[40] Urbanek K, Rota M, Cascapera S, Bearzi C, Nascimbene A, De Angelis A, Hosoda T, Chimenti S, Baker M, Limana F, Nurzynska D, Torella D, Rotatori F, Rastaldo R, Musso E, Quaini F, Leri A, Kajstura J, Anversa P, Cardiac stem cells possess growth factor-receptor systems that after activation regenerate the infarcted myocardium, improving ventricular function and long-term survival. Circ Res 97 (2005) 663-673.

[41] Aoki M, Morishita R, Taniyama Y, Kida I, Moriguchi A, Matsumoto K, Nakamura T, Kaneda Y, Higaki J, Ogihara T, Angiogenesis induced by hepatocyte growth factor in non-infarcted myocardium and infarcted myocardium: up-regulation of essential transcription factor for angiogenesis, ets. Gene Ther 7 (2000) 417-427.

[42] Jin H, Wyss JM, Yang R, Schwall R, The therapeutic potential of hepatocyte growth factor for myocardial infarction and heart failure. Curr Pharm Des 10 (2004) 2525-2533.

[43] Gonzalez A, Rota M, Nurzynska D, Misao Y, Tillmanns J, Ojaimi C, Padin-Iruegas ME, Muller P, Esposito G, Bearzi C, Vitale S, Dawn B, Sanganalmath SK, Baker M, Hintze TH, Bolli R, Urbanek K, Hosoda T, Anversa P, Kajstura J, Leri A, Activation of cardiac progenitor cells reverses the failing heart senescent phenotype and prolongs lifespan. Circ Res 102 (2008) 597-606.

[44] Linke A, Muller P, Nurzynska D, Casarsa C, Torella D, Nascimbene A, Castaldo C, Cascapera S, Bohm M, Quaini F, Urbanek K, Leri A, Hintze TH, Kajstura J, Anversa P, Stem cells in the dog heart are self-renewing, clonogenic, and multipotent and regenerate infarcted myocardium, improving cardiac function. Proc Natl Acad Sci U S A 102 (2005) 8966-8971.

[45] Lamblin N, Susen S, Dagorn J, Mouquet F, Jude B, Van Belle E, Bauters C, de Groote P, Prognostic significance of circulating levels of angiogenic cytokines in patients with congestive heart failure. Am Heart J 150 (2005) 137-143.

[46] Lamblin N, Bauters A, Fertin M, de Groote P, Pinet F, Bauters C, Circulating levels of hepatocyte growth factor and left ventricular remodelling after acute myocardial infarction (from the REVE-2 study). Eur J Heart Fail 13 (2011) 1314-1322.

[47] Rychli K, Richter B, Hohensinner PJ, Kariem Mahdy A, Neuhold S, Zorn G, Berger R, Mortl D, Huber K, Pacher R, Wojta J, Niessner A, Hulsmann M, Hepatocyte growth factor is a strong predictor of mortality in patients with advanced heart failure. Heart 97 (2011) 1158-1163.

[48] Anan F, Masaki T, Yonemochi H, Takahashi N, Nakagawa M, Eshima N, Saikawa T, Yoshimatsu H, Hepatocyte growth factor levels are associated with the results of 123I-metaiodobenzylguanidine myocardial scintigraphy in patients with type 2 diabetes mellitus. Metabolism 58 (2009) 167-173.

[49] Ueda T, Takeyama Y, Toyokawa A, Kishida S, Yamamoto M, Saitoh Y, Significant elevation of serum human hepatocyte growth factor levels in patients with acute pancreatitis. Pancreas 12 (1996) 76-83.

[50] Wang Y, Moreira MD, Khan A, Heringer-Walther S, Schultheiss HP, Wessel N, Siems WE, Walther T, Prognostic Significance of Circulating Levels of Hepatocyte Growth Factor in Patients with Chagas' Disease and Idiopathic Dilated Cardiomyopathy. Cardiology 121 (2012) 240-246.

[51] Fountoulaki K, Parissis J, Hepatocyte Growth Factor as a Prognostic Marker in Heart Failure: Promise and Challenges. Cardiology 121 (2012) 237-239.

[52] Segers VF, Lee RT, Protein therapeutics for cardiac regeneration after myocardial infarction. J Cardiovasc Transl Res 3 (2010) 469-477.

[53] Kondoh H, Sawa Y, Fukushima N, Matsumiya G, Miyagawa S, Kitagawa-Sakakida S, Imanishi Y, Kawaguchi N, Matsuura N, Matsuda H, Combined strategy using myoblasts and hepatocyte growth factor in dilated cardiomyopathic hamsters. Ann Thorac Surg 84 (2007) 134-141.

[54] Kondoh H, Sawa Y, Fukushima N, Matsumiya G, Miyagawa S, Kitagawa-Sakakida S, Memon IA, Kawaguchi N, Matsuura N, Matsuda H, Reorganization of cytoskeletal proteins and prolonged life expectancy caused by hepatocyte growth factor in a hamster model of late-phase dilated cardiomyopathy. J Thorac Cardiovasc Surg 130 (2005) 295-302.

[55] Taniyama Y, Morishita R, Aoki M, Hiraoka K, Yamasaki K, Hashiya N, Matsumoto K, Nakamura T, Kaneda Y, Ogihara T, Angiogenesis and antifibrotic action by hepatocyte growth factor in cardiomyopathy. Hypertension 40 (2002) 47-53.

[56] Li Y, Takemura G, Kosai K, Yuge K, Nagano S, Esaki M, Goto K, Takahashi T, Hayakawa K, Koda M, Kawase Y, Maruyama R, Okada H, Minatoguchi S, Mizuguchi H, Fujiwara T, Fujiwara H, Postinfarction treatment with an adenoviral vector expressing hepatocyte growth factor relieves chronic left ventricular remodeling and dysfunction in mice. Circulation 107 (2003) 2499-2506.

[57] Iwasaki M, Adachi Y, Nishiue T, Minamino K, Suzuki Y, Zhang Y, Nakano K, Koike Y, Wang J, Mukaide H, Taketani S, Yuasa F, Tsubouchi H, Gohda E, Iwasaka T, Ikehara S, Hepatocyte growth factor delivered by ultrasound-mediated destruction of microbubbles induces proliferation of cardiomyocytes and amelioration of left ventricular contractile function in Doxorubicin-induced cardiomyopathy. Stem Cells 23 (2005) 1589-1597.

[58] Esaki M, Takemura G, Kosai K, Takahashi T, Miyata S, Li L, Goto K, Maruyama R, Okada H, Kanamori H, Ogino A, Ushikoshi H, Minatoguchi S, Fujiwara T, Fujiwara H, Treatment with an adenoviral vector encoding hepatocyte growth factor mitigates established cardiac dysfunction in doxorubicin-induced cardiomyopathy. Am J Physiol Heart Circ Physiol 294 (2008) H1048-1057.

[59] Okayama K, Azuma J, Dosaka N, Iekushi K, Sanada F, Kusunoki H, Iwabayashi M, Rakugi H, Taniyama Y, Morishita R, Hepatocyte growth factor reduces cardiac fibrosis by inhibiting endothelial-mesenchymal transition. Hypertension 59 (2012) 958-965.

[60] Rastogi S, Guerrero M, Wang M, Ilsar I, Sabbah MS, Gupta RC, Sabbah HN, Myocardial transfection with naked DNA plasmid encoding hepatocyte growth factor prevents the progression of heart failure in dogs. Am J Physiol Heart Circ Physiol 300 (2011) H1501-1509.

[61] Ahmet I, Sawa Y, Iwata K, Matsuda H, Gene transfection of hepatocyte growth factor attenuates cardiac remodeling in the canine heart: A novel gene therapy for cardiomyopathy. J Thorac Cardiovasc Surg 124 (2002) 957-963.

[62] Yang ZJ, Xu SL, Chen B, Zhang SL, Zhang YL, Wei W, Ma DC, Wang LS, Zhu TB, Li CJ, Wang H, Cao KJ, Gao W, Huang J, Ma WZ, Wu ZZ, Hepatocyte growth factor plays a critical role in the regulation of cytokine production and induction of endothelial progenitor cell mobilization: a pilot gene therapy study in patients with coronary heart disease. Clin Exp Pharmacol Physiol 36 (2009) 790-796.

[63] Nakamura S, Moriguchi A, Morishita R, Aoki M, Yo Y, Hayashi S, Nakano N, Katsuya T, Nakata S, Takami S, Matsumoto K, Nakamura T, Higaki J, Ogihara T, A novel vascular modulator, hepatocyte growth factor (HGF), as a potential index of the severity of hypertension. Biochem Biophys Res Commun 242 (1998) 238-243.

[64] Morishita R, Aoki M, Hashiya N, Yamasaki K, Kurinami H, Shimizu S, Makino H, Takesya Y, Azuma J, Ogihara T, Therapeutic angiogenesis using hepatocyte growth factor (HGF). Curr Gene Ther 4 (2004) 199-206.

[65] Kulseng B, Borset M, Espevik T, Sundan A, Elevated hepatocyte growth factor in sera from patients with insulin-dependent diabetes mellitus. Acta Diabetol 35 (1998) 77-80.

[66] Fleckenstein A, Janke J, Doring HJ, Leder O, Myocardial fiber necrosis due to intracellular Ca overload-a new principle in cardiac pathophysiology. Recent Adv Stud Cardiac Struct Metab 4 (1974) 563-580.

[67] Kirchhefer U, Klimas J, Baba HA, Buchwalow IB, Fabritz L, Huls M, Matus M, Muller FU, Schmitz W, Neumann J, Triadin is a critical determinant of cellular Ca cycling and contractility in the heart. Am J Physiol Heart Circ Physiol 293 (2007) H3165-3174.

[68] Kirchhof P, Klimas J, Fabritz L, Zwiener M, Jones LR, Schafers M, Hermann S, Boknik P, Schmitz W, Breithardt G, Kirchhefer U, Neumann J, Stress and high heart rate provoke ventricular tachycardia in mice expressing triadin. J Mol Cell Cardiol 42 (2007) 962-971.

[69] Bers DM, Cardiac excitation-contraction coupling. Nature 415 (2002) 198-205.

[70] Zhang L, Kelley J, Schmeisser G, Kobayashi YM, Jones LR, Complex formation between junctin, triadin, calsequestrin, and the ryanodine receptor. Proteins of the cardiac junctional sarcoplasmic reticulum membrane. J Biol Chem 272 (1997) 23389-23397.

[71] Gyorke S, Gyorke I, Lukyanenko V, Terentyev D, Viatchenko-Karpinski S, Wiesner TF, Regulation of sarcoplasmic reticulum calcium release by luminal calcium in cardiac muscle. Front Biosci 7 (2002) d1454-1463.

[72] Shannon TR, Wang F, Bers DM, Regulation of cardiac sarcoplasmic reticulum Ca release by luminal [Ca] and altered gating assessed with a mathematical model. Biophys J 89 (2005) 4096-4110.

[73] Kobayashi YM, Alseikhan BA, Jones LR, Localization and characterization of the calsequestrin-binding domain of triadin 1. Evidence for a charged beta-strand in mediating the protein-protein interaction. J Biol Chem 275 (2000) 17639-17646.

[74] Jones LR, Suzuki YJ, Wang W, Kobayashi YM, Ramesh V, Franzini-Armstrong C, Cleemann L, Morad M, Regulation of Ca2+ signaling in transgenic mouse cardiac myocytes overexpressing calsequestrin. J Clin Invest 101 (1998) 1385-1393.

[75] Terentyev D, Viatchenko-Karpinski S, Vedamoorthyrao S, Oduru S, Gyorke I, Williams SC, Gyorke S, Protein protein interactions between triadin and calsequestrin are involved in modulation of sarcoplasmic reticulum calcium release in cardiac myocytes. J Physiol 583 (2007) 71-80.

[76] Gyorke I, Hester N, Jones LR, Gyorke S, The role of calsequestrin, triadin, and junctin in conferring cardiac ryanodine receptor responsiveness to luminal calcium. Biophys J 86 (2004) 2121-2128.

[77] Gergs U, Berndt T, Buskase J, Jones LR, Kirchhefer U, Muller FU, Schluter KD, Schmitz W, Neumann J, On the role of junctin in cardiac Ca2+ handling, contractility, and heart failure. Am J Physiol Heart Circ Physiol 293 (2007) H728-734.

[78] Maier LS, Bers DM, Role of Ca2+/calmodulin-dependent protein kinase (CaMK) in excitation-contraction coupling in the heart. Cardiovasc Res 73 (2007) 631-640.

[79] Maier LS, Zhang T, Chen L, DeSantiago J, Brown JH, Bers DM, Transgenic CaMKII-deltaC overexpression uniquely alters cardiac myocyte Ca2+ handling: reduced SR Ca2+ load and activated SR Ca2+ release. Circ Res 92 (2003) 904-911.

[80] Marx SO, Reiken S, Hisamatsu Y, Jayaraman T, Burkhoff D, Rosemblit N, Marks AR, PKA phosphorylation dissociates FKBP12.6 from the calcium release channel (ryanodine receptor): defective regulation in failing hearts. Cell 101 (2000) 365-376.

[81] Wehrens XH, Lehnart SE, Reiken S, Vest JA, Wronska A, Marks AR, Ryanodine receptor/calcium release channel PKA phosphorylation: a critical mediator of heart failure progression. Proc Natl Acad Sci U S A 103 (2006) 511-518.

[82] Terentyev D, Cala SE, Houle TD, Viatchenko-Karpinski S, Gyorke I, Terentyeva R, Williams SC, Gyorke S, Triadin overexpression stimulates excitation-contraction coupling and increases predisposition to cellular arrhythmia in cardiac myocytes. Circ Res 96 (2005) 651-658.

[83] Yuan Q, Fan GC, Dong M, Altschafl B, Diwan A, Ren X, Hahn HH, Zhao W, Waggoner JR, Jones LR, Jones WK, Bers DM, Dorn GW, 2nd, Wang HS, Valdivia HH, Chu G, Kranias EG, Sarcoplasmic reticulum calcium overloading in junctin deficiency enhances cardiac contractility but increases ventricular automaticity. Circulation 115 (2007) 300-309.

[84] Knollmann BC, Knollmann-Ritschel BE, Weissman NJ, Jones LR, Morad M, Remodelling of ionic currents in hypertrophied and failing hearts of transgenic mice overexpressing calsequestrin. J Physiol 525 Pt 2 (2000) 483-498.

[85] Golfman L, Dixon IM, Takeda N, Lukas A, Dakshinamurti K, Dhalla NS, Cardiac sarcolemmal Na(+)-Ca2+ exchange and Na(+)-K+ ATPase activities and gene expression in alloxan-induced diabetes in rats. Mol Cell Biochem 188 (1998) 91-101.

[86] Hattori Y, Matsuda N, Kimura J, Ishitani T, Tamada A, Gando S, Kemmotsu O, Kanno M, Diminished function and expression of the cardiac Na+-Ca2+ exchanger in diabetic rats: implication in Ca2+ overload. J Physiol 527 Pt 1 (2000) 85-94.

[87] Pereira L, Matthes J, Schuster I, Valdivia HH, Herzig S, Richard S, Gomez AM, Mechanisms of [Ca2+]i transient decrease in cardiomyopathy of db/db type 2 diabetic mice. Diabetes 55 (2006) 608-615.

[88] Poornima IG, Parikh P, Shannon RP, Diabetic cardiomyopathy: the search for a unifying hypothesis. Circ Res 98 (2006) 596-605.

[89] Trost SU, Belke DD, Bluhm WF, Meyer M, Swanson E, Dillmann WH, Overexpression of the sarcoplasmic reticulum Ca(2+)-ATPase improves myocardial contractility in diabetic cardiomyopathy. Diabetes 51 (2002) 1166-1171.

[90] Turan B, Vassort G, Ryanodine receptor: a new therapeutic target to control diabetic cardiomyopathy. Antioxid Redox Signal 15 (2011) 1847-1861.

[91] Fauconnier J, Thireau J, Reiken S, Cassan C, Richard S, Matecki S, Marks AR, Lacampagne A, Leaky RyR2 trigger ventricular arrhythmias in Duchenne muscular dystrophy. Proc Natl Acad Sci U S A 107 (2010) 1559-1564.

Chapter 13

Cardiomyopathy in Women: Second Heart Failure

Kenneth J. McLeod and Carolyn Pierce

Additional information is available at the end of the chapter

http://dx.doi.org/10.5772/55433

1. Introduction

Heart failure is characterized by the inability of the heart to maintain sufficient cardiac output (CO) to meet the metabolic demands of the body. Reduced CO activates compensatory mechanisms directed towards reestablishing CO, thereby initiating a cycle which can lead to cardiomyopathy. Therapeutic strategies for addressing heart failure have been developed primarily based on studies of male populations; however, heart failure in women has a distinct phenotype. In women, heart failure develops later in life, generally presents with preserved systolic function, and is less commonly attributable to ischemic heart disease. In many women, the initiating event in heart failure is extrinsic, specifically, poor venous return resulting from inadequate calf muscle (soleus) pump activity during upright posture. Such "second heart" failure has been identified in approximately half of all adult women, an observation which helps to explain the fact that while women's survival rate with heart failure is better than in men, their quality of life with heart failure is far worse. A determination that inadequate venous return is arising from calf muscle pump failure can permit effective early intervention to slow or reverse cardiomyopathy, while significantly improving quality of life in affected women.

2. Extrinsic cardiomyopathy

Cardiomyopathies are a group of diseases of the myocardium reflecting mechanical and/or electrical dysfunction of the heart [1], and can be delineated as being either intrinsic or extrinsic. Intrinsic cardiomyopathies are those which originate in the heart muscle cells, and includes both conditions which typically influence the cardiac muscle cells alone (primary cardiomyopathy) and systemic disorders which affect other tissues in the body in addition to cardiac muscle tissue (secondary cardiomyopathy). Primary cardiomyopathies are commonly genetic or acquired (e.g. inflammatory, physical stress, or physiologic stress induced). Secondary cardiomyopathies span a broad spectrum of etiologies including inflammation, toxicity, infiltrative, endocrine, nutritional, autoimmune, electrolyte imbalance, and neuromuscular.

In contrast, extrinsic cardiomyopathies arise due to conditions which do not directly produce heart muscle cell abnormalities. These include the well known conditions of ischemia, hypertension, diabetes, and alcohol abuse, but also the less commonly considered condition of insufficient venous return. Insufficient venous return results in inadequate atrial filling and a correspondingly decreased CO. Decreased CO initiates a range of compensatory responses which eventually lead to progressive heart failure. Lower limb edema, as well as ascites development, are eblematic of inadequate fluid return to the right atrium, and fatigue is common as the heart cannot maintain sufficient CO to meet the body's metabolic needs. Nausea and loss of appetite arise as blood is shifted from the gastrointestinal tract to the vital organs, and palpitations occur as the heart adapts to reduced stroke volume by increasing the heart rate [2]. This latter compensatory mechanism induces cardiac stress and systolic hypertension, eventually leading to cardiomyopathy.

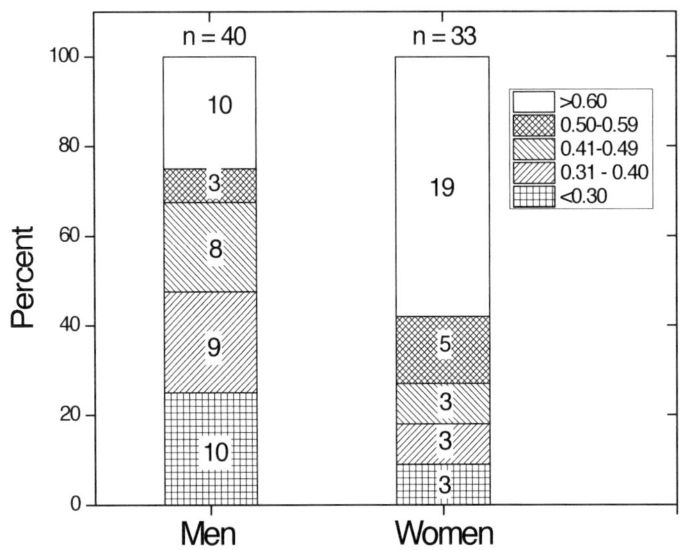

Figure 1. Left ventricular ejection fraction in men and women with congestive heart failure. *After Vasan, et al.1999.*

Heart failure arising from inadequate fluid return to the heart is most commonly experienced by women. It is well recognized that while half of heart failure patients are women [3], the characteristics of heart failure in women differ substantially from those observed in men. Specifically, heart failure develops later in life in women, is commonly associated with preserved systolic function (Figure 1) [4], less commonly involves ischemia, and, while survival rates are higher than for men, women with heart failure have a far worse quality of life [5]. The crucial link between maintaining adequate fluid return, and therefore cardiac output, and heart failure is reflected in the ability of resting heart rate to strongly and independently predict coronary events in women [6]. In a recent study of over 100,000 postmenopausal women, resting heart rate was found to predict myocardial infarction or coronary death with a risk ration of 1.6 (95% confidence interval of 1.49-1.89) when comparing the highest (>76 bpm) to the lowest (<62 bpm) quintiles of resting heart rate.

3. Anatomic and physiologic influences on venous and lymphatic return

When ventricular function is preserved, the critical factor regulating CO is end-diastolic volume, which, through the Frank-Starling mechanism provides a non-neural, non-humorally mediated, regulation of stroke volume. End-diastolic volume is a function of venous and lymphatic return to the heart, which correspondingly, are dependent on circulatory system volume and venous/lymphatic system pressure. The importance of lymphatic return is not widely appreciated in the context of maintenance of circulatory volume, and venous pressure is often considered only in the context of high venous pressure being an indicator of heart failure. However, to fully understand extrinsic heart failure it is necessary to consider the profound influence of upright posture on venous and lymphatic return.

In supine posture, fluid pressures in the arterial system are approximately 100 mmHg, and pressures in the venous system range from 15-20 mmHg in the smallest vessels to approximately 5 mmHg at the right atrium. The driving pressure to return venous blood back to the heart is therefore only 10-15 mmHg, or approximately 13-20 cm of water. Nonetheless, in the supine position this pressure is typically adequate to return venous blood from the lowest part of the body (typically the buttocks) back to the heart. In the upright position, however, hydrostatic forces (i.e. gravitational forces operating on the venous fluid column) add significantly to arterial, venous, and capillary pressures. At the right atrium, fluid pressure drops to zero. Above the atrium, venous pressures become negative, venous blood readily flows back to the heart and the veins collapse. At the same time, hydrostatic forces serve to reduce arterial pressures by 40mmHg at the top of the head, and if this reduces arterial pressure below 60 mmHg, regulation of cerebral perfusion can be significantly affected [7].

Below the heart, venous pressure increases progressively with distance below the heart such that at the level of the feet venous pressure can exceed 100 mmHg; yet the driving return pressure (i.e. capillary pressure) remains at approximately 20 mmHg. Moreover, blood return to the heart must take place through the highly distensible venous system so that the volume of the venous system has the potential to increase significantly in upright posture. Hydrostatic effects also increase pressures in the arterial system below the heart, though the thick walled structure of arteries prevents significant dilation. However, the increased pressures in the capillaries result in increased extravasation, resulting in significant pooling of interstitial fluid until interstitial fluid pressures increase to match capillary pressures (Figure 2) [8].

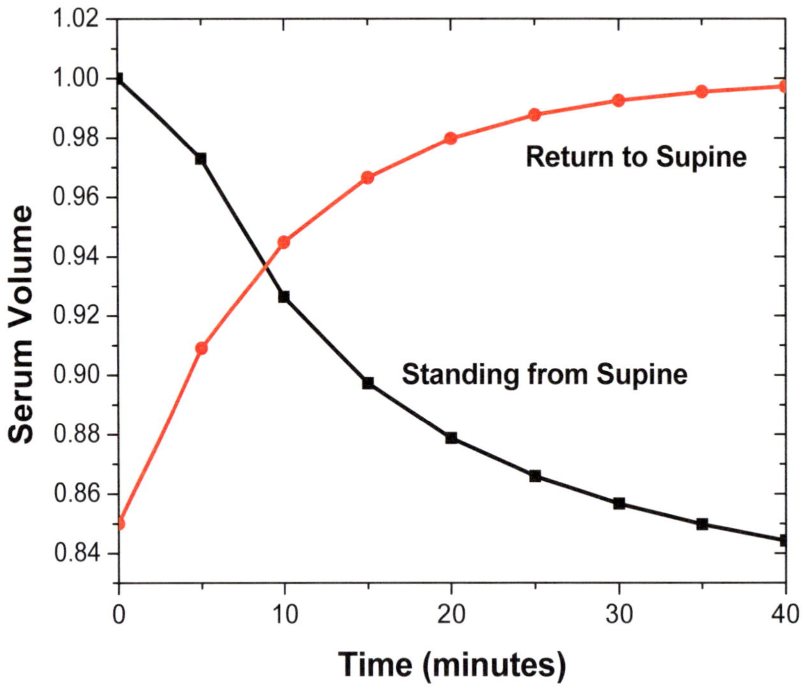

Figure 2. Fractional blood volume changes associated with postural shifts in young adult men. *After Hagan, et al., (1978) J. Appl. Physiol. 45:414-417*

The net effect of these various processes is that 500-600 ml of blood pools into the lower limb veins within 2-3 minutes after attaining upright posture, while increased filtration from the capillaries reduces blood fluid volume by an additional 750 ml over the following 30-40 minutes, resulting in well over 1L decrease in effective circulatory system volume. The upright human therefore is confronted with three significant challenges with respect to maintaining adequate CO. First, fluid pooling into the lower limb veins and dependent tissues rapidly reduces effective blood fluid volume. Second, the fluid pressure available to return blood to the heart from the lower extremities remains at little more than 20 mmHg, which is incapable of overcoming the 80 mmHg of hydrostatic pressure created by the venous fluid column. Third, the high compliance of human skin allows these conditions to become exacerbated over the course of the day through interstitial fluid build up. This stress of upright posture is particularly challenging for women in that they have both more compliant veins [9], and somewhat more compliant skin [10].

4. Soleus muscle anatomy/physiology

The cardiovascular challenges of upright posture are, in part, overcome by neuro-humorally mediated venoconstriction which limits venous pooling, though vasoconstriction has essentially no effect on interstitial fluid pooling nor on venous and lymphatic return pressures. Further, during locomotion it is well recognized that skeletal muscle pumping serves to drive venous blood back to the heart; however, for most people, for the vast majority of the time they are in upright posture, they are either standing or sitting quietly, not in ambulation. Correspondingly, the essential features of human physiology which permits long-term upright posture are the second heart (soleus muscle) combined with competent venous and lymphatic valves. In upright posture (sitting or standing) venous pressure alone is sufficient to pump blood only one-third of the distance up the lower leg. This blood then collects in the venous sinuses of the soleus muscle. These sinuses are large, thin-walled veins which have the capacity to hold large volumes of blood and the soleus muscle can have up to 18 such sinuses [11]. While the sinuses themselves are valveless, the indirect perforating veins feeding the sinuses are valved, as well as the posterior tibial and peroneal veins into which the soleus sinuses drain. These valves play a crucial role in the effectiveness of the calf muscle pump (CMP), providing an opportunity for the pump to incrementally force venous blood back to the heart. Importantly, the soleus is a deep postural muscle, and correspondingly is composed of more than 70% slow-twitch muscle fibers [12]. Moreover, the soleus originates on the posterior tibia and fibula such that when either standing or seated the muscle is able to be active, producing slow, continuous rhythmic, involuntary contractions. During contraction, the soleus can generate venous driving forces exceeding 200 mmHg, more than sufficient to force the blood in the sinuses back to the heart [13].

The soleus also plays an essential role in ensuring lymphatic drainage back to the heart. Collecting lymphatics, which appear downstream in the lymphatic system, contain smooth muscle cells in the media and therefore the ability for spontaneous contractions sufficiently large to pump lymph fluid back to the heart (fluid pressures in the collecting lymphatics is relatively low as the fluid column is not continuous) [14]. However, the initial lymphatics, which are the site of interstitial fluid absorption, are non-muscular, and so require an extrinsic force in the surrounding tissue to create a periodic driving pressure gradient. This force can arise from arterial pressure pulsations and arteriolar vasomotion, and muscle contraction. In the lower limbs, the involuntary contractile activity of the soleus, which typically is the sole active muscle in the lower leg during quiet sitting or standing, therefore provides a critical extrinsic periodic compression of these lymphatics, driving the lymph fluid in the initial lymphatics upward toward the collecting lymphatics, relying on endothelial microvalves to ensure unidirectional flow.

5. Second heart failure in women

The essential role of non-locomotory based calf muscle pumping (i.e. second heart activity) in maintaining CO when individuals are in quiet upright posture, raises the question of the extent to which second heart activity varies within the population. Recent studies in our laboratory have focused on identifying the extent of second heart insufficiency in adults, with a particular focus on the prevalence of second heart failure in women. The predictive ability of resting heart rate in identifying women at greatest risk of experiencing coronary events suggests that tracking heart rate during the transition from standing to quiet sitting should be an effective means to quantify second heart capability. Moving from a standing to seated position represents a decrease in both physical stress on the cardiovascular system (i.e. a reduction in the hydrostatic forces operating on the venous fluid column and therefore a reduction in pooling forces), and a reduction in physiologic stress (i.e. reduced metabolic activity). Quiet sitting, therefore, should result in a decrease in heart rate in otherwise healthy individuals.

We monitored heart rate in adult women (N=20) for 20 minutes following a transition from standing to quiet sitting [15]. Initial heart rate in this population of self-reported healthy women (average age = 52±4 years) was 77.5±3.5 bpm. In nine of these women (45%), heart rate decreased 1-8 bpm as expected (Figure 3) [15]. However, in 55% of the tested women (N=11), 20 minutes of quiet sitting led to a 6-12 bpm increase in heart rate (avg. 8.3 ± 0.5 bpm). Consistent with this increase in resting heart rate, brachial systolic blood pressure in this group of women was observed to fall by average 9.5 ± 1.8mmHg from an initial average pressure of 122.4 mmHg (±3.6 mmHg).

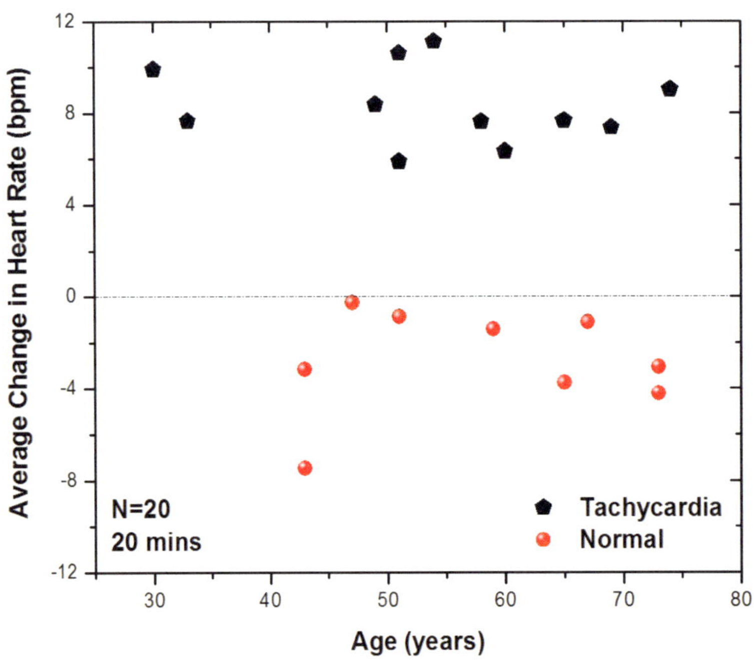

Figure 3. Change in systolic blood pressure in healthy adult women following 20 minutes of quiet sitting. *From Madhavan, et al., 2005.*

Though approximately 50 percent of women appear to be able to maintain adequate fluid return from the lower limbs to support CO during 20 minutes of quiet sitting, 20 minutes is a

http://dx.doi.org/10.5772/55433

relatively short time period in the context of typical durations of sitting which most individuals experience during the day, and so does not directly address the challenge women face during extended upright posture given the high venous and skin compliances previously discussed. To address the impact of extended orthostatic stress, we have monitored beat-to-beat blood pressure changes during quiet sitting periods of over 30 minutes [16]. This research was motivated by recent reports of delayed orthostatic hypotension (DOH), a condition observed in 40% of individuals with symptoms of orthostatic intolerance, but with no evidence of acute orthostatic hypotension as assessed through traditional tilt-table testing [17]. We have observed that among women who appear to be able to maintain CO during quiet sitting, for approximately 30% of such women this capability is transient. We observe in these women that following 20-30 minutes of sustained quiet sitting, fluid return to the heart rapidly falls and resting blood pressure cannot be maintained (Figure 4) [16]. This inability to maintain resting blood pressure is particularly striking with respect to diastolic pressure as the average diastolic pressure in this group was found to fall to an average of 53 mmHg (±0.9mmHg) after 30 minutes of quiet sitting (Figure 5) [16], a value well below that necessary to adequately regulate cerebral perfusion.

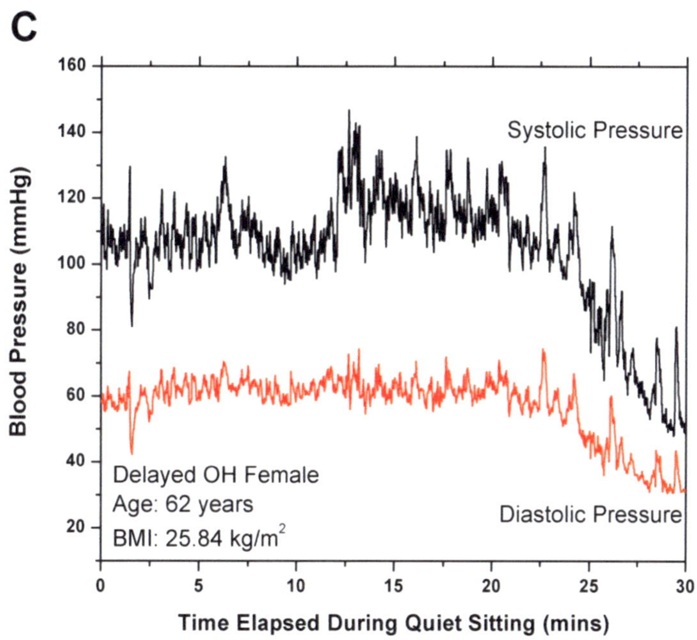

Figure 4. Typical blood pressure response to 30 minutes of quiet sitting in an adult woman with delayed orthostatic hypotension. *From Madhavan et al., 2008.*

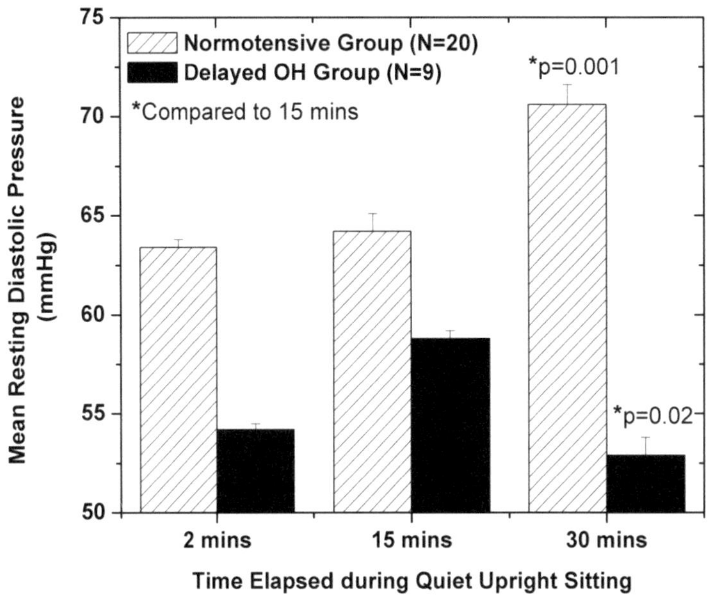

Figure 5. Time dependent changes in resting diastolic blood pressure in 29 adult women capable of maintaining HR and BP for the first 20 minutes of quiet sitting. Twenty women (70%) demonstrated a normotensive response to 30 minutes of the orthostatic stress of quiet sitting, while 9 (30%) demonstrated a distinct delayed orthostatic hypotensive response. *From Madhavan, et al., 2008.*

Similarly, a large fraction of women have been observed to experience extensive interstitial fluid pooling during quiet sitting. The high compliance of human skin, and women's skin in particular, creates a scenario in which extended duration orthostatic stress can permit extensive extravasation from the blood supply without the development of high tissue pressures which would inhibit this flow. To determine the extent to which this phenomenon could play a significant role in reducing fluid return to the heart, and correspondingly, maintaining CO, we utilized air plethysmography to follow calf volume over time in healthy adult women sitting quietly [18]. Fifty-four adult women (average age 46.7 ± 1.5 years) were recruited. After being placed in the supine position, the right calf was instrumented for air-pleythsmographic recording and the recording system was allowed to equilibrate to body temperature (approximately 30 minutes). The subject was then transitioned to the upright seated position and calf

http://dx.doi.org/10.5772/55433

volume was continuously monitored for another 30 minutes. Two distinct subpopulations could be readily delineated according to their interstitial pooling behavior (Figure 6) [18]. Approximately half of the women experienced a significant decrease in calf fluid volume during the 30 minutes of quiet sitting at a median rate of 8 ml/hour, while half demonstrated significant calf swelling at a median rate of 12 ml/hour under these conditions.

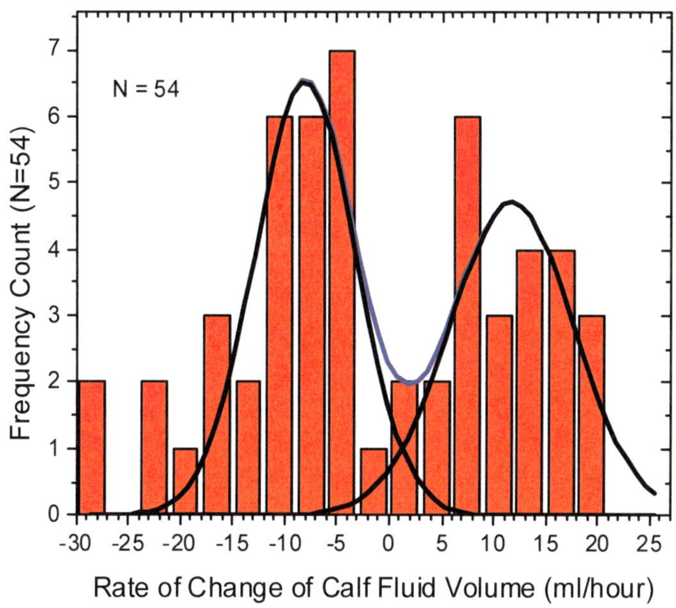

Figure 6. Interstitial fluid swelling of the calf during quiet sitting in a population (N=54) of healthy adult women. Bimodal distribution of pooling responses indicates that 55% of the subjects experienced decreased calf fluid volume while 45% were found to pool interstitial fluid into the calf at an average rate of 12ml/Hr. *From Goddard et al., 2008.*

While women who experience increased venous and interstitial pooling tend to be somewhat heavier, on average, than those that maintained their HR, BP, and calf volume during extended sitting, no significant differences in age, weight, or BMI have been identified. Moreover, these individuals do not demonstrate any frank failure of the circulatory system as measured by microvascular filtration rate, venous ejection fraction, venous filling index, or calf venous volume. Importantly, these responses do not reflect the behavior of just a small subset of women, but rather 50% or more of an otherwise healthy population of women. The most likely explanation for these observations appears to be inadequate calf muscle pump (second heart) activity, though this can only be confirmed through direct intervention by second heart stimulation.

6. Intervention for second heart failure

The soleus muscle operates primarily as an involuntary postural muscle whose activity is mediated by two different reflex arcs. In addition to the stretch reflex associated with venous sinus filling and emptying, the soleus is the primary lower leg muscle supporting upright stance. As such, its activity is mediated by a postural reflex arc originating on the frontal plantar surface. That is, pressure on the frontal aspect of the plantar surface during standing results in contraction of the soleus which pulls the body in the posterior direction; this unloads the frontal plantar surface, resulting in the soleus relaxing, and the body stops its posterior motion and begins to sway forward. While the stretch reflex appears to fail in a large fraction of adult women, very few of these individuals have any difficulty standing upright, indicating that the postural reflex arc controlling soleus activity is intact. This observation sets the stage for a convenient method to exogenously activate the soleus muscle.

We have pursued this hypothesis that the postural reflex arc regulating soleus activity is intact in women with inadequate fluid return from the lower limbs, and our experimental results support both the contention that this postural reflex is operational, and that exogenous activation of this soleus reflex arc is sufficient to significantly increase venous and lymphatic return from the lower limbs. Initial work focused on identifying the characteristics of the stimulus necessary to activate the soleus reflex and we observed that a micromechanical stimulation of plantar surface at 45 Hz, with a magnitude of 10 micrometers or greater was sufficient. This observation is consistent with the activated mechanoreceptors on the foot being the Meisner corpuscles [19]. A stimulus of this nature applied to the frontal plantar surface was found to completely block the drop in BP and increase in HR observed in women who could not maintain fluid return from the lower limbs during quiet sitting (Figure 7) [15]. Further studies on the mechanism underlying these clinical observations have shown that the plantar reflex stimulation has no effect on lymphatic microfiltration rate, but rather increases the isovolumetric lymphatic pressure, as well as significantly enhancing perfusion in the lower leg, pelvic, and thoracic segments of the body [20].

As importantly, activation of the second heart (soleus) has been found to effectively inhibit interstitial fluid pooling in adult women [17]. Following a 30 minute quiet sitting period during which a population of women (N=24) were observed to pool extensively (using air plethysmography), the subjects were exposed to 20 minutes of continuous plantar stimulation sufficient to activate the soleus muscle. Activation of the stimulus was found to result in an immediate drop in calf volume, which is interpreted to be due to the rapid decrease in venous volume (Figure 8) [17]. This rapid volume decrease was then followed by a sustained slower decrease in calf volume consistent with interstitial fluid migration to the initial lymphatics with subsequent ejection to the collecting lymphatics and back to the heart. Sustained stimulation with continuous blood pressure monitoring confirms that the ejected fluid is returning to the heart per the associated increase in systolic blood pressure (Figure 9) [21].

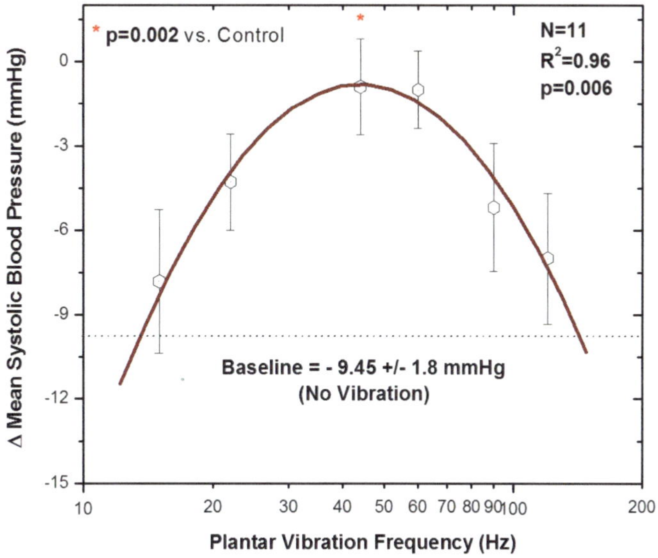

Figure 7. Efficacy of soleus muscle activation, through its postural reflex arc, to prevent blood pressure drop in adult women. *From Madhavan, et al., 2005.*

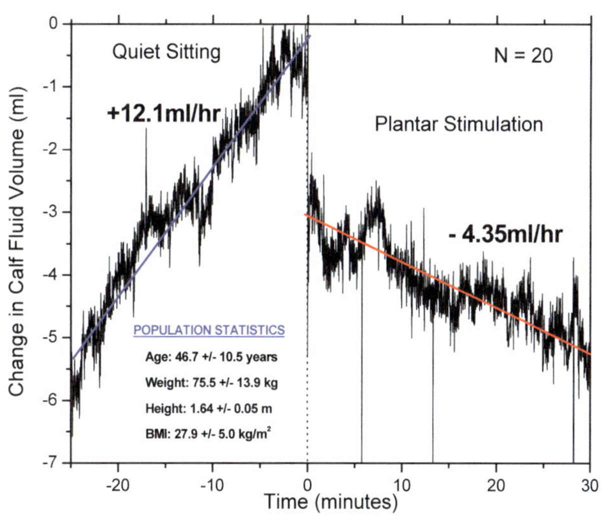

Figure 8. Efficacy of second heart stimulation, through the plantar reflex, to reverse interstitial fluid pooling in adult women. *From Goddard, et al., 2008.*

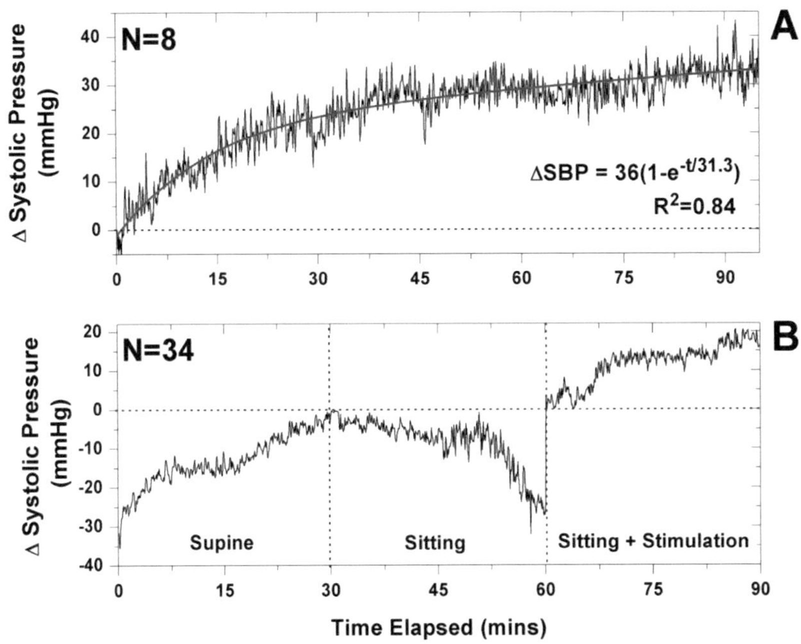

Figure 9. Influence of sustained second heart stimulation via the plantar reflex on systolic blood pressure during extended orthostatic stress associated with extended sitting. A) Time course of change in systolic blood pressure with transition from sitting to supine position. Time constant of 30 minutes suggests that close to three hours are necessary for interstitial fluid in the lower limbs to be recovered into the circulatory system following a transition to a supine position. B) Ability of second heart stimulation to accelerate fluid recovery from the lower limbs. Left panel: recovery rate associated with supine rest; Middle panel: Pooling associated with quiet sitting; Right panel: Influence of plantar reflex stimulation of the second heart. *From Madhavan, et al., 2009.*

The potential for second heart stimulation to assist individuals with diastolic heart failure, and at stage NYHA III has been tested in a pilot clinical study wherein individuals were provided with a plantar reflex stimulation device to use in their home for a four week period of time [22]. Three men and three women (average age 68 years) were recruited into the study with a group average LVEF of 49.8%. Lower limb water content was assessed using Dual Energy X-ray Absorptiometry (DXA). The average daily use of second heart stimulation ranged from 0.2 hours per day to 1.8 hours per day, and the change in retained lower limb water over the one month study period was associated with daily stimulation use (Figure 10). On average, a significant ($p=0.03$) decrease in lower limb water mass of 0.5Kg was observed, ranging from no decrease to over 1 liter.

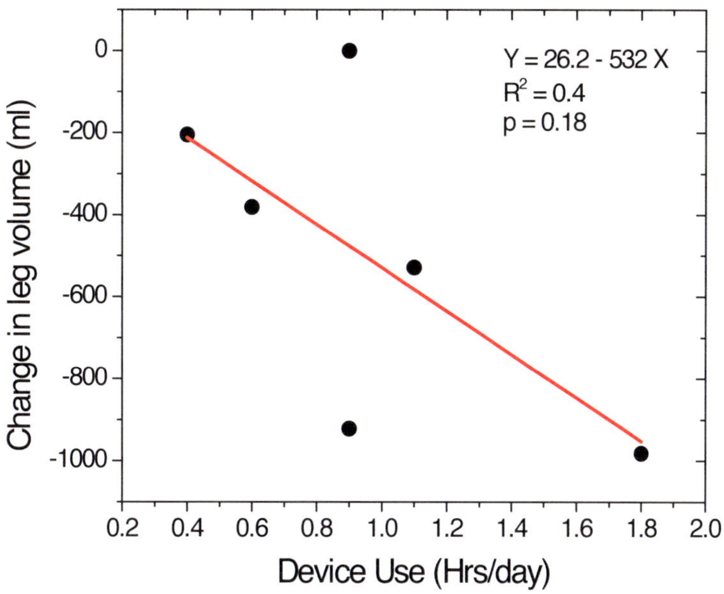

Figure 10. Change in lower limb body fluid over a one month time period as a function of average daily use of plantar reflex stimulation of the second heart. *After Pierce & McLeod, 2009.*

7. Differential diagnosis

The recent research on second heart activity has largely relied on measurements such as continuous (beat-to-beat) blood pressure monitoring, air plethysmography, electrical impedance plethysmography, and strain-gage plethysmography. However, none of these techniques represent a practical technique for the clinical environment. We would suggest that the critical factors in diagnosing inadequate second heart activity are the creation of an extended time period of orthostatic stress coupled with blood pressure monitoring and HR determination. These can be readily accomplished utilizing either upright standing or extended sitting, though as many older individuals have difficulty standing quietly for extended time periods, an extended sitting protocol is likely the most practical. A useful approach would be to obtain the BP and HR from a patient upon entering the examining room and first sitting down, then having them continue to sit for another 30 minutes or more with BP and HR obtained at the 15 and 30 minute time points. HR increases of more than 5 bpm, coupled to BP decreases of more than 10 mmHg, or more specifically, a diastolic BP dropping below 60 mmHg, should be considered a strong indication of inadequate fluid return to the heart, with long term implications for heart health and the development of extrinsic cardiomyopathy.

8. Summary and conclusions

Second heart failure, which occurs in close to 50% of women, represents a common etiology in extrinsic heart failure and cardiopathy. Clinical recognition of this condition opens the opportunity for early diagnosis and intervention, reducing the long term risk for this substantial subpopulation of women, with the potential to maintain a much higher quality of life into old age. Simple office tests of temporal changes in blood pressure and heart rate over 30 minutes of quiet sitting can reveal significant pooling associated with failed second heart activity. Augmenting venous return to the right heart to improve atrial refilling will allow for improved stroke volume and thus improved peripheral and cerebral blood flow. Early interventions can include specific exercises to train up the soleus muscle, lifestyle changes which challenge the postural reflexes; or utilization of extrinsic stimulation technology.

Acknowledgements

The authors acknowledge the support of the Clinical Science and Engineering Research Center at Binghamton University.

Author details

Kenneth J. McLeod[1] and Carolyn Pierce[2]

*Address all correspondence to: kmcleod@binghamton.edu

1 Clinical Science and Engineering Research Center Watson School of Engineering and Applied Science, USA

2 Decker School of Nursing, Binghamton University, Binghamton, NY, U.S.A.

References

[1] Maron, B. J. The 2006 American Heart Association classification of cardiomyopathies is the gold standard. Circ Heart Fail (2008). , 1, 72-76.

[2] Kemp, C. D, & Conte, J. V. The pathophysiology of heart failure. Cardiovasc Pathol (2012). , 21, 365-371.

[3] Hsich, E. M, & Pina, I. L. Heart failure in women: A need for prospective data. J Am Coll Cardiol (2009). , 54, 491-498.

[4] Vasan, R. S, Larson, M. G, Benhamin, E. J, Evans, J. C, Reiss, C. K, & Levy, D. Congestive heart failure in subjects with normal versus reduced left ventricular ejection fraction: Prevalence and morality in a population based cohort. J Am Coll Cardiol (1999). , 33, 1948-1955.

[5] Scardovi, A. B, Petruzzi, M, Rosana, A, & Demaria, R. Heart failure phenotype in women. G Ital Cardio (Rome) (2012). , 13, 6-100.

[6] Hsia, J, Larson, J. C, Ockene, J. K, et al. Resting heart rate as a low tech predictor of coronary events in women: Prospective cohort study. BMJ (2009). , 338, 219-225.

[7] Heistad, D. D, & Kontos, H. A. Cerebral circulation. In Shepherd JT and Abboud FM, eds Handbook of Physiology. The Cardiovascular System: Peripheral Circulation and Organ Blood Flow (1983). sec 2, vol III, part I Am Physiol Soc. Bethesda, MD., 137-182.

[8] Hagan, R. D, Diaz, F. J, & Horvath, S. M. Plasma volume changes with movement to supine and standing positions. J Appl Physiol (1978). , 45, 414-417.

[9] Monahan, K. D, & Ray, C. A. Gender affects calf venous compliance at rest and during baroreceptor unloading in humans. Am J Phsyiol Heart Circ Physiol (2004). HH901., 895.

[10] Firooz, A, Sadr, B, Babakoohi, S, et al. Variation of biophysical parameters of the skin with age, gender, and body region. Sci Word J (2012).

[11] Moneta, G. L, & Nehler, M. R. The lower extremity venous system: Anatomy and physiology of normal venous function and chronic venous insufficiency. In Gloviczki P, Yao JST, eds. Handbook of Venous Disorders. Guidelines of the American Venous Forum. London: Chapman & Hall Medical, (1996). , 1996, 3-26.

[12] Edgerton, Y. R, Smith, J. L, & Simpson, D. R. Muscle fibre type populations of human leg muscles. Histochem J (1975). , 7, 259-266.

[13] Rowell, L. B. Human Cardiovascular Control. Oxford University Press, New York, (1993). , 1993, 29-30.

[14] Schmid-schonbein, G. W. Microlymphatics and lymph flow. Physiol Rev (1990). , 70, 987-1028.

[15] Madhavan, G, Stewart, J. M, & Mcleod, K. J. Effect of plantar micromechanical stimulation on cardiovascular responses to immobility. Am J Phys Med Rehabil (2005). , 84, 338-345.

[16] Madhavan, G, Goddard, A. A, & Mcleod, K. J. Prevalence and etiology of delayed orthostatic hypotension in adult women. Arch Phys Med Rehabil (2008). , 89, 1788-1794.

[17] Gibbons, C. H, & Freeman, R. Delayed orthostatic hypotension: A frequent cause of orthostatic intolerance. Neurology (2006). , 67, 28-32.

[18] Goddard, A. A, Pierce, C. S, & Mcleod, K. J. Reversal of lower limb edema by calf muscle pump stimulation. J Cardiopulm Rehabil Prev (2008). , 28, 174-179.

[19] Kennedy, P. M, & Inglis, J. T. Distribution and behavior of glabrous cutaneous receptors in the human foot sole. J Physiol (2002). , 538, 995-1002.

[20] Stewart, J. M, Karman, C, Montgomery, L. D, & Mcleod, K. J. Plantar vibration improves leg fluid flow in perimenopausal women. Am J Physiol Integr Comp Physiol 1005; , 288, 623-629.

[21] Madhavan, G, Nemcek, M. A, Martinez, D. G, & Mcleod, K. C. Enhancing hemodialysis efficacy through neuromuscular stimulation. Blood Purif (2009). , 27, 58-63.

[22] Pierce, C. S, & Mcleod, K. J. Feasibility of treatment of lower limb edema with calf muscle pump stimulation in chronic heart failure. Eur Cardiovasc Nurs (2009). , 5, 345-348.

Chapter 14

Pediatric Cardiomyopathies

Aspazija Sofijanova and Olivera Jordanova

Additional information is available at the end of the chapter

http://dx.doi.org/10.5772/55820

1. Introduction

1.1. Development of the cardiovascular system

The development of the cardiovascular system is an early embryological event. From fertilization, it takes eight weeks for the human heart to develop into its definitive fetal structure. During this period the system develops so it can 1) **supply nutrients and oxygen to the fetus,** and 2) **immediately start functionining after birth.**

1.2. Early development of the circulatory system

1.2.1. Blood islands

During the third week of gestation angioblastic blood islands of mesoderm (angiogenic clusters) appear in the yolk sac, chorion and body stalk. The innermost cells of these blood islands are hematopoietic cells that give rise to the blood cell lines. The outermost cells give rise to the endothelial cell layer of blood vessels. A series of blood islands eventually coalesce to form blood vessels (fig 1).

1.2.2. Heart tube

By the middle of the third week of gestation angioblastic blood islands from the splanchnic mesoderm appear and form a plexus of vessels lying deep into the horseshoe-shaped prospective pericardial cavity (fig 2). These small vessels develop into paired endocardial heart tubes. The splanchnic mesoderm proliferates and develops into the myocardial mantle, which gives rise to the myocardium. The epicardium develops from cells that migrate over the myocardial mantle from areas adjacent to the developing heart (fig 3,4).

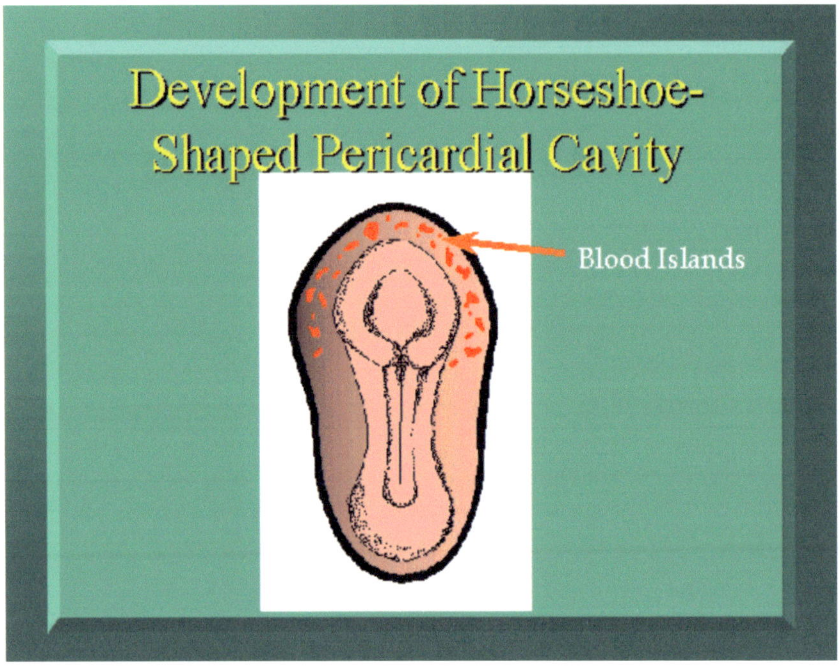

Figure 1. Angioblastic blood islands of mesoderm

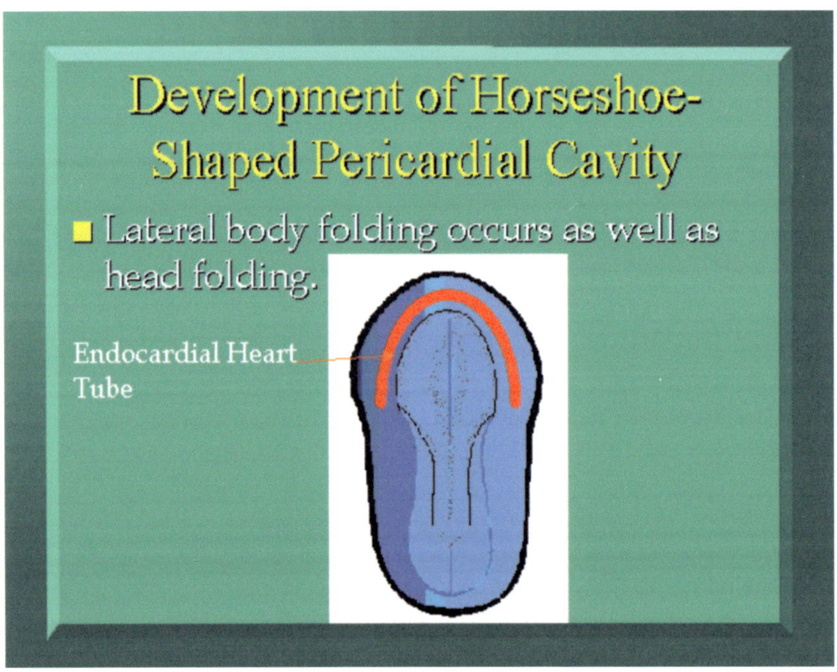

Figure 2. Horseshoe-shaped prospective pericardial cavity

http://dx.doi.org/10.5772/55820

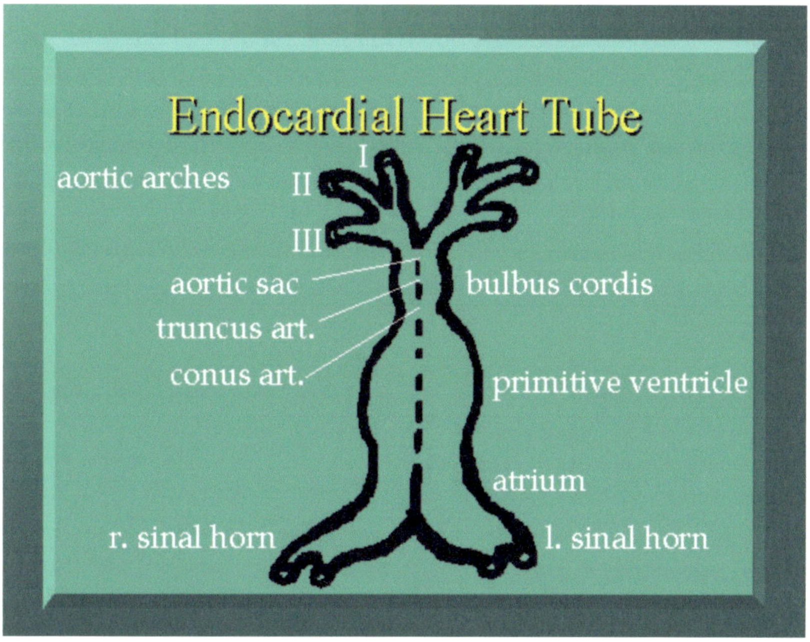

Figure 3. Endocardial heart tubes

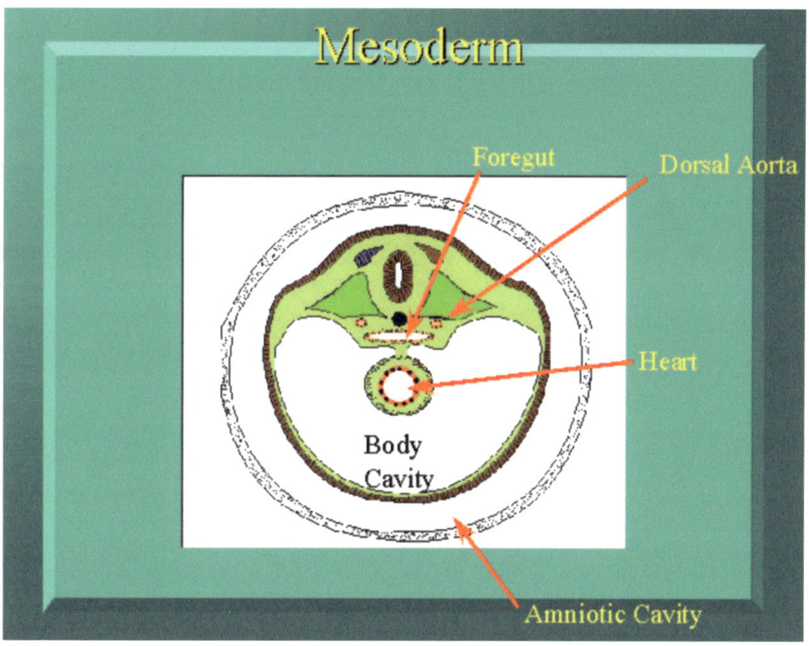

Figure 4. Splanchnic mesoderm

The bilateral endocardial heart tubes continue to develop and connect with a pair of vessels, the dorsal aortae, located on either side of the midline. As the embryo develops, the lateral folding and cephalic growth of the embryo shift the endocardial heart tubes medially, ventrally and caudally. They fuse in the midline as a single endocardial heart tube. The endocardial heart tube is surrounded by the myocardial mantle and between these two layers is the cardiac jelly. The resulting heart tube is kept suspended in the pericardial cavity through the dorsal mesocardium. When the single heart tube is formed, the embryo is in the fourth week of gestation, is about 3 mm in length, has 4 - 12 somites, and the neural tube is beginning to form. The heart now begins to beat (fig 5).

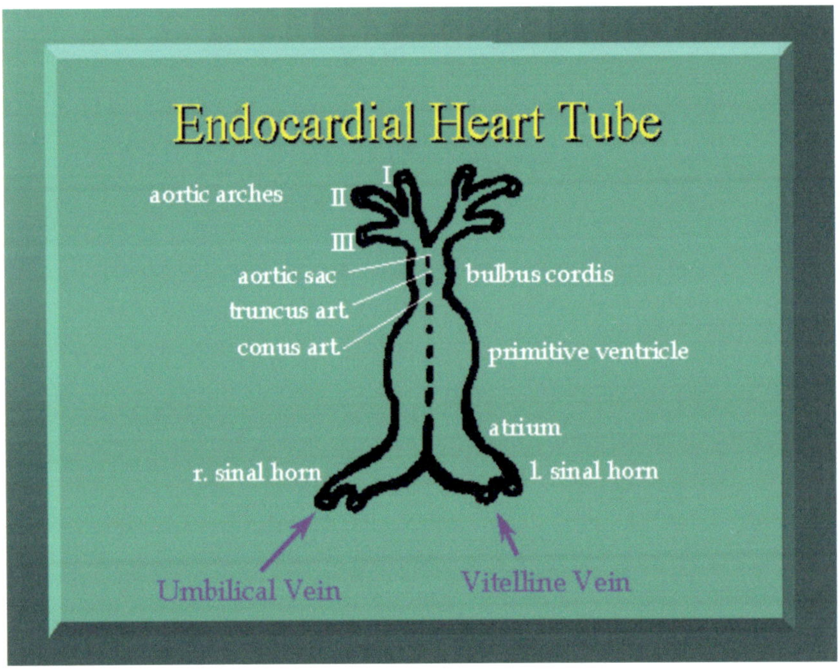

Figure 5. Endocardial heart tube

1.2.3. Vascular circuits

As the heart begins to beat, three sets of blood islands coalesce to form three vascular circuits. Within the embryo an embryonic circuit forms (fig 6.)It consists of paired dorsal aortae that arise from the endocardial heart tube and break up into capillary networds that supply blood to the developing embryonic tissues. Blood is drained from these tissues byanterior and posterior cardinal veins that drain into common cardinal veins, which in turn drain into the endocardial heart tube.

Two extraembryonic circuits also form. The first is the vitelline (omphalomesenteric, yolk sac) circuit. In this circuit blood from the dorsal aortae drain into vitelline arteries that in turn

http://dx.doi.org/10.5772/55820

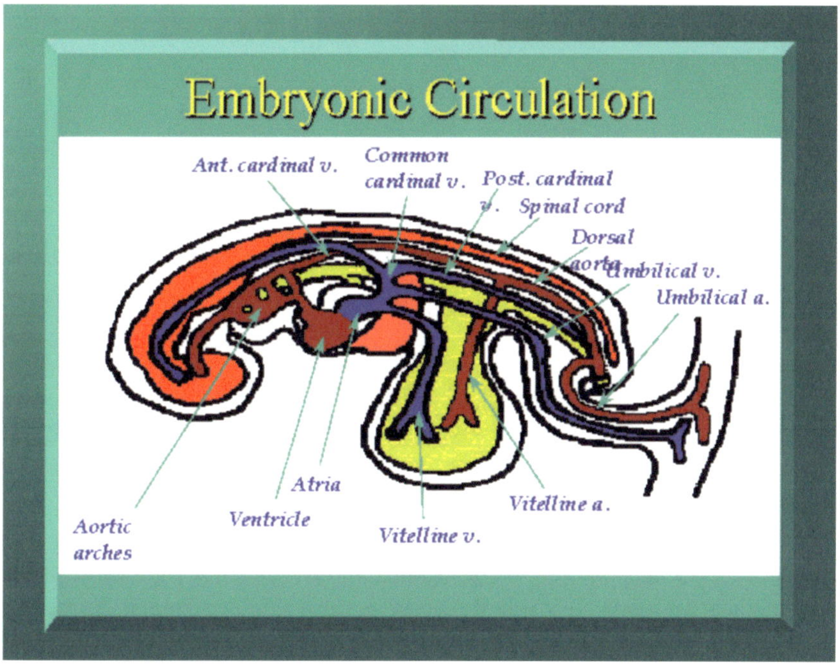

Figure 6. Embryonic circuit forms

supply the yolk sac. The blood drains back to the heart tube via paired vitelline veins. The second circuit is the umbilical (allantoic, placental) extraembryonic circuit. In this instance, the dorsal aortae supply blood to umbilical arteries that in turn bring this now unoxygenated blood back to the placenta. Blood from the placenta is carried to the heart tube via umbilical veins.

1.3. Formation of the primitive four chambered heart

As the endocardial heart tubes fuse, several bulges and sulci appear. From the cephalic end, the bulges are the bulbus cordis (truncus arteriosus and the conus arteriosus), the primitive ventricle, the primitive atrium and the sinus venosus (fig 7.) The veins connect to the heart tube via the sinus venosus, while the paired dorsal aortae arise from aortic arches that in turn arise from the aortic sac. The aortic sac is at the most cephalic end of the bulbus cordis. The sulci are present as the bulboventricular sulcus, between the bulbus cordis and the ventricle, and the atrioventricular sulcus, between the atrium and the ventricle.

Then, a rapid growth of the heart tube takes place, and the heart begins to convolute. With this convolution the dorsal mesocardium begins to degenerate. During the process of convolution, the first flexure seen is between the bulbus cordis and the ventricle. The bulbo-ventricular loop that is formed shifts this region of the heart to the right and ventrally. The second flexure, the atrioventricular loop, is between the atrium and the ventricle and this region of the heart is shifted to the left and dorsally. As growth continues the atria shift cephalically.

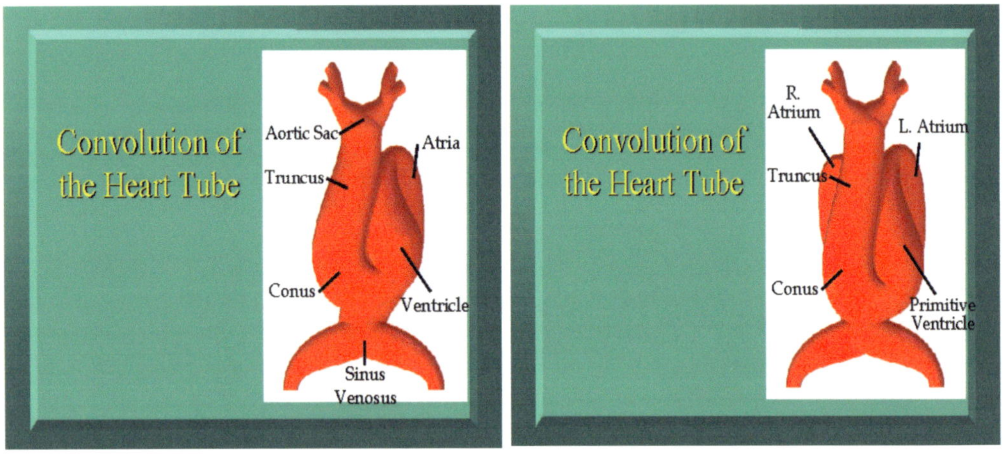

Figure 7. Convolution of the Heart Tube

The sinus venosus gradually shifts to the right to empty into the right atrium. The bulbo-ventricular sulcus is represented inside the heart as the bulbo-ventricular flange. The bulbo-ventricular flange and the muscular interventricular septum begin to separate the primitive ventricle (which will become the left ventricle) from the proximal bulbus cordis (which will become the definitive right ventricle). The atria continue to grow, and bulge forward on either side of the bulbus cordis, and shift the bulbus medially. With increased blood flow the bulbo-ventricular flange regresses. Thus, the primitive four-chambered heart is formed and blood flows from the veins to sinus venosus, to atria, to ventricles, to conus, to truncus, to aortic sac, to dorsal aorta.

Now the enlarging liver encroaches upon the developing vitelline and umbilical veins and gradually all the blood will drain to the proximal right vitelline vein. The distal vitelline veins will give rise to the portal system. The left umbilical vein remains and drains into the ductus venosus, a shunt which allows blood to bypass the developing liver.

1.4. Septation of the heart

During the second month, the heart begins to septate into two atria, two ventricles, the ascending aorta and the pulmonary trunk.

1.4.1. Atrial septation

Endocardial cushions develop in the dorsal (inferior) and ventral (superior) walls of the heart. These grow toward each other as the cardiac jelly mesenchyme proliferates deep to the endocardium. These cushions fuse and divide the common AV canal into the left and right AV canals.

At the same time there is a developing septum from the dorsocranial atrial wall that grows toward the cushions. This is the septum primum, and the intervening space is called the

http://dx.doi.org/10.5772/55820

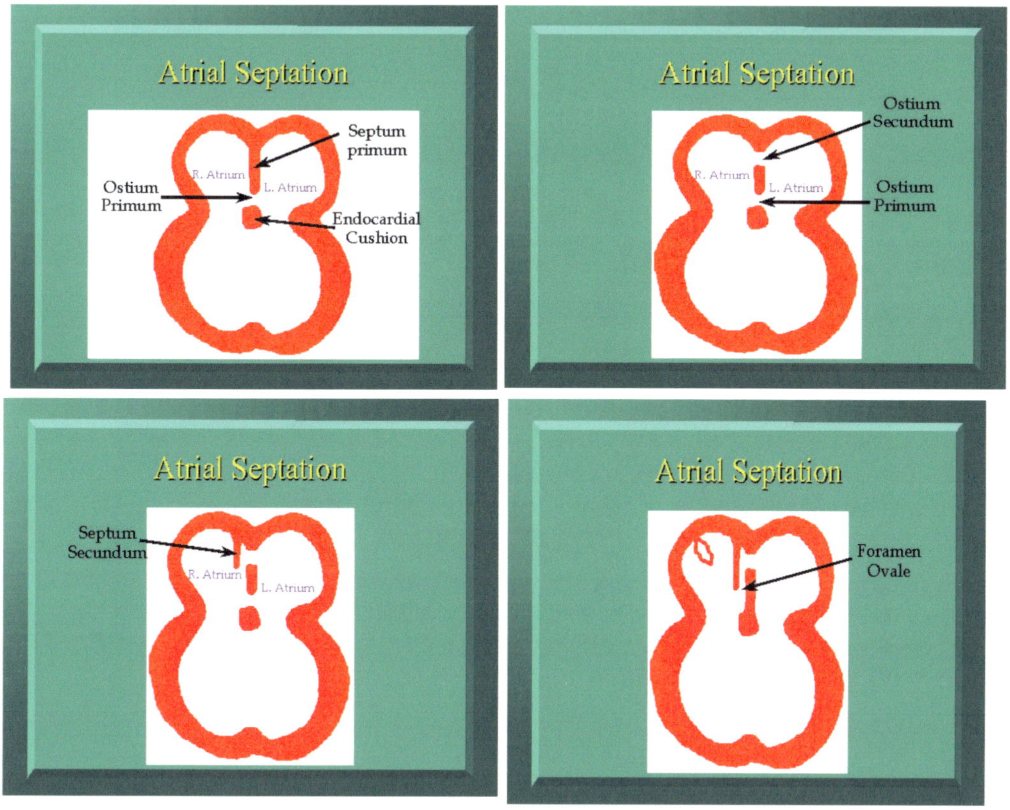

Figure 8. Atrial Septation

foramen primum. As the septum reaches the endocardial cushions closing foramen primum, a second opening, foramen secundum appears in septum primum. As foramen secundum enlarges, a second septum, septum secundum forms to the right of septum primum. Septum secundum forms an incomplete partition (lying to the right of foramen secundum) which leaves an opening, the foramen ovale. The remaining portions of septum primum become the valve of foramen ovale (fig 8).

Concurrently, the sinus venosus has shifted to the right as the proximal portions of the left vitelline and umbilical veins are obliterated by the liver. The right sinus venosus becomes incorporated into the right atrium forming the smooth portion of the right atrium. The primitive right atrium is seen in the adult as the rough portion (auricle) of the right atrium. The remainder of the left sinus horn is the coronary sinus and the oblique vein (of Marshall) in the adult heart (fig 9).

On the left side, the primitive atrium is enlarged by the incorporation of tissue from the original, single pulmonary vein and its proximal branches. This incorporated tissue is the adult smooth left atrial wall through which four pulmonary veins empty independently. The trabeculated left atrial appendage originated from the primitive left atrium.

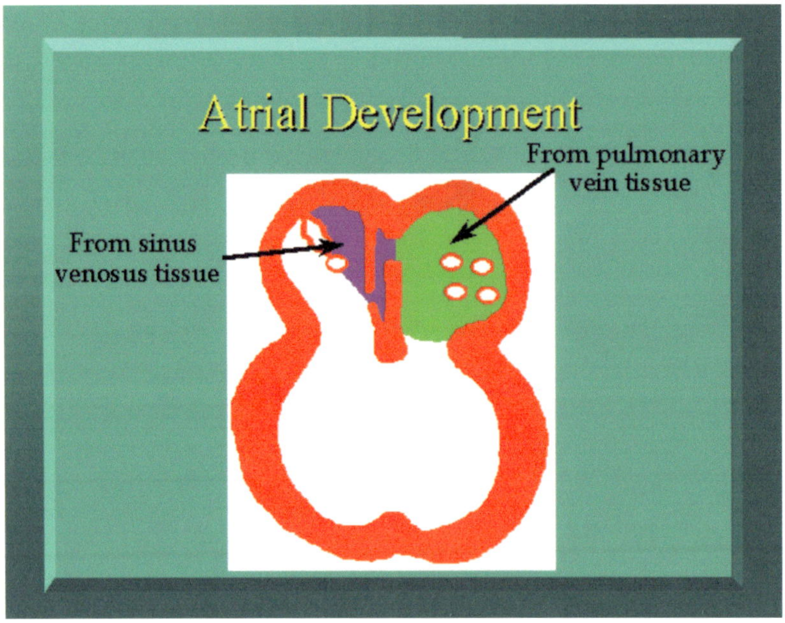

Figure 9. Atrial Development

1.4.2. Ventricular septation

The muscular interventricular septum grows as a ridge of tissue from the caudal heart wall toward the fused endocardial cushions. The remaining opening is the interventricular (IV) foramen. The IV foramen is closed by the conal ridges, outgrowth of the inferior endocardial cushion, the right tubercle, and connective tissue from the muscular interventricular septum. This portion of the I.V. septum is called the membranous part of the interventricular septum (fig 10).

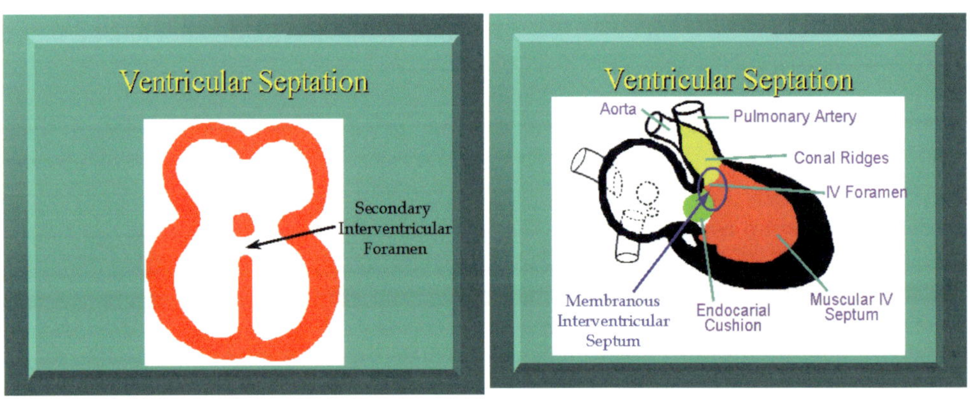

Figure 10. Ventricular Septation

1.4.3. Septation of the bulbus cordis

Truncal swellings (ridges) appear first as bulges in the truncus on the right superior and the left inferior walls. They enlarge and fuse in the midline to form the truncal (aorticopulmonary) septum. This septum spirals as it develops distally, separating the distal pulmonary artery from the aorta. At the same time, right dorsal and left ventral conal ridges form and fuse in the midline. The conal septum helps dividing the proximal aorta from the pulmonary artery and contributes to the membranous IV septum. The truncal and conal septa fuse to form a 180° spiral and together definitively form the aorta and the pulmonary artery. Cells that contribute to the conal and the truncal septa are in part derived from neural crest cells that migrate into these regions (fig 11).

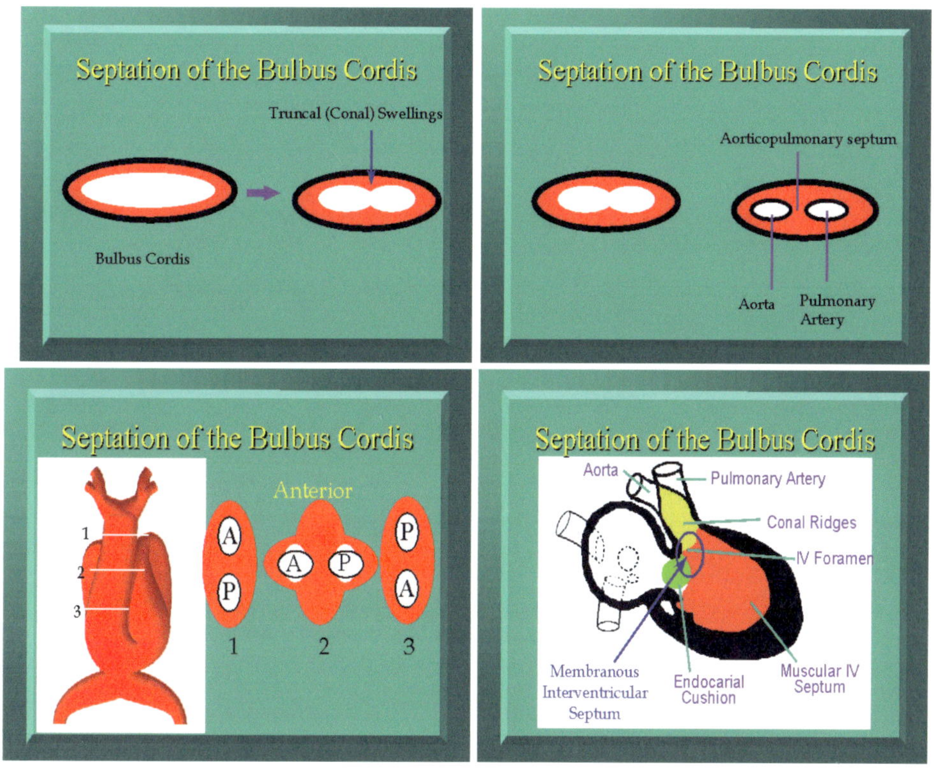

Figure 11. Septation of the Bulbus Cordis

1.4.4. Cardiac valve fromation

Semilunar valves develop in the aorta and pulmonary artery as localized swellings of endocardial tissue. The atrioventricular valves develop as subendocardial and endocardial tissues and project into the AV canal. These bulges are excavated from the ventricular side and invaded by muscle. Eventually, all the muscle, except that remaining as papillary muscle, disappear and three cusps of the right AV (tricuspid) valve, and two cusps of the left AV (mitral) valve remain as fibrous structures.

1.4.5. Development of the major arteries

The six pairs of aortic arches, develop in a cephalocaudal direction and interconnect the ventral aortic roots and the dorsal aorta. They are never all present in the developing human heart. Of the six pairs of aortic arches, most of the first, second and fifth arches disappear (fig 12).

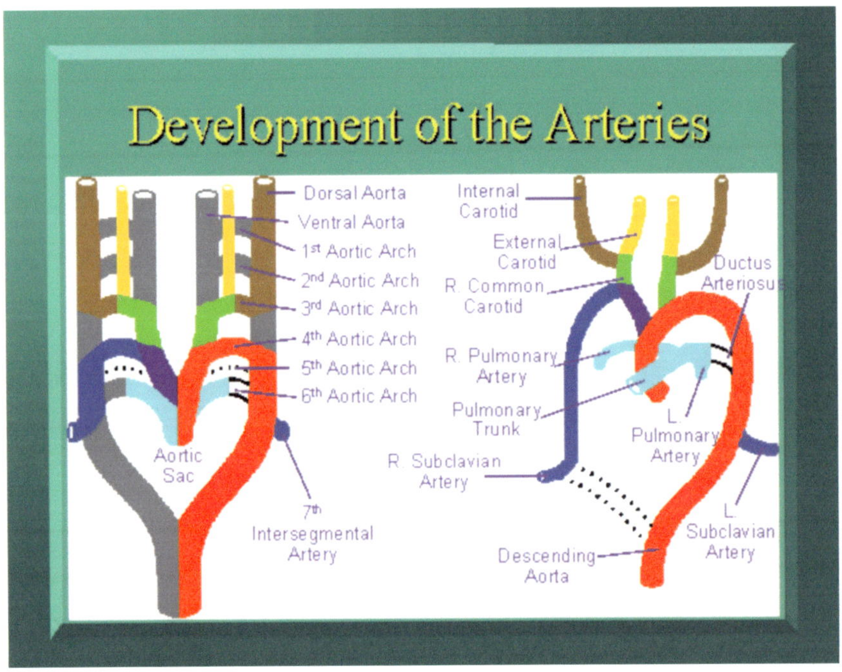

Figure 12. Development of the Major Arteries

1.4.6. Development of the veins

The veins develop from the three major vascular circuits. As with the arteries they develop in a cephalocaudal direction and as a consequence the precursors to the veins are never all present at the same time. In addition, as new structures develop the course of veins changes.

In considering the development of the veins, the veins to the head are derived from the anterior cardinal veins. New channels also develop such as the thymicothyroid anastomoses and the external jugular veins and give rise to veins of the head and neck (fig 13).

http://dx.doi.org/10.5772/55820

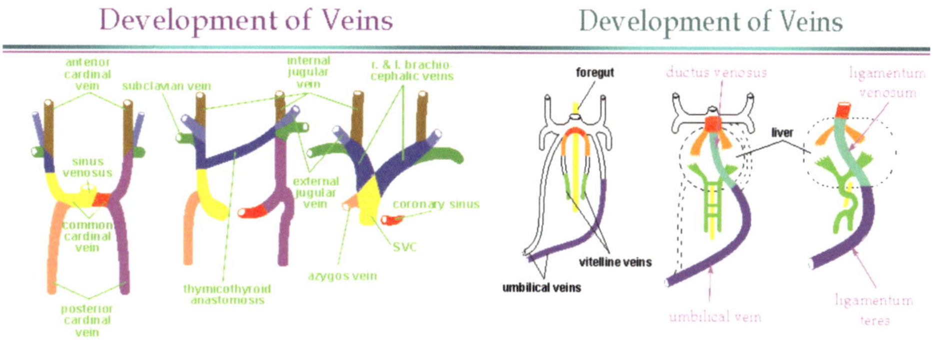

Figure 13. Development of the Veins

In the trunk, one set of veins develops from the posterior cardinal veins and veins that develop from it later in development, such as the subcardinal, supracardinal, and sacrocardinal veins. These veins will give rise to the inferior vena cava, the renal, adrenal and gonadal veins, as well as the azygos and hemiazygos viens (fig 14).

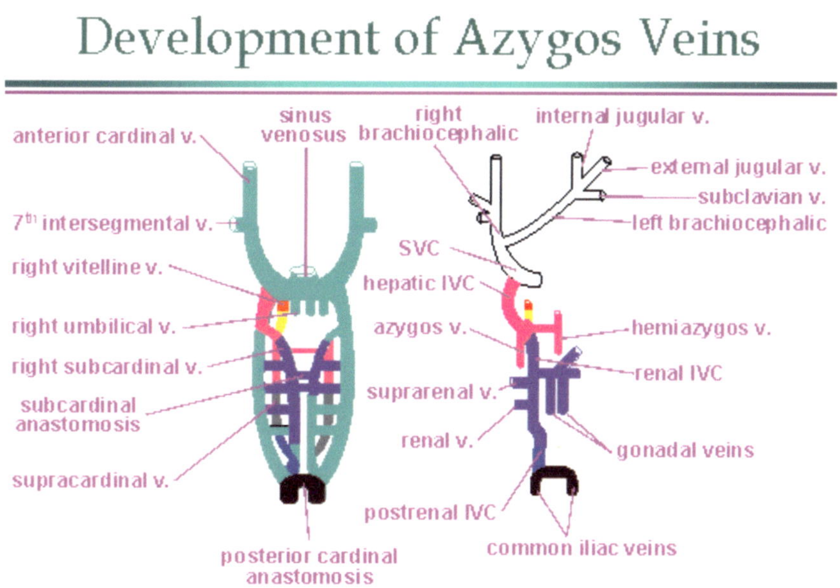

Figure 14. Development of Azygos Veins

The superior mesenteric vein (and perhaps the splenic vien) as well as the veins to the liver develop from the vitelline (omphlomesenteric) veins. The ductus venosus develops as a new structure that connects the left umbilical vein with the inferior vena cava (fig 12).

2. The cardiomyopathies

Cardiomyopathy is a chronic disease of the heart muscle (myocardium), in which the muscle is abnormally enlarged, thickened, and/or stiffened. The weakened heart muscle loses the ability to pump blood effectively, resulting in irregular heartbeats (arrhythmias) and possibly even heart failure. Cardiomyopathy, a disease of the heart muscle, primarily affects the left ventricle, which is the main pumping chamber of the heart. Usually, cardiomyopathy begins in the heart's lower chambers (the ventricles), but in severe cases can affect the upper chambers, or atria.The disease is often associated with inadequate heart pumping and other heart function abnormalities. Cardiomyopathy is not common but it can be severely disabling or fatal. Most people are only mildly affected by cardiomyopathy and can lead relatively normal lives.However, people who have severe heart failure may need a heart transplant.Cardiomyopathy is a heart condition that not only affects middle-aged and elderly persons, but can also affect infants, children, and adolescents. Cardiomyopathy is classified as either "ischemic" or "nonischemic". All cases related to children and teenagers are considered "nonischemic" cardiomyopathy. Non-ischemic cardiomyopathy predominately involves the heart's abnormal structure and function. It does not involve the hardening of arteries on the heart surface typically associated with ischemic cardiomyopathy. Nonischemic cardiomyopathy can then be broken down into: 1) "primary cardiomyopathy" where the heart is predominately affected and the cause may be due to infectious agents or genetic disorders and 2) "secondary cardiomyopathy" where the heart is affected due to complications from another disease affecting the body (i.e. HIV, cancer, muscular dystrophy or cystic fibrosis).Cardiomyopathy is nondiscriminatory in that it can affect any adult or child at any stage of their life. It is not gender, geographic, race or age specific. It is a particularly rare disease when diagnosed in infants and young children. Cardiomyopathy continues to be the leading reason for heart transplants in children.Pediatric cardiomyopathy is a rare heart condition that affects infants and children. Specifically, cardiomyopathy means disease of the heart muscle (myocardium). Several different types of cardiomyopathy exist and the specific symptoms vary from case to case. In some cases, no symptoms may be present (asymptomatic); in many cases, cardiomyopathy is a progressive condition that may result in an impaired ability of the heart to pump blood; fatigue; heart block; irregular heartbeats (tachycardia); and, potentially, heart failure and sudden cardiac death.There are numerous causes for a complex disease such as cardiomyopathy. For the majority of diagnosed children, the exact cause remains unknown (termed "idiopathic"). In some cases, it may be related to an inherited condition such as a family history of cardiomyopathy or a genetic disorder such as fatty acid oxidation, Barth syndrome, orNoonan syndrome. Cardiomyopathy can also be a consequence of another disease or toxin where other organs are affected. Possible causes include viral infections (Coxsackie B - CVB), auto-immune diseases during pregnancy, the build-up of proteins in the heart muscle (amyloidosis), and an excess of iron in the heart (hemochromatosis). Excessive use of alcohol, contact with certain toxins, complications from AIDS, and the use of some therapeutic drugs (i.e. doxorubicin) to treat cancer can also contribute to the development of the disease.

http://dx.doi.org/10.5772/55820

3. Pediatric cardiomyopathies

Pediatric cardiomyopathy is a rare heart condition that affects infants and children.There is a vast amount of literature on adult cardiomyopathy but not all of the information is relevant to children diagnosed with the disease. Unfortunately, there has been little research and focus on pediatric cardiomyopathy over the years. Consequently, the causes are not well understood. Pediatric cardiomyopathy is more likely to be due to genetic factors while lifestyle or environmental factors play a greater role in adult cardiomyopathy.

In rare cases, pediatric cardiomyopathy may be a symptom of a larger genetic disorder that may not be immediately detected. For example, when an infant or young child is diagnosed with dilated cardiomyopathy, a rare genetic heart disease called Barth Syndrome or a mitochondrial defect (i.e. Kearns-Sayre syndrome) may be the cause. Similarly, a child with severe hypertrophic cardiomyopathy may actually have Noonan Syndrome, Pompe disease (type II glycogen storage disease), a fatty acid oxidation disorder, or mitochondrial HCM. It is therefore important for any diagnosed child to be properly evaluated for other suspected genetic disorders. A thorough evaluation remains a complicated and expensive process due to the large number of rare genetic causes, the broad range of symptoms and the existence of many specialized biochemical, enzymatic and genetic tests. Verifying a diagnosis may require getting additional blood, urine or tissue tests and consulting other specialists such as a neurologist and geneticist.

Cardiomyopathy in children may also present differently from diagnosed teenagers or adult. It is considered unusual when an infant or a child is diagnosed with symptoms at such a young age. Typically, symptoms are not apparent until the late teens or adult years when most patients are diagnosed. With hypertrophic cardiomyopathy, the disease commonly develops in association with growth and is detected when a child progresses through puberty. Even in genetically affected family members, a child that carries the muted gene from birth may appear to have a normal heart and be asymptomatic until puberty.

A diagnosis at a young age usually, but not always, signifies a serious heart condition that requires aggressive treatment. The concern lies in the uncertainty of how the heart muscle will respond with each additional growth spurt. With some older children, the condition may stabilize over time with the aid of certain medications or surgery. In severe cases, small children may experience progressive symptoms quickly leading to heart failure. This presentation contrasts with most diagnosed adults who may only have minor symptoms without serious limitations or major problems for years.Aside from differences in the cause and manifestation, cardiomyopathy may also progress differently in children than adults. When children are diagnosed at an early age, the prognosis may be poor depending on the form of cardiomyopathy and the stage of the disease. For example, dilated cardiomyopathy can progress quite rapidly when diagnosed in young children. Up to 40% of diagnosed children with dilated cardiomyopathy fail medical management within the first year of diagnosis and of those that survive many have permanently impaired heart function. Children diagnosed with hypertrophic cardiomyopathy seem to fare better but the outcome is highly variable.Mortality and heart transplant rates of childhood cardiomyopathies are much higher than in adults due to the rarity and uncertainty of the disease. Less than optimal outcomes may be attributed to the more fragile state of infants and young children or it may be a function of the disease's advanced progression associated with another genetic disorder. Another unfortunate reason is that cardiomyopathy is not usually detected until the end stage when obvious symptoms of heart failure are apparent. Cardiomyopathy can be easily missed in routine check-ups when there are no obvious symptoms (i.e heart murmur) or when there is no reason for diagnostic testing (i.e. no family history of the disease).

3.1. What causes cardiomyopathy?

Although pediatric cardiomyopathy is one of the leading causes of cardiac death in children, an explanation for why it occurs remains unknown. Most cases are familial conditions that are genetically transmitted, but the disease can also be acquired during childhood. The most common cause for acquired cardiomyopathy is myocarditis, a viral infection that weakens the heart muscle. Other causes for acquired cardiomyopathy include: 1) cardiovascular conditions (i.e. Kawasaki disease, congenital heart defect, hypertension, cardiac transplantation or surgery), 2) infectious or inflammatory diseases, 3) immunologic diseases (i.e. HIV), 4) obesity or dietary deficiencies, 5) toxin reactions (i.e. drug, alcohol, radiation exposure), 6) connective tissue and autoimmune diseases, 7) endocrine diseases and 8) pregnancy related complications. Persistent rhythm problems or problems of the coronary arteries, either congenital or acquired, can also lead to a weakening of the heart.

It is being increasingly recognized that certain genetic mutations are the primary cause for pediatric cardiomyopathy. Mutations are defects in the DNA spiral, the protein structure of many genes. The abnormalities in DNA involve a displacement in the sequence of one or more of the amino acids that make up a gene protein. The disease is either inherited through one parent who is a carrier (autosomal dominant transmission with a 50% chance of recurrence) or through both parents who each contribute a defective gene (autosomal recessive transmission with a 25% chance of recurrence). Cardiomyopathy can also be inherited by maternal transmission (X-linked). Research continues to focus on identifying the specific genes that cause cardiomyopathy and better understanding how these genetic abnormalities contribute to the disease. However, it is a complex process with multiple diverse genes producing extremely variable outcomes. Many children with hypertrophic cardiomyopathy (50-60%) and to a lesser degree with dilated cardiomyopathy (20-30%) have a family history of the disease. Recent advancements in genetic research show that hypertrophic cardiomyopathy involves defects in the sarcomere genes and can be inherited in an autosomal dominant manner. Dilated cardiomyopathy involves defects in the cytoskeleton genes and can be inherited autosomal dominant, autosomal recessive or X-linked. In some cases, cardiomyopathy can be related to another inherited metabolic or congenital muscle disorder such as Noonan syndrome, Pompe disease, fatty acid oxidation defect or Barth syndrome. Most often, symptoms of these disorders present early in life.Although there is a long list of possible causes for cardiomyopathy, few of them are directly treatable and most therapy is aimed at treating the secondary effects on the heart.

http://dx.doi.org/10.5772/55820

According to the Pediatric Cardiomyopathy Registry, cardiomyopathies can be grouped into five categories based on the specific genetic cause of the disease:

- myocarditis and other viral infections (27%),
- familial inherited cardiomyopathies (24%),
- neuromuscular disorders associated with cardiomyopathy (22%),
- metabolic disorders (16%),
- malformation syndromes associated with cardiomyopathy (10%).

3.2. Myocarditis and other viral infections

This a leading cause in children with cardiomyopathy and is more commonly associated with DCM. It is caused by viral infections that cause the body's immune system to malfunction damaging/inflaming the heart muscle tissue while attacking the invading virus. At this point, it is unknown whether certain children have a certain genetic makeup that may make them more susceptible to contracting myocarditis.

3.3. Familial inherited cardiomyopathies

Isolated familial cardiomyopathy is considered when the child does not show features of metabolic or muscular disorders, and there is a known family history of cardiomyopathy. In affected families with HCM, ARVD, DCM, and RM, the condition is predominately inherited in an autosomal dominant manner where an affected parent has a 50% chance of passing the defective gene to his/her offspring. In rare cases, ARVC, DCM and HCM can be inherited through autosomal recessive or maternal transmission where unaffected parent(s) have a 25% chance of an affected child with each pregnancy.

Although the genetic defect is the same in all members of an individual family, there are variable outcomes and severity of the disease in different family members. The disease's manifestation can range from minimal abnormality and no symptoms to severe complications within the same family. In some families it may appear that the mutated gene skips a generation but in reality the defective gene may not have expressed itself fully in a particular family member, and therefore echocardiograms may appear normal.

3.3.1. Neuromuscular disorders associated with cardiomyopathy

Neuromuscular diseases associated with cardiomyopathy include those that affect the nerve or skeletal muscles. These include muscular dystrophies (i.e. Duchenne and Becker), congenital myopathies, metabolic myopathies, and ataxias (i.e. Friedreich Ataxia). Common symptoms are decreased muscle tone, weakness beginning after infancy, loss of motor control, decreased muscle relaxation and decreased muscle bulk. Almost all of the neuromuscular diseases associated with cardiomyopathy have a genetic basis.

3.3.2. Metabolic disorders

Inborn errors of metabolism consist of numerous infiltrative storage diseases, abnormal energy production, biochemical deficiencies and disorders related to toxic substances accumulating in the heart. This category also includes mitochondrial abnormalities (i.e. MELAS, MERRF, respiratory chain diseases, mitochondrial myopathies), fatty acid oxidation defects (carnitine deficiency, VCHAD, LCHAD, LCAD, MCAD), Pompe disease and Barth syndrome. When the demand for energy exceeds what the body can supply (i.e. during illness, physical stress or decreased oral intake), patients with impaired energy metabolism are unable to maintain their body's biochemical stability. This may lead to low blood sugar, excessive acidity in the blood and/or high ammonia levels that put additional strain on the heart.Metabolic disorders are inherited by autosomal recessive transmission (each parent contributes a defective gene) or X-linked transmission (mother contributes defective gene). Usually patients appear to be physically normal in early childhood but as the body's energy production continues to be impaired, toxic substances may accumulate throughout the body leading to multiple organ failure. Common symptoms include muscle weakness, decreased muscle tone, growth retardation, developmental delays, failure to thrive, constant vomiting and lethargy. In critical states, the child may exhibit stroke like symptoms, seizures, have low blood sugar, and be unable to use the body's fuel correctly.

In contrast, patients with storage diseases such as Pompe, Cori, and Andersen disease cannot break down glycogen, the storage form of sugar. These syndromes are characterized by problems with growth, brain dysfunction, decreased muscle tone, muscle weakness, and symptoms of heart failure.

3.3.3. Malformation syndromes associated with cardiomyopathy

Malformation syndromes are characterized by minor and major physical abnormalities with distinctive facial features. It is caused by genetic mutations through autosomal dominant, autosomal recessive, or X-linked recessive inheritance. It can also be cause by a chromosomal defect where a specific chromosome is deleted or duplicated. Noonan syndrome is the most common form associated with pediatric cardiomyopathy. Common symptoms include short stature, webbed neck, wide set eyes, low set ears and extra skin folds.

3.4. Forms of cardiomyopathy

There are four main types of nonischemic cardiomyopathy that are recognized by the World Health Organization: dilated (DCM), hypertrophic (HCM), restrictive (RCM) and arrhythmogenic right ventricular (ARVC). Each form is determined by the nature of muscle damage. With some patients, cardiomyopathy may be classified as more than one type or may change from one type to another over time. According to the pediatric cardiomyopathy survey, dilated cardiomyopathy is the most common (58%), followed by hypertrophic cardiomyopathy (30%) and a few cases of restrictive cardiomyopathy (5%) and arrhythmogenic right ventricular cardiomyopathy (5%). Although not formally categorized by the World Health Organization, left ventricular non-compaction cardiomyopathy (LVNC) is increasingly being recognized.

http://dx.doi.org/10.5772/55820

With each type of cardiomyopathy, symptoms and reactions to pharmaceutical or surgical therapies may vary widely among patients.

4. Dilated cardiomyopathy

Dilated or congestive cardiomyopathy (DCM) is diagnosed when the heart is enlarged (dilated) and the pumping chambers contract poorly (usually left side worse than right). A diagram and echocardiogram comparing a normal heart and a heart with DCM (fig. 15)

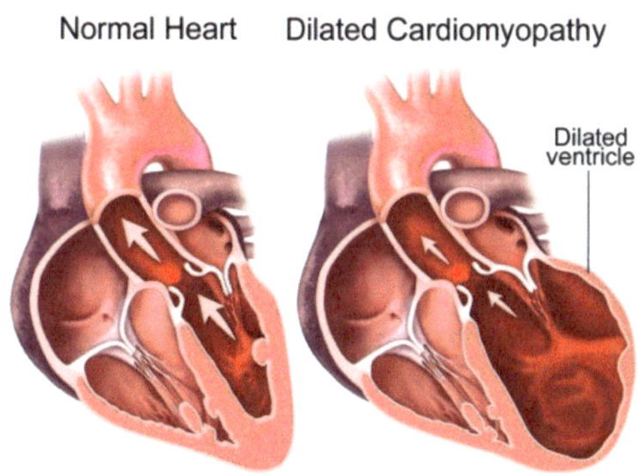

Figure 15. A normal heart is shown on the left compared to a heart with dilated cardiomyopathy on the right.

This condition is the most common form of cardiomyopathy and accounts for approximately 55–60% of all childhood cardiomyopathies. It can have both genetic and infectious/environmental causes.It is more commonly diagnosed in younger children with the average age at diagnosis being 2 years. Dilated cardiomyopathy can be familial (genetic), and it is estimated that 20–30% of children with DCM have a relative with the disease, although they may not have been diagnosed or have symptoms.

4.1. Signs and symptoms of DCM

Dilated cardiomyopathy can appear along a spectrum of no symptoms, subtle symptoms or, in the more severe cases, congestive heart failure (CHF), which occurs when the heart is unable to pump blood well enough to meet the body tissue needs for oxygen and nutrients.When only subtle symptoms exist, infants and young children are sometimes diagnosed with a viral upper respiratory tract infection or recurrent "pneumonia" without realizing that a heart problem is the basis for these symptoms. Older children and adolescents are less likely to be diagnosed with viral syndromes and more likely to present with decreased exercise capacity or easy fatigability. With CHF, babies and young children will usually have more noticeable clinical changes such as irritability, failure to thrive (poor gain weight), increased sweating especially with activities, pale color, faster breathing and/or wheezing. In older children, congestive heart failure can manifest as difficulty breathing and/or coughing, pale color, decreased urine output and swelling, excessive sweating, and fatigue with minimal activities. Until the diagnosis is made in many children, chronic coughing and wheezing, particularly during activities, can be misinterpreted as asthma.Some patients with DCM caused by viral myocarditis (weakened, enlarged heart muscle usually due to a viral infection) can have a rapid increase in the number and severity of CHF symptoms such that within 24–48 hours the child can become very ill requiring emergency hospitalization, and occasionally, advanced life support.Symptoms due to heart rhythm problems (or arrhythmias, which means irregular, fast or slow heart rates) can also be either the first symptom or a symptom that appears after other symptoms have led to a diagnosis of DCM. Symptoms of rhythm problems include palpitations (feeling of funny or fast heart beats), syncope (fainting), seizures (convulsions), or even sudden cardiac arrest (heart stops beating effectively requiring resuscitation). These symptoms can occur at any age and with any stage of cardiomyopathy, even if other more severe symptoms of congestive heart failure have not yet appeared.

4.2. Diagnosis of DCM

Once there is clinical suspicion based on the patient history and physical exam, the diagnosis of DCM is primarily based on echocardiography. With this test, will be using ultrasound beams to evaluate the heart looking for dilated chambers and decreased pump function. Along with the echocardiogram, there are other tests that will likely be done to confirm the diagnosis or provide clues as to the cause.A chest X-ray will show the heart size and can be used as a reference to follow increases in heart size that may occur over time. An electrocardiogram, or EKG, records the electrical conduction through the heart and is used to look for evidence of thickened or enlarged chambers as well as abnormal heart beats that can occur in children with this diagnosis. To more completely evaluate for the presence or absence of these abnormal heart rhythms, which may effect treatment, your doctor may also order a Holter monitor which records heart beats over a 24–48 hour period. A treadmill test can also be useful in some children (beyond age 5–7 years) who can cooperate with this study. This exercise test is used to assess the energy reserve child's heart and, in cases when children do not respond adequately to medicines, this test may also help predict the need for heart transplantation.Depending on child's age, a battery of blood tests may be done in order to identify treatable causes for the cardiomyopathy. This may include testing for certain viral infections such as adenovirus and the Coxsackie viruses as they have been associated with DCM especially in younger children. In many cases, no cause is discovered, and the cardiomyopathy may be referred to as "idiopathic" (cause unknown). Many heart failure specialists believe this "idiopathic" form of the cardiomyopathy is genetic. While genetic screening has not yet become a standard procedure, some physicians may send blood to molecular testing labs located in a few centers around the country so that limited genetic testing can be performed looking for possible mutations currently known to cause dilated cardiomyopathy. evaluation, usually with echo, of other family members is recommended to rule out presence of this disease in other close relatives (parents, siblings).

Finally, in more advanced cases of DCM, cardiac catheterization may be performed. During this procedure, a catheter (thin plastic tube) will be slowly advanced through an artery or vein into the heart (while watching its course on a TV monitor) so that pressures within the heart chambers can be measured. A cardiac biopsy, which involves removing tiny pieces of heart muscle for inspection under the microscope, may be performed to help distinguish between infectious and genetic causes.

4.3. Current treatment

Currently, there are no therapies that can "cure" DCM; however, many treatments are available that can improve symptoms and decrease risk in children with DCM. The choice of a specific therapy depends on the clinical condition of the child, the risk of dangerous events and the ability of the child to tolerate the therapy. In the following sections, current medical and non-medical therapies for DCM are summarized.

4.4. Medical therapy

The majority of children with DCM have signs and symptoms of heart failure. The most common types of medications used to treat heart failure include diuretics, inotropic agents, afterload reducing agents and beta-blockers.

Diuretics, sometimes called "water pills," reduce excess fluid in the lungs or other organs by increasing urine production. The loss of excess fluid reduces the workload of the heart, reduces swelling and helps children breathe more easily. Diuretics can be given either orally or intravenously. Common diuretics include furosemide, spironolactone, bumetanide and metolazone. Common side effects of diuretics include dehydration and abnormalities in the blood chemistries (particularly potassium loss).

Inotropic Agents are used to help the heart contract more effectively. Inotropic medications and are most commonly used intravenously to support children who have severe heart failure and are not stable enough to be home. Common types of inotropic medications include:

- Digoxin (taken by mouth): improves the contraction of the heart. Side effects include low heart rate, and, with high blood levels, vomiting and abnormal heart rhythm.
- Dobutamine, dopamine, epinephrine, norepinephrine (intravenous medications given in the hospital): medications that increase blood pressure and the strength of heart contractions. Side effects include increased heart rate, arrhythmias and for some, constriction of the arteries.
- Vasopressin (intravenous medication): increases blood pressure and improves blood flow to the kidneys. Side effects include excessive constriction of the arteries and low sodium.
- Milrinone (intravenous medication): improves heart contraction and decreases the work of the heart by relaxing the arteries. Side effects include low blood pressure, arrhythmias and headaches.

Afterload Reducing Agents reduce the work of the heart by relaxing the arteries and allowing the blood to flow more easily to the body. Common afterload reducing medications include:

- Angiotensin converting enzyme inhibitors (ACE inhibitors): captopril, enalapril, lisinopril, monopril (taken by mouth). Side effects include low blood pressure, low white blood cell count, high potassium levels and kidney or liver abnormalities.
- Angiotensin I Blocker: Losartan (taken by mouth). Side effects include diarrhea, muscle cramps and dizziness.
- Milrinone is an inotropic agent (see above) that also relaxes the arteries.

Beta-blockers slow the heartbeat and reduce the work needed for contraction of the heart muscle. Slowing down the heart rate can help to keep a weakened heart from overworking. In some cases, beta-blockers allow an enlarged heart to become more normal in size. Common beta-blockers (taken by mouth) include carvedilol, metoprolol, propanolol and atenolol. Side effects include dizziness, low heart rate, low blood pressure, and, in some cases, fluid retention, fatigue, impaired school performance and depression.In addition to improving the symptoms of heart failure, ACE inhibitors and beta-blockers have been shown to return the heart size toward normal and lessen the number of deaths and hospitalizations in adult patients with dilated cardiomyopathy without symptoms. An ACE inhibitor is recommended in children with dilated cardiomyopathy even in the absence of symptoms. Currently, no firm recommendations are available for beta-blockers in children.

4.5. Anticoagulation medications

In children with a heart that does not contract well, there is a risk of blood clots forming inside the heart possibly leading to a stroke. Anticoagulation medications, also known as blood thinners are often used in these situations. The choice of anticoagulation drug depends on how likely it is that a blood clot will form. Less strong anticoagulation medications include aspirin and dipyridamole. Stronger anticoagulation drugs are warfarin, heparin, and enoxaparin; these drugs require careful monitoring with regular blood testing. While variable, common side effects of anti-coagulants include excessive bruising or bleeding from otherwise minor skin injuries, interaction with other medications and, for warfarin, fluctuations in anticoagulation blood levels caused by changes in daily dietary intake.

4.6. Anti-arrhythmia medications

In some DCM patients, especially those with very dilated and poorly contractile ventricles, there may be a higher risk of an abnormal, life-threatening heart rhythm (ventricular tachycardia), and medications are used to prevent or control this abnormal rhythm which then keeps the heart beating in a regular pattern. Common anti-arrhythmia medications include: amiodarone, procainamide and lidocaine. General side effects may include slower heart rate, lower blood pressure, GI upset (nausea/constipation), headache, depressed mood, difficulties concentrating, dizziness, and skin rash among others. Consult your cardiologist for drug-specific side effects once a particular anti-arrhythmic medicine has been prescribed.

4.7. Pacing therapies for DCM

4.7.1. Pacemakers

Pacemakers are small, battery-operated devices that are placed under the skin of the chest or abdomen and attached to electrical wires (leads) which are threaded to the heart. Depending on which type of pacemaker is used, these leads are attached to muscle tissue either on the inside or outside of the heart. The devices monitor the heartbeat and help maintain a regular rhythm in children who are prone to have abnormal heartbeats.In some patients with DCM, the heart rate can become too slow either due to abnormally slow conduction of impulses through the heart or as a side effect of medications. In those instances, a "back-up" pacemaker can be implanted to help maintain an appropriate heart rate.Conversely, as mentioned above, patients with DCM can develop abnormally fast, life-threatening arrhythmias (ventricular tachycardia and/or fibrillation). Implantable cardioverter defibrillators (ICDs) can be used in those children to convert these arrhythmias to a normal rhythm.Finally, a bi-ventricular pacing system has recently become part of the standard therapy in adults with end-stage heart failure associated with DCM, and this treatment modality is currently being evaluated in children.

4.7.2. Implantable Cardioverter Defibrillator (ICD)

ICDs are designed to prevent sudden death from a serious arrhythmia known as ventricular tachycardia or fibrillation. An ICD constantly monitors heart rate, and when ventricular tachycardia or fibrillation is detected, the ICD delivers a shock to the heart that restores normal rhythm. ICDs are used in patients with hypertrophic cardiomyopathy who are felt to be at high risk for a sudden death and in children with dilated cardiomyopathy who have serious ventricular arrhythmias.

4.7.3. Biventricular pacemaker

In recent promising studies in adult patients with dilated cardiomyopathy, a special pacemaker that can pace both the right and left ventricles has been designed. This system, which has to be specially timed, allows the two ventricles to contract together and improves the synchrony of contraction between the walls of the left ventricle. Study results have shown that, when added to other medical treatments, this mode of pacing has helped some patients live longer with fewer hospitalizations and, in some cases, has decreased the need for transplantation. At the time of this publication, use of bi-ventricular pacing in children is in the early stages of development. It is not yet known which children may benefit most from this form of pacing or the best way to implant the system

4.8. Surgical options for DCM

No surgery has been effective in improving the heart function in dilated cardiomyopathy. In a few patients with a severely dilated left ventricle and a very leaky (regurgitant) mitral valve, surgery to repair or replace the mitral valve may help the heart function improve temporarily.

Heart transplantation is the only effective surgery offered for patients with DCM who have severe heart failure that does not respond to medications or other treatments.

4.9. Cardiac assist devices (Mechanical hearts)

Cardiac assist devices are machines that do the work of the heart using a mechanical pump to deliver blood to the body. Cardiac assist devices are implanted when all other therapies have failed and the heart failure is severe. They improve blood flow to the body and allow other organs to recover from the stress of heart failure. These devices are typically used as bridges to transplantation. That is, they are used to support a child either until the heart function has recovered enough to effectively circulate blood through the body or until a suitable donor organ can be found. In pediatric patients, they are designed as a temporary means of support and cannot be used as a permanent alternative to the child's own heart or a transplanted heart. Potential complications of cardiac assist devices include infection, blood clots, stroke and mechanical problems with the devices themselves. There are a variety of cardiac assist devices available. The type of cardiac assist device that is used for an individual child depends on body size and also the type of assist support needed.

4.10. Heart transplantation

Dilated cardiomyopathy is one of the leading reasons for heart transplantation in children. Heart transplant is only considered in children who have such serious heart disease that there are no other medications or support devices available to sustain the child. A heart transplant offers the child with DCM the chance to return to a normal lifestyle.

While a donor heart can cure the symptoms of heart failure and greatly improve survival, it is a major operation with considerable risks and long-term complications. Once a transplant is done, other concerns arise, such as infection, organ rejection, coronary artery disease, and the side effects of medications.

5. Hypertrophic cardiomyopathy

Most often diagnosed during infancy or adolescence, hypertrophic cardiomyopathy (HCM) is the second most common form of heart muscle disease, is usually genetically transmitted, and comprises about 35–40% of cardiomyopathies in children. A diagram and echocardiogram comparing a normal heart and a heart with HCM (fig.16).

"Hypertrophic" refers to an abnormal growth of muscle fibers in the heart. In HCM, the thick heart muscle is stiff, making it difficult for the heart to relax and for blood to fill the heart chambers. While the heart squeezes normally, the limited filling prevents the heart from pumping enough blood, especially during exercise.Although HCM can involve both lower chambers, it usually affects the main pumping chamber (left ventricle) with thickening of the septum (wall separating the pumping chambers), posterior wall or both. With hypertrophic obstructive cardiomyopathy (HOCM), the muscle thickening restricts the flow of blood out of

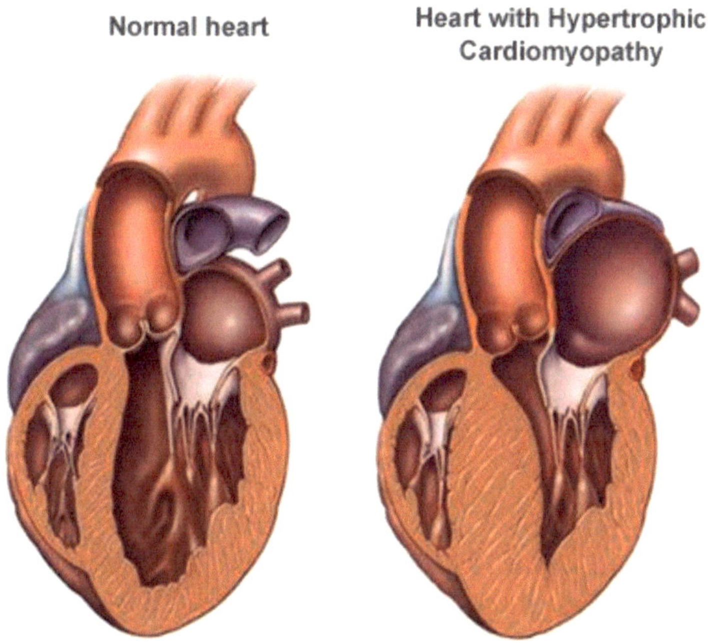

Figure 16. A normal heart is shown on the left compared to a heart with a hypertrophic cardiomyopathy on the right.

the heart. Often, leakage of the mitral valve causes the blood in the lower chamber (left ventricle) to leak back into the upper chamber (left atrium). In less than 10% of patients, the disease may progress to a point where the heart muscle thins and the left ventricle dilates resulting in reduced heart function similar to that seen in DCM.HCM is most often diagnosed during infancy or adolescence. Gene defects can be familial, and it is estimated that 50–60% of children with HCM have a relative with the disease, although they may not have been diagnosed or have symptoms.

5.1. Signs and symptoms of HCM

There is tremendous variation in how HCM presents and progresses. While some children have no or mild symptoms, others may have more severe symptoms including heart failure. Some patients develop abnormal heart rhythms (arrhythmias) that may put them at increased risk for sudden cardiac death. Children under 1 year of age often have symptoms of congestive heart failure whereas older children may be symptom free and, therefore, may be unaware that HCM is present. Onset of symptoms often coincides with the rapid growth and development of late childhood and early adolescence. The strenuous exercise of competitive sports has also been known to make symptoms of HCM more apparent. Disease severity and symptoms are related to the extent and location of the hypertrophy and whether there is obstruction to blood leaving the heart or valve leakage from the left-sided pumping chamber back into the left atrium above. The first sign of HCM may be a murmur, although this is usually absent in the non-obstructive form of HCM. Symptoms in children with HCM can include dyspnea (shortness of breath during exercise), angina (chest pain), presyncope (light-headedness or dizziness), syncope (fainting), exercise intolerance or palpitations/arrhythmias (irregular heartbeats). Symptoms in infants may be more difficult to detect but include difficulty breathing, poor growth, excessive sweating (diaphoresis) or crying and agitation during feeding thought to be due to chest pain Children with severe HCM may have symptoms of heart failure such as difficulty breathing, swelling around the eyes and legs (edema), tiredness or weakness, coughing, abdominal pain and vomiting. Mild symptoms of heart failure can also resemble asthma. Children with HCM may also develop an abnormal heartbeat (arrhythmia), either beating too fast (tachycardia) or too slow (bradycardia). Symptoms resulting from rhythm problems can appear without a child having congestive heart failure or other more obvious symptoms of HCM. The risk of sudden death from arrhythmia is higher with this form of cardiomyopathy compared with other forms of pediatric myopathy especially among adolescent patients. Finally, in some cases of HCM (especially those with extreme wall thickness), the disease evolves towards progressive wall thinning and LV chamber dilation until theheart appears to have all the features of DCM. In these cases, a family history of HCM, a prior echocardiogram that showed HCM or a cardiac biopsy may help differentiate between the two.

5.2. Diagnosis of HCM

Once suspected, the diagnosis of hypertrophic cardiomyopathy is established with an echocardiogram (or ultrasound of the heart) looking for abnormally thick walls predominantly in the left pumping chamber (left ventricle). In addition, the extent of obstruction or muscular narrowing through the outlet of the left ventricle to the aorta (main vessel which carries blood to the body) will be assessed. This diagnosis can only be made after other potential causes of abnormal wall thickening (i.e., aortic valve stenosis, coarctation of the aorta, high blood pressure, etc.) are eliminated either by physical exam or echocardiogram. An electrocardiogram, or EKG, which records the electrical impulses sent through the heart, may show evidence of thickened pumping chambers. Many cardiologists will order a Holter monitor to record you child's heartbeats over a 24–48 hour period. This will allow your physician to check for abnormal, and sometimes life-threatening, heart rhythms, which can occur more often in children with HCM. To further estimate child's risk for developing these abnormal heart rhythms, some cardiologists may ask, in children old enough to cooperate, to perform an exercise treadmill test.Since the cause of this form of cardiomyopathy varies and depends on child's age, additional laboratory testing may be requested. In some cases, an accumulation of abnormal proteins or sugars (glycogen) may occur in the heart causing the increased wall thicknesses. In others, genetic mutations or abnormalities in the mitochondria (powerhouses of the cells) produce this effect. Genetic testing is available for some but not all forms of HCM. In the next decade, as more genetic bases for HCM are identified, genetic testing may become a routine part of the HCM evaluation.

5.3. Current treatment for HCM

Currently, there are no therapies that can "cure" HCM; however, many treatments are available that can improve symptoms and potentially decrease risk in children with HCM. The choice of a specific therapy depends on the clinical condition of the child, the risk of dangerous events and the ability of the child to tolerate the therapy. In the following sections, treatments for HCM are summarized.

5.4. Medical therapies

Medications are used to treat children with HCM who have symptoms such as difficulty breathing, chest pain, decreased activity tolerance or fatigue and generally include beta-blocking and calcium channel-blocking medicines. Beta-blocking medications are used to slow the heartbeat and allow the heart to fill more completely when the thick muscle in the ventricular septum narrows the outflow of blood from the heart. These medications can cause excessive slowing of the heart rate, low blood pressure, dizziness, and in some cases, fluid retention, fatigue, impaired school performance and depression. Calcium channel blockers improve the filling of the heart by reducing the stiffness of the heart muscle, and are used in patients with chest pain or breathlessness. Side effects can include excessive slowing of the heart rate and lower blood pressure. Common calcium channel blockers are verapamil and diltiazem. Diuretics, which must be used with caution in this disease, are used to decrease fluid accumulation (when present) from the lungs in children with severe hypertrophic cardiomyopathy. In the case of HCM which has progressed into a myopathy with DCM features (occurs relatively infrequently as a later stage of HCM - see previous discussion of HCM), therapies used to treat HCM will no longer be effective, and standard medicines for the treatment of DCM will be substituted.

5.5. Pacing therapies for HCM

5.5.1. Implantable Cardioverter Defibrillator (ICD)

ICDs are designed to prevent sudden death from a serious arrhythmia known as ventricular tachycardia or fibrillation. An ICD constantly monitors heart rate, and when ventricular tachycardia or fibrillation is detected, the ICD delivers a shock to the heart that restores normal rhythm. ICDs are used in patients with hypertrophic cardiomyopathy who are felt to be at high risk for a sudden death or have documented serious ventricular arrhythmias.

5.6. Surgery for HCM

Septal myomectomy is a surgery that is performed in patients with hypertrophic cardiomyopathy when symptoms of heart failure have developed because the thickened muscle of the septum (the wall dividing the two sides of the heart) has narrowed (obstructed) the blood flow out of the heart, and medical therapy has not been effective. The surgery involves removing the muscle that has obstructed the blood flow. While septal myomectomy is effective in controlling symptoms, it does not stop hypertrophy from progressing, nor does it treat the life-threatening abnormal rhythms associated with HCM.

5.7. Heart transplantation

Currently, transplantation for HCM is not routinely performed. Two exceptions include medically refractory ventricular arrhythmias, and HCM which has developed features of DCM not responsive to standard DCM therapy. A heart transplant will offer that child the chance to return to a normal lifestyle. While a donor heart can cure the symptoms of heart failure and greatly improve survival, it is a major operation with considerable risks and long-term complications. Once a transplant is done, other concerns arise, such as infection, organ rejection, coronary artery disease, and the side effects of medications.

6. Restrictive cardiomyopathy

Restrictive cardiomyopathy (RCM) is a rare form of heart muscle disease that is characterized by restrictive filling of the ventricles. In this disease the contractile function (squeeze) of the heart and wall thicknesses are usually normal, but the relaxation or filling phase of the heart is very abnormal. This occurs because the heart muscle is stiff and poorly compliant and does not allow the ventricular chambers to fill with blood normally. This inability to relax and fill with blood results in a "back up" of blood into the atria (top chambers of the heart), lungs and body causing the symptoms and signs of heart failure(fig.17).

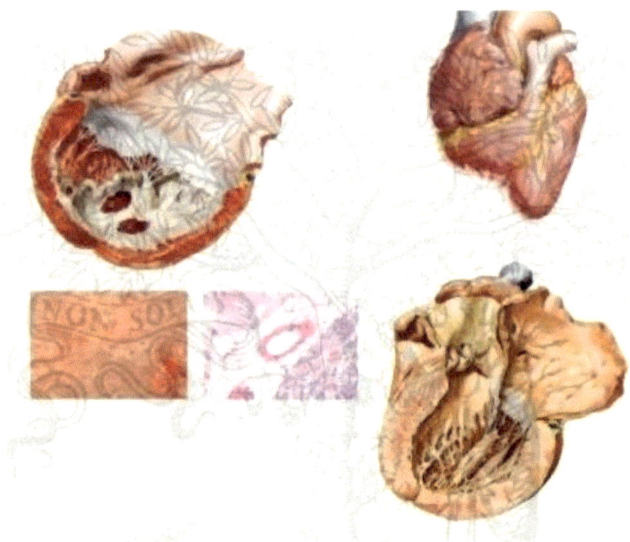

Figure 17. Restrictive Cardiomyopathy (RCM)

Within the broad category of cardiomyopathy, RCM is the least common in children, accounting for 2.5–5% of the diagnosed cardiomyopathies The average age at diagnosis is 5 to 6 years. RCM appears to affect girls somewhat more often than boys. There is a family history of cardiomyopathy in approximately 30% of cases. In most cases the cause of the disease is unknown (idiopathic), although a genetic cause is suspected in most cases of pediatric RCM.

6.1. Signs and symptoms of RCM

In children the first symptoms of RCM often seem related to problems other than the heart. The most common symptoms at first may appear to be lung related. Children with RCM frequently have a history of "repeated lung infections" or "asthma." In these cases, referral to a cardiologist eventually occurs when a large heart is seen on chest x-ray. The second most common reason for referral is an abnormal physical finding during a doctor's examination. Children who have ascites (fluid in the abdomen), hepatomegaly (enlarged liver) and edema (fluid causing puffy looking feet, legs, hands or face) are often sent to see a gastroenterologist first. Referral to a cardiologist is made when additional cardiac signs or symptoms occur, a chest x-ray is found to be abnormal or no specific gastrointestinal cause is found for the edema or enlarged liver. When the first sign of the disease is an abnormal heart sound, or signs of heart failure are recognized, then earlier referral to a cardiologist occurs. In approximately 10% of cases, fainting is the first symptom causing concern. Unfortunately, sudden death has been the initial presentation in some patients.

6.2. Diagnosis of RCM

Restrictive cardiomyopathy is among the rarest of childhood cardiomyopathies. Its diagnosis is difficult to establish early in the clinical course due to the lack of symptoms. Therefore, in many cases, this diagnosis is made only after presentation with symptoms such as decreased exercise tolerance, new heart sound (gallop), syncope (passing out) or chest pain with exercise.Once suspected, there are certain tests that can help confirm this diagnosis. An electrocardiogram, or EKG, which records the electrical conduction through the heart, can be very helpful. This can show abnormally large electrical forces from enlargement of the atria (upper chambers) of the heart. An echocardiogram, or ultrasound of the heart, can provide additional clues to help make this diagnosis. Generally, in children with RCM, the echocardiogram shows marked enlargement of the atria (upper chambers), normal sized ventricles (lower chambers) and normal heart function. In more advanced disease states, pulmonary artery pressure (blood pressure in the lungs) will be increased and can often be estimated during the echocardiogram.Cardiac catheterization is usually the next procedure done to confirm the diagnosis. During this procedure, a catheter (thinplastic tube) will be slowly advanced through an artery or vein into the heart (while watching its course on a TV monitor) so that pressures within the heart chambers can be measured. These measurements often show significantly elevated pressures during the relaxation period of the heart (when it fills with blood before the next beat) and varying degrees of increased pulmonary artery pressure (which can confirm the echo estimates) in the absence of any other structural heart disease. In very rare cases, based on clinical symptoms and prior laboratory evaluation, a cardiac biopsy may be performed. This involves removing tiny pieces of heart muscle for inspection under the microscope to search for potential causes of this condition (such as amyloidosis or sarcoidosis, which are common causes of RCM in adults but rarely in pediatric patients). Finally, since childhood RCM is often genetic and in many cases will be inherited, once this diagnosis is established, your doctor will likely request that parents, siblings of the patient and sometimes other close relatives be screened with an echocardiogram to rule out the presence of this disease in other family members.

6.3. Current treatment

Currently, there are no therapies that can "cure" RCM; however, some treatments are available that can improve symptoms in children with RCM. The choice of a specific therapy depends on the clinical condition of the child, the risk of dangerous events and the ability of the child to tolerate the therapy.

6.4. Medical therapies to treat RCM and associated heart failure

Some children with RCM have signs and symptoms of heart failure due to the abnormal relaxation properties of the heart muscle. The most common types of medications used to treat heart failure under these circumstances include diuretics, beta-blockers and occasionally afterload reducing agents.

Diuretics, sometimes called "water pills," reduce excess fluid in the lungs or other organs by increasing urine production. Diuretics can be given either orally or intravenously. Common diuretics include furosemide, spironolactone, bumetanide and metolazone. Common side effects of diuretics include dehydration and abnormalities in the blood chemistries (particularly potassium loss). In patients with RCM, diuretics must be used very carefully and given only in doses to treat extra lung and abdominal fluid without inducing excessive fluid loss as this may cause symptomatically low blood pressure.

Beta-blockers slow the heartbeat and increase the relaxation time of the heart. This may allow the heart to fill better with blood before each heart beat and decrease some of the symptoms created by the stiff pumping chambers. Common beta-blockers (taken by mouth) include carvedilol, metoprolol, propanolol and atenolol. Side effects include dizziness, low heart rate, low blood pressure, and, in some cases, fluid retention, fatigue, impaired school performance and depression.

6.5. Anticoagulation medications

In children with a heart that does not relax well, there is a risk of blood clots forming inside the heart possibly leading to a stroke. Anticoagulation medications, also known as blood thinners, are often used in these situations. The choice of anticoagulation drug depends on how likely it is that a blood clot will form. Less strong anticoagulation medications include aspirin and dipyridamole. Stronger anticoagulation drugs are warfarin, heparin, and enoxaparin; these drugs require careful monitoring with regular blood testing. While variable, common side effects of anticoagulants include excessive bruising

http://dx.doi.org/10.5772/55820

or bleeding from otherwise minor skin injuries, interaction with other medications and, for warfarin, fluctuations in anticoagulation blood levels caused by changes in daily dietary intake. Information regarding which food groups can significantly affect warfarin levels can be obtained from your cardiologist.

6.6. Surgery for restrictive cardiomyopathy

No surgery has been effective in improving the heart function in restrictive cardiomyopathy. Heart transplantation is the only effective surgery offered for patients with RCM, particularly those who already have symptoms at the time of diagnosis or in whom reactive pulmonary hypertension exists.

6.7. Heart transplantation

Since there are no proven effective therapies for children with RCM, transplantation is the only known intervention for this disease. This is especially true in cases where evaluation has demonstrated the presence of pulmonary hypertension, which can be fatal if not treated. For children with RCM, heart transplantation can address both the abnormal heart function as well as associated pulmonary hypertension. A heart transplant offers the child with RCM the chance to return to a normal lifestyle. While a donor heart can cure the symptoms of heart failure and greatly improve survival, it is a major operation with considerable risks and long-term complications. Once a transplant is done, other concerns arise, such as infection, organ rejection, coronary artery disease, and the side effects of medications.

7. Miscellaneous (Rare) cardiomyopathies

There are other forms of cardiomyopathy which comprise only a very small percentage of the total (~2–3%) number of cardiomyopathies in children. These cardiomyopathies may have overlapping features with any of the previous types described and include arrhythmogenic right ventricular dysplasia (ARVD), mitochondrial and left ventricular non-compaction cardiomyopathies (LVNC).Patients with ARVD have dilated, poorly functioning right ventricles which have fatty deposits within the walls and are at risk for abnormally fast, life-threatening heart rhythms (ventricular tachycardia). This myopathy can be diagnosed (usually due to the abnormal rhythms) either in early infancy or later in adolescence/adulthood by echocardiogram or MRI, and its prognosis depends, in part, on the age at presentation.Mitochondrial myopathies are rare and often present early in life. Hearts in the affected patients are often thick-walled (hypertrophic), although dilated hearts with poor function can also occur with this type of myopathy. This cardiomyopathy is caused by abnormalities in the mitochondria of the cells, which are small structures within each cell responsible for generating the energy the cell uses for its normal activities. These cardiomyopathies are often associated with other muscle, liver, neurologic and/or developmental abnormalities and are usually genetically passed from an affected mother to her children.Finally, left ventricular non-compaction (LVNC) cardiomyopathy is characterized by deep trabeculations (or crevices) within muscle of the left ventricular walls. These hearts may have features of both dilated and/ or hypertrophic cardiomyopathy. Conditions associated with LVNC include mitochondrial and metabolic disorders as well as systemic (whole body) processes such as Barth syndrome. Barth syndrome has a constellation of abnormalities including cyclic neutropenia or periodic fluctuations in the white blood cell count (which may not be apparent in early infancy), hypotonia (weak muscles) and LVNC cardiomyopathy. Barth syndrome has recently been linked to an abnormality in the X-chromosome and is passed from mother to son.

7.1. Symptoms of ARVD, mitochondrial and LVNC cardiomyopathies

Symptoms (the problems noted by the child and/or family) and signs (the problems detected by your physician) of cardiomyopathy in children are dependent on several factors including the type, cause and severity of the specific cardiomyopathy, the age when the problems started, and the effects of treatment. Since patients with ARVD generally have symptoms consistent with DCM, and patients with mitochondrial or LVNC cardiomyopathies can have symptoms seen with either HCM or DCM, families are encouraged to review the relevant sections written for dilated and hypertrophic cardiomyopathies within this brochure to become familiar with the pertinent symptoms for each of these cardiomyopathy types.

7.2. Diagnosis of ARVD, mitochondrial and LVNC cardiomyopathies

As with presenting symptoms, the clinical diagnosis of these rare forms of cardiomyopathy will depend on the features of the specific cardiomyopathy. That is, the diagnostic criteria in a child with ARVD will generally follow that of DCM while the mitochondrial and LVNC myopathies will follow that of either DCM or HCM depending on the clinical manifestations of the myopathy. In addition to what is discussed in the diagnostic sections written for the dilated and hypertrophic forms of cardiomyopathy found elsewhere in this brochure, the following comments highlight a few details specific for the diagnosis of each of these rare cardiomyopathies.

The diagnosis of ARVD can be difficult especially in children given its low incidence. However, opposed to the usual form of DCM, which involves the left ventricle to a greater extent, ARVD typically involves the right ventricle preferentially and often times, the clinical suspicion for ARVD can be further explored with MRI (Magnetic Resonance Imaging) which, in many cases, can differentiate fatty deposits from muscle tissue within the wall of the right ventricle that are commonly seen with this disease. The diagnosis can usually be confirmed with visualization of significant fatty deposition within the right ventricular walls (where muscle should be) from biopsy specimens obtained during cardiac catheterization.

Patients with mitochondrial cardiomyopathy often have other associated medical problems such as hearing or vision problems, skeletal muscle weakness in the arm and leg muscles and/ or central nervous system issues including learning problems, developmental delay or loss of developmental milestones. Once suspected, in addition to the cardiac assessment (for DCM or HCM) outlined elsewhere in this brochure, a muscle biopsy performed to evaluate both structure and function of the mitochondria can help verify this diagnosis. A cardiac biopsy is generally not useful because the volume of muscle tissue necessary to perform the mitochondrial analyses can only be safely obtained from arm or leg muscles.

The diagnosis of LVNC can often by strongly suspected when deep crevices or trabeculations are noted with the walls of the left ventricle during an echocardiogram. Very few other cardiac diagnoses have these specific findings. Genetic testing may become more available in the near future to assess identified causes of LVNC especially among male children and those suspected of having Barth syndrome (see following discussion on the G4.5 mutation testing).

7.3. Current treatment

Currently, there are no therapies that can "cure" cardiomyopathy; however, many treatments are available that can improve symptoms and decrease risk in children with cardiomyopathy. The choice of a specific therapy depends on the type of cardiomyopathy, the clinical condition of the child, the risk of dangerous events and the ability of the child to tolerate the therapy.

8. Living with cardiomyopathy

The diagnosis of cardiomyopathy affects many areas of a child's life. The following sections outline the general approaches to living with cardiomyopathy. It is important that specific recommendations are developed by the team caring for the child with cardiomyopathy

9. Diet

All children with cardiomyopathy should follow a healthy diet. Certain types of cardiomyopathy are associated with an inability to digest certain types of food, and in these cases, a special diet is developed in consultation with metabolic specialists. In children with the dilated subtype of cardiomyopathy and heart failure, a low salt diet is recommended to avoid fluid retention. Some children with heart failure may not grow well. In these cases, a diet that increases calories is recommended. Children who are taking some medications may have low levels of magnesium or potassium and a diet that has a higher amount of one or both of these two electrolytes may be recommended. Some children with severe heart failure can retain extra body fluid, and it may be necessary to limit the amount that a child can drink to prevent fluid from accumulating in the lungs.

10. Long term prognosis

The long-term outlook of pediatric cardiomyopathy continues to be unpredictable because it occurs with such a wide spectrum of severity and outcome. Even if a child has a family history of the disease, the degree to which he or she is affected can vary considerably from his/her parents or siblings. The overall prognosis for a child also depends on the type of cardiomyopathy and the stage the disease is first diagnosed. Although there is no cure for the disease, symptoms and complications can be managed and controlled with regular monitoring. Some children will stabilize with treatment and lead a relatively normal lifewith fewphysical activity restrictions. Other children with a more serious form of cardiomyopathy may face more limitations, need specialized care and encounter minor developmental delays. Occasionally children with certain types of cardiomyopathy do improve, but the majority do not show any recovery in heart function. For the most severe cases, a heart transplant may be necessary. Children diagnosed with DCM or RCM are more likely to require a transplant; it is less common with HCM. Post transplant survival continues to improve with two year survival rates at 80 percent and ten-year survival rates near 60 percent. Longer-term survival remains to be determined but is expected to improve with more medical progress and research.

Author details

Aspazija Sofijanova[1] and Olivera Jordanova[2]

1 Medical Director of University Children's Hospital,Skopje, Macedonia

2 University Children's Hospital,Skopje, Macedonia

References

[1] Anderson PAW (1995) The molecular genetics of cardiovascular disease. Curr Opin Cardiol 10:33–43.

[2] Bartelings MM (1989) The outflow tract of the heart—embryologic and morphologic correlations. Int J Cardiol 22:289–300.

[3] Bartelings MM (1990) The Outflow Tract of the Heart - embryologic and morphholayre correlations. Fnt. J Condcol 22:289–300.

[4] Bartelings MM, Gittenberger-deGroot AC (1988) The arterialorifice level in the early human embryo. Anat Embryol 177:537–542.

[5] Bartelings MM, et al. (1986) Contribution of the aortopulmonary septum to the muscular outlet septum in the humanheart. Acta Morphol Neerl-Scand 24:181–192.

[6] Becker AE, Anderson RH (1984) Cardiac embryology. In:Nora JJ, Talao A(Eds.), Congenital Heart Disease: Causes andProcesses. Futura, New York, pp 339–358.

[7] Benson DW, et al. (1996) New understanding in the genetics ofcongenital heart disease. Curr Opin Pediatr 8:505–511.

[8] R. Abdulla et al.: Cardiovascular Embryology 19913. Bolender D, Holterman ML (2001) Animated thoughts onteaching human development. FASEB J 15:Abstract 793.1.

[9] Burn J, Goodship J (1996) Developmental genetics of theheart. Curr Opin Genet Dev 6:322–326.

[10] Clark EB (1984) Hemodynamic control of the chick embryocardiovascular system. In: Nora JJ, Talao A(Eds.), CongenitalHeart Disease: Causes and Processes. Futura, New York, pp337–386.

[11] Colvin EV (1998) Cardiac embryology. In: Garson AJr (Eds.),The Science and Practice of Pediatric Cardiology, 2nd ed.Williams & Wilkins, Baltimore, pp 91–126.

[12] Creazzo TL, et al. (1998) Role of cardiac neural crest in cardiovascular development. Ann Rev Physiol 60:267–286.

[13] Hay DA(1978) Development and fusion of the endocardialcushion. In: Rosenquist GC, Bergsma D (Eds.), Morphogenesisand Malformations of the Cardiovascular System. Liss, NewYork, pp 69–90.

[14] Kathiriya IS, Srivastava D (2000) Left–right asymmetry andcardiac looping: implications for cardiac development andcongenital heart disease. Am J Med Genet 97:271–279.

[15] Kirby ML (1989) Plasticity and predetermination of mesencephalic and trunk neural crest transplanted into the region ofthe cardiac neural crest. Dev Biol 134:402–412Los JA(1978) Cardiac septation and development of the aorta,pulmonary trunk, and pulmonary veins. In: Rosenquist GC,Bergsma D (Eds.), Morphogenesis and Malformations of theCardiovascular System. Liss, New York, pp 109–138.

[16] McBride RE (1981) Development of the outflow tract andclosure of the interventricular septum. Am J Anat 106:309–331.

[17] McGowan Jr FX (1992) Cardiovascular and airway interactions. Int Anesthesiol Clin 30:21–44.

[18] Moorman AF, de Jong F, Denyn MM, et al. (1998) Development of the cardiac conduction system. Circ Res 82:629–644.

[19] Pexieder T (1978) Development of the outflow tract of theembryonic heart. In: Rosenquist GC, Bergsma D (Eds.),Morphogenesis and Malformation of the Cardiovascular System.Liss, New York, pp 29–68.

[20] Steding G, Seidl W (1984) Cardiac septation in normal development. In: Nora JJ, Talao A(Eds.), Congenital HeartDisease: Causes and Processes. Futura, New York, pp 481–500.

[21] Thompson RP (1985) Morphogenesis of human cardiac out-flow. Anat Rec 213:578–586.

[22] Van Mierop LHS (1986) Cardiovascular anomalies in DiGeorge syndrome and importance of neural crest as a possiblepathogenetic factor. Am J Cardiol 58:133–137.

[23] Elliott P, Andersson B, Arbustini E, Bilinska Z, Cecchi F, Charron P, Dubourg O, Kühl U, Maisch B, McKenna WJ, Monserrat L, Pankuweit S, Rapezzi C, Seferovic P, Tavazzi L, Keren A. Classification of the cardiomyopathies: a position statement from the European Society Of Cardiology Working Group on Myocardial and Pericardial Diseases. Eur Heart J. 2008 Jan;29(2):270-6.

[24] Mogensen J, Arbustini E. Restrictive cardiomyopathy. Curr Opin Cardiol. 2009 May; 24(3):214-20.

[25] Sen-Chowdhry S, Syrris P, McKenna WJ. Genetics of restrictive cardiomyopathy. Heart Fail Clin. 2010 Apr;6(2):179-86. doi: 10.1016/j.hfc.2009.11.005.

[26] Xu Q, Dewey S, Nguyen S, Gomes AV. Malignant and benign mutations in familial cardiomyopathies: insights into mutations linked to complex cardiovascular phenotypes. J Mol Cell Cardiol. 2010 May;48(5):899-909. doi: 10.1016/j.yjmcc.2010.03.005. Epub 2010 Mar 16.

[27] Ly HQ; Greiss I; Talakic M; Guerra PG; Macle L; Thibault B; Dubuc M; Roy D, Clinical Electrophysiology Service, Department of Medicine, Montreal Heart Institute, University of Montreal, Montreal, et al. Sudden death and hypertrophic cardiomyopathy: a review. Can J Cardiol. 2005; 21(5):441-8 (ISSN: 0828-282X).

[28] Colombo MG, Botto N, Vittorini S, Paradossi U, Andreassi MG. Clinical utility of genetic tests for inherited hypertrophic and dilated cardiomyopathies. Cardiovasc Ultrasound. Dec 19 2008;6:62. [Medline].

[29] Morimoto S. Sarcomeric proteins and inherited cardiomyopathies. Cardiovasc Res. Mar 1 2008;77(4):659-66.

[30] Soor GS, Luk A, Ahn E, Abraham JR, Woo A, Ralph-Edwards A, et al. Hypertrophic cardiomyopathy: current understanding and treatment objectives. J Clin Pathol. Mar 2009;62(3):226-35.

[31] Van Driest SL, Ackerman MJ, Ommen SR, Shakur R, Will ML, Nishimura RA, et al. Prevalence and severity of "benign" mutations in the beta-myosin heavy chain, cardiac troponin T, and alpha-tropomyosin genes in hypertrophic cardiomyopathy. Circulation. Dec 10 2002;106(24):3085-90.

[32] Gersh BJ, Maron BJ, Bonow RO, et al. 2011 ACCF/AHA Guideline for the Diagnosis and Treatment of Hypertrophic Cardiomyopathy: Executive Summary: A Report of the American College of Cardiology Foundation/American Heart Association Task Force on Practice Guidelines. Circulation. Nov 8 2011;

[33] [Guideline] Gersh BJ, Maron BJ, Bonow RO, et al. 2011 ACCF/AHA Guideline for the Diagnosis and Treatment of Hypertrophic Cardiomyopathy: a report of the American College of Cardiology Foundation/American Heart Association Task Force on

Practice Guidelines. Developed in collaboration with the American Association for Thoracic Surgery, American Society of Echocardiography, American Society of Nuclear Cardiology, Heart Failure Society of America, Heart Rhythm Society, Society for Cardiovascular Angiography and Interventions, and Society of Thoracic Surgeons. J Am Coll Cardiol. Dec 13 2011;58(25):e212-60.

[34] [Guideline] Maron BJ, McKenna WJ, Danielson GK, Kappenberger LJ, Kuhn HJ, Seidman CE, et al. American College of Cardiology/European Society of Cardiology clinical expert consensus document on hypertrophic cardiomyopathy. A report of the American College of Cardiology Foundation Task Force on Clinical Expert Consensus Documents and the European Society of Cardiology Committee for Practice Guidelines. J Am Coll Cardiol. Nov 5 2003;42(9):1687-713.

[35] Maron BJ, Peterson EE, Maron MS, Peterson JE. Prevalence of hypertrophic cardiomyopathy in an outpatient population referred for echocardiographic study. Am J Cardiol. Mar 15 1994;73(8):577-80.

[36] Maron BJ, Gardin JM, Flack JM, et al. Prevalence of hypertrophic cardiomyopathy in a general population of young adults. Echocardiographic analysis of 4111 subjects in the CARDIA Study. Coronary Artery Risk Development in (Young) Adults. Circulation. Aug 15 1995;92(4):785-9.

[37] Maron BJ. Hypertrophic cardiomyopathy: a systematic review. JAMA. Mar 13 2002;287(10):1308-20.

[38] Elliott PM, Gimeno JR, Thaman R, Shah J, Ward D, Dickie S, et al. Historical trends in reported survival rates in patients with hypertrophic cardiomyopathy. Heart. Jun 2006;92(6):785-91.

[39] Minami Y, Kajimoto K, Terajima Y, et al. Clinical implications of midventricular obstruction in patients with hypertrophic cardiomyopathy. J Am Coll Cardiol. Jun 7 2011;57(23):2346-55.

[40] DeRose JJ Jr, Banas JS Jr, Winters SL. Current perspectives on sudden cardiac death in hypertrophic cardiomyopathy. Prog Cardiovasc Dis. May-Jun 1994;36(6):475-84.

[41] Maron BJ, Roberts WC, Epstein SE. Sudden death in hypertrophic cardiomyopathy: a profile of 78 patients. Circulation. Jun 1982;65(7):1388-94.

[42] Musat D, Sherrid MV. Echocardiography in the treatment of hypertrophic cardiomyopathy. Anadolu Kardiyol Derg. Dec 2006;6 Suppl 2:18-26.

[43] Peteiro J, Bouzas-Mosquera A, Fernandez X, et al. Prognostic value of exercise echocardiography in patients with hypertrophic cardiomyopathy. J Am Soc Echocardiogr. Feb 2012;25(2):182-9.

[44] Bruder O, Wagner A, Jensen CJ, Schneider S, Ong P, Kispert EM. Myocardial scar visualized by cardiovascular magnetic resonance imaging predicts major adverse

events in patients with hypertrophic cardiomyopathy. J Am Coll Cardiol. Sep 7 2010;56(11):875-87.

[45] Soor GS, Luk A, Ahn E, Abraham JR, Woo A, Ralph-Edwards A, et al. Hypertrophic cardiomyopathy: current understanding and treatment objectives. J Clin Pathol. Mar 2009;62(3):226-35.

[46] Schaff HV, Dearani JA, Ommen SR, Sorajja P, Nishimura RA. Expanding the indications for septal myectomy in patients with hypertrophic cardiomyopathy: Results of operation in patients with latent obstruction. J Thorac Cardiovasc Surg. Feb 2012;143(2):303-9.

[47] [Guideline] Epstein AE, Dimarco JP, Ellenbogen KA, Estes NA 3rd, Freedman RA, Gettes LS, et al. ACC/AHA/HRS 2008 guidelines for Device-Based Therapy of Cardiac Rhythm Abnormalities: executive summary. Heart Rhythm. Jun 2008;5(6): 934-55.

[48] Topilski I; Sherez J; Keren G; Copperman I, Department of Cardiology, Tel-Aviv Sourasky Medical Center, Tel Aviv, Israel. talitop@biu.013.net.il. Long-term effects of dual-chamber pacing with periodic echocardiographic evaluation of optimal atrioventricular delay in patients with hypertrophic cardiomyopathy >50 years of age. Am J Cardiol. 2006;97(12):1769-1775.

[49] Galve E, Sambola A, Saldaña G, Quispe I, Nieto E, Diaz A, et al. Late benefits of dual-chamber pacing in obstructive hypertrophic cardiomyopathy. A 10-year follow-up study. Heart. May 28 2009;

[50] Silva LA, Fernández EA, Martinelli Filho M, Costa R, Siqueira S, Ianni BM, et al. Cardiac pacing in hypertrophic cardiomyopathy: a cohort with 24 years of follow-up. Arq Bras Cardiol. Oct 2008;91(4):250-6, 274-80.

[51] Hagège AA, Desnos M. New trends in treatment of hypertrophic cardiomyopathy. Arch Cardiovasc Dis. May 2009;102(5):441-7.

[52] Jassal DS; Neilan TG; Fifer MA; Palacios IF; Lowry PA; Vlahakes GJ; Picard MH; Yoerger DM, Cardiac Ultrasound Laboratory, Cardiology Division, Massachusetts General Hospital, Boston, MA 02114, et al. Sustained improvement in left ventricular diastolic function after alcohol septal ablation for hypertrophic obstructive cardiomyopathy. Eur Heart J. 2006; 27(15):1805-10 (ISSN: 0195-668X).

[53] Streit S, Walpoth N, Windecker S, Meier B, Hess O. Is alcohol ablation of the septum associated with recurrent tachyarrhythmias?. Swiss Med Wkly. Dec 1 2007;137(47-48):660-8.

[54] You JJ, Woo A, Ko DT, Cameron DA, Mihailovic A, Krahn M. Life expectancy gains and cost-effectiveness of implantable cardioverter/defibrillators for the primary prevention of sudden cardiac death in patients with hypertrophic cardiomyopathy. Am Heart J. Nov 2007;154(5):899-907.

[55] Maron BJ, Isner JM, McKenna WJ. 26th Bethesda conference: recommendations for determining eligibility for competition in athletes with cardiovascular abnormalities. Task Force 3: hypertrophic cardiomyopathy, myocarditis and other myopericardial diseases and mitral valve prolapse. J Am Coll Cardiol. Oct 1994;24(4):880-5.

[56] Thompson PD, Franklin BA, Balady GJ, Blair SN, Corrado D, Estes NA 3rd, et al. Exercise and acute cardiovascular events placing the risks into perspective: a scientific statement from the American Heart Association Council on Nutrition, Physical Activity, and Metabolism and the Council on Clinical Cardiology.Circulation. May 1 2007;115(17):2358-68.

[57] Counihan PJ, McKenna WJ. Low-dose amiodarone for the treatment of arrhythmias in hypertrophic cardiomyopathy. J Clin Pharmacol. May 1989;29(5):436-8.

[58] Fananapazir L, Leon MB, Bonow RO, et al. Sudden death during empiric amiodarone therapy in symptomatic hypertrophic cardiomyopathy. Am J Cardiol. Jan 15 1991;67(2):169-74.

[59] Mason JW, O'Connell JB, Herskowitz A, Rose NR, McManus BM, Billingham ME, et al. A clinical trial of immunosuppressive therapy for myocarditis. The Myocarditis Treatment Trial Investigators. N Engl J Med. Aug 3 1995;333(5):269-75.

[60] van Spaendonck-Zwarts KY, van Tintelen JP, van Veldhuisen DJ, van der Werf R, Jongbloed JD, Paulus WJ, et al. Peripartum cardiomyopathy as a part of familial dilated cardiomyopathy. Circulation. May 25 2010;121(20):2169-75.

[61] McKee PA, Castelli WP, McNamara PM, Kannel WB. The natural history of congestive heart failure: the Framingham study. N Engl J Med. Dec 23 1971;285(26):1441-6.

[62] La Vecchia L, Mezzena G, Zanolla L, Paccanaro M, Varotto L, Bonanno C, et al. Cardiac troponin I as diagnostic and prognostic marker in severe heart failure. J Heart Lung Transplant. Jul 2000;19(7):644-52.

[63] Peacock WF, Emerman CE, Doleh M, Civic K, Butt S. Retrospective review: the incidence of non-ST segment elevation MI in emergency department patients presenting with decompensated heart failure.Congest Heart Fail. Nov-Dec 2003;9(6):303-8.

[64] Wang CS, FitzGerald JM, Schulzer M, Mak E, Ayas NT. Does this dyspneic patient in the emergency department have congestive heart failure?. JAMA. Oct 19 2005;294(15):1944-56.

[65] Hunt SA, Abraham WT, Chin MH, Feldman AM, Francis GS, Ganiats TG, et al. 2009 Focused update incorporated into the ACC/AHA 2005 Guidelines for the Diagnosis and Management of Heart Failure in Adults A Report of the American College of Cardiology Foundation/American Heart Association Task Force on Practice Guidelines Developed in Collaboration With the International Society for Heart and Lung Transplantation. J Am Coll Cardiol. Apr 14 2009;53(15):e1-e90.

[66] van Veldhuisen DJ, Genth-Zotz S, Brouwer J, Boomsma F, Netzer T, Man In 'T Veld AJ, et al. High- versus low-dose ACE inhibition in chronic heart failure: a double-

blind, placebo-controlled study of imidapril. J Am Coll Cardiol. Dec 1998;32(7): 1811-8.

[67] Effects of enalapril on mortality in severe congestive heart failure. Results of the Co-operative North Scandinavian Enalapril Survival Study (CONSENSUS). The CONSENSUS Trial Study Group. N Engl J Med. Jun 4 1987;316(23):1429-35.

[68] Effect of enalapril on survival in patients with reduced left ventricular ejection fractions and congestive heart failure. The SOLVD Investigators. N Engl J Med. Aug 1 1991;325(5):293-302.

[69] Packer M, Poole-Wilson PA, Armstrong PW, Cleland JG, Horowitz JD, Massie BM, et al. Comparative effects of low and high doses of the angiotensin-converting enzyme inhibitor, lisinopril, on morbidity and mortality in chronic heart failure. ATLAS Study Group. Circulation. Dec 7 1999;100(23):2312-8.

[70] Pfeffer MA, Braunwald E, Moyé LA, Basta L, Brown EJ Jr, Cuddy TE, et al. Effect of captopril on mortality and morbidity in patients with left ventricular dysfunction after myocardial infarction. Results of the survival and ventricular enlargement trial. The SAVE Investigators. N Engl J Med. Sep 3 1992;327(10):669-77.

[71] Poole-Wilson PA, Swedberg K, Cleland JG, Di Lenarda A, Hanrath P, Komajda M, et al. Comparison of carvedilol and metoprolol on clinical outcomes in patients with chronic heart failure in the Carvedilol Or Metoprolol European Trial (COMET): randomised controlled trial. Lancet. Jul 5 2003;362(9377):7-13.

[72] Waagstein F, Bristow MR, Swedberg K, Camerini F, Fowler MB, Silver MA, et al. Beneficial effects of metoprolol in idiopathic dilated cardiomyopathy. Metoprolol in Dilated Cardiomyopathy (MDC) Trial Study Group. Lancet. Dec 11 1993;342(8885): 1441-6.

[73] Packer M, Bristow MR, Cohn JN, Colucci WS, Fowler MB, Gilbert EM, et al. The effect of carvedilol on morbidity and mortality in patients with chronic heart failure. U.S. Carvedilol Heart Failure Study Group. N Engl J Med. May 23 1996;334(21): 1349-55.

[74] Effect of metoprolol CR/XL in chronic heart failure: Metoprolol CR/XL Randomised Intervention Trial in Congestive Heart Failure (MERIT-HF). Lancet. Jun 12 1999;353(9169):2001-7.

[75] Hjalmarson A, Goldstein S, Fagerberg B, Wedel H, Waagstein F, Kjekshus J, et al. Effects of controlled-release metoprolol on total mortality, hospitalizations, and well-being in patients with heart failure: the Metoprolol CR/XL Randomized Intervention Trial in congestive heart failure (MERIT-HF). MERIT-HF Study Group. JAMA. Mar 8 2000;283(10):1295-302.

[76] The Cardiac Insufficiency Bisoprolol Study II (CIBIS-II): a randomised trial. Lancet. Jan 2 1999;353(9146):9-13.

[77] Packer M, Fowler MB, Roecker EB, Coats AJ, Katus HA, Krum H, et al. Effect of carvedilol on the morbidity of patients with severe chronic heart failure: results of the carvedilol prospective randomized cumulative survival (COPERNICUS) study. Circulation. Oct 22 2002;106(17):2194-9.

[78] Pitt B, Segal R, Martinez FA, Meurers G, Cowley AJ, Thomas I, et al. Randomised trial of losartan versus captopril in patients over 65 with heart failure (Evaluation of Losartan in the Elderly Study, ELITE). Lancet. Mar 15 1997;349(9054):747-52.

[79] Pitt B, Poole-Wilson P, Segal R, Martinez FA, Dickstein K, Camm AJ, et al. Effects of losartan versus captopril on mortality in patients with symptomatic heart failure: rationale, design, and baseline characteristics of patients in the Losartan Heart Failure Survival Study--ELITE II. J Card Fail. Jun 1999;5(2):146-54.

[80] Pitt B, Zannad F, Remme WJ, Cody R, Castaigne A, Perez A, et al. The effect of spironolactone on morbidity and mortality in patients with severe heart failure. Randomized Aldactone Evaluation Study Investigators. N Engl J Med. Sep 2 1999;341(10): 709-17.

[81] Bertram Pitt, M.D., Willem Remme, M.D., Faiez Zannad, M.D., et al. Eplerenone, a Selective Aldosterone Blocker, in Patients with Left Ventricular Dysfunction after Myocardial Infarction (The EPHESUS Trial). N Engl J Med. April 2003;348(14): 1309-1321:

[82] Zannad F, McMurray JJ, Krum H, van Veldhuisen DJ, Swedberg K, Shi H, et al. Eplerenone in patients with systolic heart failure and mild symptoms. N Engl J Med. Jan 6 2011;364(1):11-21.

[83] Jaeschke R, Oxman AD, Guyatt GH. To what extent do congestive heart failure patients in sinus rhythm benefit from digoxin therapy? A systematic overview and meta-analysis. Am J Med. Mar 1990;88(3):279-86.

[84] Rich MW, McSherry F, Williford WO, Yusuf S. Effect of age on mortality, hospitalizations and response to digoxin in patients with heart failure: the DIG study. J Am Coll Cardiol. Sep 2001;38(3):806-13.

[85] Felker GM, Lee KL, Bull DA, Redfield MM, Stevenson LW, Goldsmith SR, et al. Diuretic strategies in patients with acute decompensated heart failure. N Engl J Med. Mar 3 2011;364(9):797-805.

[86] Cohn JN, Archibald DG, Ziesche S, Franciosa JA, Harston WE, Tristani FE, et al. Effect of vasodilator therapy on mortality in chronic congestive heart failure. Results of a Veterans Administration Cooperative Study. N Engl J Med. Jun 12 1986;314(24): 1547-52.

[87] Taylor AL, Ziesche S, Yancy C, Carson P, D'Agostino R Jr, Ferdinand K, et al. Combination of isosorbide dinitrate and hydralazine in blacks with heart failure. N Engl J Med. Nov 11 2004;351(20):2049-57.

[88] Intravenous nesiritide vs nitroglycerin for treatment of decompensated congestive heart failure: a randomized controlled trial. JAMA. Mar 27 2002;287(12):1531-40.

[89] Burger AJ, Horton DP, LeJemtel T, Ghali JK, Torre G, Dennish G, et al. Effect of nesiritide (B-type natriuretic peptide) and dobutamine on ventricular arrhythmias in the treatment of patients with acutely decompensated congestive heart failure: the PRECEDENT study. Am Heart J. Dec 2002;144(6):1102-8.

[90] Packer M, Carver JR, Rodeheffer RJ, Ivanhoe RJ, DiBianco R, Zeldis SM, et al. Effect of oral milrinone on mortality in severe chronic heart failure. The PROMISE Study Research Group. N Engl J Med. Nov 21 1991;325(21):1468-75.

[91] Xamoterol in severe heart failure. The Xamoterol in Severe Heart Failure Study Group. Lancet. Jul 7 1990;336(8706):1-6.

[92] Baker DW, Wright RF. Management of heart failure. IV. Anticoagulation for patients with heart failure due to left ventricular systolic dysfunction. JAMA. Nov 23-30 1994;272(20):1614-8.

[93] Bristow MR, Saxon LA, Boehmer J, Krueger S, Kass DA, De Marco T, et al. Cardiac-resynchronization therapy with or without an implantable defibrillator in advanced chronic heart failure. N Engl J Med. May 20 2004;350(21):2140-50.

[94] Van Bommel RJ, Mollema SA, Borleffs CJ, Bertini M, Ypenburg C, Marsan NA, et al. Impaired renal function is associated with echocardiographic nonresponse and poor prognosis after cardiac resynchronization therapy. J Am Coll Cardiol. Feb 1 2011;57(5):549-55.

[95] Moss AJ, Hall WJ, Cannom DS, Daubert JP, Higgins SL, Klein H, et al. Improved survival with an implanted defibrillator in patients with coronary disease at high risk for ventricular arrhythmia. Multicenter Automatic Defibrillator Implantation Trial Investigators. N Engl J Med. Dec 26 1996;335(26):1933-40.

[96] Moss AJ. Implantable cardioverter defibrillator therapy: the sickest patients benefit the most. Circulation. Apr 11 2000;101(14):1638-40.

[97] Suma H. Partial left ventriculectomy. Circ J. Jun 2009;73 Suppl A:A19-22.

[98] Caspi O, Huber I, Kehat I, Habib M, Arbel G, Gepstein A, et al. Transplantation of human embryonic stem cell-derived cardiomyocytes improves myocardial performance in infarcted rat hearts. J Am Coll Cardiol. Nov 6 2007;50(19):1884-93.

[99] Patel AN, Genovese JA. Stem cell therapy for the treatment of heart failure. Curr Opin Cardiol. Sep 2007;22(5):464-70.